Praise fo**r** *T**h**e* **U**lti**m**ate ***a****te* ***nde***

KT-430-989

"**Dr. Gary Richter** has given us a remarkable book that brings together the best information available for us to use in caring for our dogs and cats. It helps us understand how our pets are dealing with diseases and the conventional and complementary ways to help them."

— **Dr. Gladys McGarey**, cofounder of the American Holistic Medicine Association and internationally recognized as the Mother of Holistic Medicine

"This book on integrative medicine is a must-read. There are practical approaches to diagnosis, management, and therapy for a variety of animal conditions. It's simply outstanding!"

— **W. Jean Dodds, D.V.M.**, founder of Hemopet and Hemolife Diagnostics, and winner of the Holistic Veterinarian of the Year Award from the American Holistic Veterinary Medical Association

"The impact of **Dr. Gary Richter**'s work excited me to support his mission by creating the 50 holistic recipes contained within this book. Miracles are being achieved through whole-food nutrition and veterinary medicine."

— **Susan Lauten**, M.A. in Animal Nutrition and Ph.D. in Biomedical Science

"*The Ultimate Pet Heath Guide* by **Dr. Gary Richter** is a wonderful book. It contains excellent information on how to holistically approach medical care for dogs and cats. I recommend this book to all caregivers who wish for their pets to have longer and healthier lives."

— **Huisheng Xie, D.V.M., Ph.D.**, founder and dean of the Chi Institute of Traditional Chinese Veterinary Medicine

SWANSEA LIBRARIES

6000306701

THE Ultimate Pet Health Guide

To my wife, Lee, the loving warrior who makes things happen that no one else would believe possible.

To my daughter, Abbey, the magical light in my life.

To my parents, Michael and Priscilla, whose love and support allowed me to achieve my dreams.

And to all animal-health professionals, who spend countless hours in pursuit of improving the lives of animals. It is our good fortune to be in the presence of these wondrous creatures.

THE Ultimate Pet Health Guide

Breakthrough Nutrition and Integrative Care for Dogs and Cats

Gary Richter, M.S., D.V.M.

HAY HOUSE, INC.
Carlsbad, California • New York City
London • Sydney • Johannesburg
Vancouver • New Delhi

Copyright © 2017 by Gary Richter

Published and distributed in the United States by: Hay House, Inc.: www.hayhouse.com® • *Published and distributed in Australia by:* Hay House Australia Pty. Ltd.: www.hayhouse.com.au • *Published and distributed in the United Kingdom by:* Hay House UK, Ltd.: www.hayhouse.co.uk • *Published and distributed in the Republic of South Africa by:* Hay House SA (Pty), Ltd.: www.hayhouse.co.za • *Distributed in Canada by:* Raincoast Books: www.raincoast.com • *Published in India by:* Hay House Publishers India: www.hayhouse.co.in

Interior design: Nick C. Welch • *Indexer:* Jay Kreider

All rights reserved. No part of this book may be reproduced by any mechanical, photographic, or electronic process, or in the form of a phonographic recording; nor may it be stored in a retrieval system, transmitted, or otherwise be copied for public or private use—other than for "fair use" as brief quotations embodied in articles and reviews—without prior written permission of the publisher.

The author of this book does not dispense medical advice or prescribe the use of any technique as a form of treatment for physical, emotional, or medical problems without the advice of a physician, either directly or indirectly. The intent of the author is only to offer information of a general nature to help you in your quest for emotional, physical, and spiritual well-being. In the event you use any of the information in this book for yourself, the author and the publisher assume no responsibility for your actions.

**Cataloging-in-Publication Data is on file
with the Library of Congress**

ISBN: 978-1-4019-5350-8

10 9 8 7 6 5 4 3 2 1
1st edition, August 2017

Printed in Great Britain by TJ International, Padstow, Cornwall.

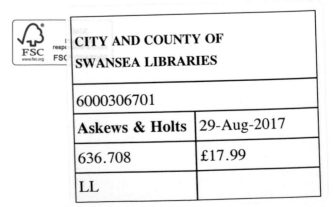

CITY AND COUNTY OF SWANSEA LIBRARIES	
6000306701	
Askews & Holts	29-Aug-2017
636.708	£17.99
LL	

CONTENTS

FOREWORD

by Ian Somerhalder

I haven't written a book since I was eight years old. Aside from writing a few movie scripts or giving notes on countless TV pilots, I wouldn't necessarily call myself a writer. I'm an actor and now a producer, which means I spend my life reading the words of others. But today I'm writing my own words down, because of how important this book has been to me.

Two of my passions are holistic health care and the love of animals. Some friends of mine knew this, so they got me an advanced copy of Dr. Gary Richter's book, *The Ultimate Pet Health Guide*. They told me that this was the guidebook that finally brings together these two incredibly important worlds.

Almost immediately, I couldn't put the book down. It explores a ton of what I already knew about nutrition and helped me see how Western, Eastern, and holistic medicine translate to dogs and cats. It is the book I knew could exist but, until now, simply had not.

The content blew me away, and I decided to connect with Dr. Richter personally. This world-renowned veterinarian could be famous. In fact, he's turned down the offer of a veterinarian TV show because he wanted to focus on his work. Fame and a TV show aren't what drive him. What drives him is what drives me, and so many of us: the desire for all to enjoy every possible day with their healthy pet's unconditional love.

Gary knows what alternative medicines and therapies can turn around cancer, epilepsy, arthritis, and common itching. Dr. Richter even had 50 unique natural recipe formulations created for our furry family members so they can live healthier, happier, and longer lives.

As the founder of the Ian Somerhalder Foundation (ISF), it is my goal to find people around the world who use their skills and passions to make a difference. I immediately recognized that Dr. Richter has the same dedication to animal health, spay and neuter education and action, rescue programs, and programs like ISF's Emergency Medical Animal Grants. I invited him to join ISF as the Veterinarian Medical Advisor to our foundation. We absolutely wanted to be involved to help pet parents get these life-changing insights from "America's Favorite Veterinarian," a man who has dedicated his life and career to helping creatures and informing us.

The Ultimate Pet Health Guide has the potential to start a global healthy pet movement, and I truly hope it does. I hope that you enjoy this book, share it with your friends, and use the important advice within to ensure you have as much time as possible with your furry loved ones. These amazing creatures enrich our lives, our souls, and our families. Let's take care of them and learn along the way.

Ian Somerhalder
actor, founder of the Ian Somerhalder
Foundation (www.isfoundation.com)

PREFACE

Ask any child what they want to be when they grow up and the most likely answer you will hear is: "I want to be a veterinarian." People have an innate connection with animals that starts from the earliest stages of life. We enjoy their appearance (they are super cute), their behavior (they are super funny), and overall we connect with them on an emotional level. In many cases this connection transcends those we have with people. There is purity to the relationship that cannot exist between two humans.

Because of this our instinct is to protect them in every way possible. This reflex shows up in the way we care for our pets as well as in larger forums such as animal rescue, wildlife habitat preservation, and even to extremes such as activists ramming whaling vessels. When animals are unnecessarily harmed or killed, there is an inevitable outcry from concerned humans. So we can all agree that animals are special. Why else would you be reading this book?

Growing up, I always felt a connection with animals. There is something about the unspoken nature of how they go about their lives that appealed to me long before I could verbalize the concept. Being the owner and medical director of two veterinary hospitals means I get to explore that connection nearly every day while challenging medical boundaries in the quest for more and better treatments for my patients. As a veterinarian, I understand the strength and depth of the emotional connection every dedicated pet owner has with animals. After all, I've got three dogs and two cats myself. My dogs are family members. My cats are family members. I love my pets, and my pets love me.

This human–animal bond is so strong that most pet owners would do anything in their power to keep their companions healthy. So pet owners rely on their veterinarian to provide them with medical care and guidance regarding what is best for their pet.

Finding the Magic in Medicine

Like all branches of medicine, veterinary medicine is an evolving science. As a profession, we are getting better at treating illness, curing disease, and promoting quality of life. When it comes to preventing disease, however, conventional medicine has a way to go. I came to this troubling professional realization after almost a decade in a small animal and emergency veterinary practice.

Like everything else in life, you don't know what you don't know. After some nine years in practice, I realized the conventional Western medical care I was providing was great when it came to dealing with trauma, surgery, infection, etc.; however, for patients with longer-term chronic problems, treatment options were far more limited, and sometimes long-term side effects were almost as bad as the condition we were treating. The brand of medicine I was practicing felt incomplete. It's in my nature to be a problem solver, and when it comes to medicine, science is the cornerstone to problem-solving. So I set off to increase my knowledge by furthering my education and filling in the gaps. To be clear, my formal veterinary education was thorough and complete. The shortcoming was not with school or the instructors but with the Western paradigm itself.

Medical and veterinary schools around the world provide the doctors of the future with a solid foundation in anatomy, physiology, and the principles of modern medicine. They do a good job at this. Very few of them, however, offer students a glimpse into forms of medicine that lie outside the boundaries of surgery and modern pharmacology. Physicians and veterinarians in search of a broader medical knowledge must embark on a different voyage and set sail away from the conventional and into a different but closely related realm.

There has been some collateral damage with the advent of modern medicine. The unfortunate victim has been thousands of years of accumulated knowledge on how to use naturally occurring substances to treat disease. The origins of medicine are all about the natural world. By necessity, healers utilized the materials available to them such as plants, minerals, fungi, and animals combined with prayer to treat and cure illness. People practicing medicine in ancient days were often considered "magical." Were they? It depends on your definition of the word. In the sense that they were (unbeknownst to them) utilizing science to heal people who otherwise would have died, perhaps they were magic.

As modern medicine gained prominence, treatments that were commonplace even in the early 20th century became maligned and demonized by the rapidly growing population of modern doctors and pharmaceutical companies. When we became a "take two pills and call me in the morning" culture, the hubris of modern society turned its back on a wealth of medical knowledge that still has the power to save lives—often in ways and circumstances our modern forms of medicine are unable to. Western society is only just now rediscovering the ancient magic.

Before we begin to explore the strange and wonderful lands on our voyage of medical discovery, I'd like to give you, the reader, a glimpse of how and why I practice integrative health care. By sharing my experiences, you will begin to see how ancient and modern medical techniques can not only co-exist but also complement one another with powerful synergy.

The "Hopeless" Case of Sly the Horse

In 1996, as a veterinary student, I was assigned to care for a sick horse named Sly. He was hospitalized in the isolation ward, meaning everyone in contact with him was required to wear a disposable gown, cap, mask, and shoe covers. Sly was isolated because no one knew what was wrong and he was literally dying before our eyes. It must have been terrifying for him to feel so sick and be given medication by so many strange, oddly dressed people.

As the student on the case, I saw firsthand how Sly was declining. Every day he was worse. I saw his white blood cells plummet on his lab work, indicating his immune system was becoming depleted. I remember talking with the faculty clinicians on the case, and they were convinced he was going to die. (In hindsight, I now realize this is because they had exhausted their list of treatment options with no positive results.) At the owner's request, a veterinary acupuncturist, Dr. Huisheng Xie, came in to consult on the case.

The internists on faculty were not particularly interested in what Dr. Xie had to offer, so they sent the student (me) to assist. Although I had no knowledge of traditional Chinese medicine (TCM) at the time, I remember being excited to see and learn something new. Also, I had grown fond of Sly and it was difficult to see him wasting away. I wanted to see him get better.

Dr. Xie almost exactly matched my idea at the time of what an acupuncturist would look like: a quiet, professorial man with a thick Chinese accent. Although he knew I was a student with no knowledge of TCM, he was very respectful toward me. I held Sly's head while Dr. Xie treated him with a combination of electroacupuncture and an herbal remedy that we administered through a tube into his stomach. These treatments continued for several days, and Sly began to improve. He became more energetic and started eating again. His white blood cell count improved dramatically, his diarrhea resolved, and he started gaining weight. Within a week, it was clear he was on the mend, and ultimately Sly went home "healthy as a horse," so to speak.

Sly's case had a profound effect on the faculty at the veterinary college. The seemingly miraculous recovery of this horse at the hands of Dr. Xie eventually played a part in the creation of an alternative medicine internship at the University of Florida. It's difficult to overstate the significance of this: A respected veterinary school began allowing acupuncture and alternative forms of medicine to be taught within its walls. This was groundbreaking! Since then, Dr. Xie has taught thousands of veterinarians to practice TCM through his own school, the Chi Institute, just minutes away from the University of Florida College of Veterinary Medicine.

Years after my experience, I enrolled in Dr. Xie's course to learn TCM. On the first day of the course, he recounted the story of Sly. I had not seen or spoken with Dr. Xie since I assisted him nine years earlier. As he was recounting the tale and walking around the classroom, he stopped at my desk and looked at me. "I know you," he said. "It was you who helped me with

Sly." The thought still gives me chills. The ripple effect caused by Sly's recovery has, in many ways, led to the training of a new facet of veterinary medicine that embraces complementary and alternative medicine (CAM).

A More Personal Matter

The case of Sly is an excellent example of how alternative forms of medicine can succeed when Western medicine falls short. In other circumstances, the integration of Western and alternative medicine is required to achieve optimal results. In many ways, I wish this next story were not mine to tell. One of our great lessons in life, however, is learning from adversity.

May 4, 2001, began as just another day. I was working at a veterinary hospital in Berkeley, California, when the front desk paged me and let me know my wife, Lee, was on the phone and it was an emergency. When I picked up the phone, the background noise alone filled me with dread. Sirens.

The entire conversation exists in my memory as a surreal, almost out-of-body experience. I remember Lee telling me she had been in a car accident. Someone hit her head-on. She told me her arm and both her legs were broken. She was pinned and firefighters were working on cutting her out of the car. She was going to be airlifted to a trauma center.

I stood there in the treatment room of Berkeley Dog & Cat Hospital in shock and disbelief. Did I just hear this correctly? If this were true, how was my wife calling me to tell me this? None of it seemed possible. Needless to say, I raced home to collect a few things on my way to the hospital. While I was at home, I tried to call Lee on her cell phone. I didn't really expect an answer, but what happened was one of the most surreal experiences of my life.

Somehow the call picked up. I later found out the phone was on her front seat, and perhaps something leaned on the phone at that moment and allowed the call to be picked up. No one knew I was on the line. No one could hear me on that end. What I heard was the sound of firefighters extracting my wife from the car with the Jaws of Life. It was the most helpless feeling I have ever experienced. Based on what I heard, things did not sound good.

When I arrived at the hospital, I was only able to see Lee for a few seconds as they took her into surgery. While that moment is seared into my memory, I will not recount it here. Suffice it to say, the doctors did not know if she would survive. If she did survive, they were not sure they could save her leg.

After several hours of surgery, a doctor spoke with me. Lee had, in fact, survived the operation, and all of her limbs were intact (barely). In addition to her broken legs and arm, her back was broken. She was going to be in the hospital for a long time.

The next four months were a series of battles, victories, and setbacks. Anyone who has ever experienced a major medical event will know what I mean. Through the greatest of fortunes, the spinal fracture narrowly missed Lee's spinal cord and would not cause paralysis. That said, at least 15 bones were broken. (Honestly, we stopped counting at 15.) After a fight with the doctors, I convinced them not to surgically fuse her spine where it was fractured. I knew this would cause major problems years later. She was going to be bedridden for months anyway with the two broken legs. The spinal fracture would heal.

Fast-forward through four months of hospitalization, multiple surgeries, and in-patient physical therapy. Lee finally came home and was learning to walk again. There was no question Western medical care literally saved her life and limbs. But what now? Outside of ongoing physical therapy, the only thing Western medicine had to offer was pain medication. It's not as though she was 100 percent better on the day she was discharged from the hospital.

You would have to know Lee to understand the level of drive she has. After the hospital came ongoing physical therapy, Pilates, acupuncture, herbal therapy, chiropractic, and spiritual work. Much of this is ongoing even today. Fifteen years later, people who meet her have no idea how close she came to death, paralysis, and/or a prosthetic leg. Doctors look at her and marvel at how she even walks at all. She accomplished this Herculean feat through a combination of integrative care and sheer force of will. Western medicine brought Lee back from the brink of death (literally), and complementary/alternative care gave Lee her life back. It took both to bring her back.

The Practice of Integrative Veterinary Medicine

The story of Sly the horse and of Lee's car accident and subsequent recovery are two examples of how alternative medicine and integrative care can lead to more successful outcomes than conventional medicine alone. In addition, these experiences played a significant part in my journey toward becoming an integrative medicine practitioner. Everyone is ultimately a product of his or her life experiences, and these two moments were pivotal in my personal and professional life.

In addition to these profound experiences showing me the power of integrative health care, there is something else that drives me: a deep-seated desire for answers. As a medical professional, I want all of my patients to get better. While intellectually I know this is not possible, it doesn't mean I don't try. In the quest to find answers to difficult medical problems, looking outside the box is a necessity. Western medicine does not have all the answers. No one claims it does. While the same can be said for every form of alternative care, a lot more answers are available for patients if we take the time to look.

Anyone who has been faced with a serious medical condition within themselves or a loved one knows about the search for answers. This quest has been going on since the dawn of time. Through the ages, people have searched for cures through prayer, the witch doctor, wise men, magicians, faith healers, and oracles. Today we have a new kind of oracle—the Internet. While not always the repository of legitimate or reliable medical knowledge, the Internet has democratized medicine. It means that pet owners have access to much of the same information their veterinarians do. The challenge we all face is separating fact from fantasy when it comes to medical solutions. That is where I come in.

As a veterinarian trained in conventional Western medicine, traditional Chinese medicine, chiropractic, and a variety of other holistic modalities, one of my responsibilities to my clients is separating fact from fiction. My mission is to offer the most effective combination of treatment options for my patients. I learn through research, from professional colleagues, and from pet owners. All the information that I encounter must pass my own litmus test for legitimacy before I recommend something as a treatment option. That said, I am not proud. I will take information any way it chooses to come to me.

Not a week goes by when I don't learn something from a client. This is due, in part, to the nature of my practice. Sometimes my lesson is medical, sometimes it's personal or spiritual. While my conventional medical office, Montclair Veterinary Hospital (MVH), attracts the usual clientele, having an office called Holistic Veterinary Care (HVC) certainly attracts pet owners who are searching for more than they are getting from their general-practice veterinarian. The purpose of having both facilities is to be able to offer the full spectrum of integrative health care. It is very common for a patient being seen at MVH to be referred over to HVC and vice versa. I consider the offices as two sides of the same coin, and we will see the patient at whichever office can provide them with what they need on any given visit.

When it comes to HVC patients, clients tend to bring their pets to my clinic as either their first or their last stop. Clients who are very holistically minded come to us for preventive care or for solutions to recently diagnosed problems. More of them come with a very sick pet after all of their other options have been exhausted. Regardless, many people come in with questions (and sometimes answers) regarding how best to care for their pet.

Through years of practicing integrative medicine, I have learned volumes from my patients and clients. Clients have shown me the strength of the bond that forms between pets and their owners. People will often go to lengths to treat their pet that they might not pursue even for themselves. Few things please me more as a veterinarian than providing a successful treatment solution where there was none before. The satisfaction that comes from this is immeasurable. And while not every medical condition is curable, we can still provide pets with a soft landing. When a beloved pet's life transitions smoothly, everyone can ultimately find peace.

While clients are providing their lessons, pets have other things to teach. An animal's response to medical therapy is a pure vision. There is no placebo effect. Either they improve or they do not. Real-world experience treating animals is the best education for how to continually improve as a health-care practitioner. In addition, they show us how to live in the moment.

As I have said, many of my patients come to me with serious, sometimes terminal, diseases. Guess what? They don't care. Pets wake up every morning and go about their day. As long as their pain is not excessive, pets will find a way to get through the day. They have no use for self-pity. They never ask, "Why me?" There is no greater lesson we humans can learn. Carpe diem—seize the day.

INTRODUCTION

What Integrative Health Care Means for You and Your Pets

The concept of integrative health care is still in its evolution. As the field of medicine currently stands, there is conventional Western care and "everything else." Everything else, or complementary and alternative medicine, is a pretty big tent that encompasses modalities such as traditional Chinese medicine (TCM) as well as all other forms of indigenous medicine, chiropractic, homeopathy, energy healing, and many others. The evolution of integrative health care is away from the viewpoint of "Western versus everything else" and toward the effective combination of multiple modalities beginning with the earliest stages of health care.

The magic of integrative health care is in how well Western care and complementary and alternative medicine (CAM) augment one another. They are related much like TCM describes yin and yang as two inseparable parts of a whole. Each excels where the other is wanting.

Think about it this way: If you break your arm, develop an infection, or are in an accident, what kind of medical care do you think of? I hope you are thinking about conventional doctors and hospitals. Western care came into its own as a means of treating the previously untreatable and thus is fantastic at surgery and treating injury, infection, and acute illness.

On the other paw, if you or your pet has long-term chronic pain, long-standing gastrointestinal issues, allergies, or other nagging health problems, you may not have had enormous success with Western care. CAM is much better suited to treating long-term conditions or conditions whose underlying causes are somewhat vague. This synergy is no accident. Just as Western medicine is better designed for acute care, CAM evolved in an era where long-term care was critical.

During the times that many indigenous and natural medical techniques were being developed, Western medicine did not exist. Because of this, many people died from conditions that would now be considered routine. Minor infections, trauma, even appendicitis, all were life-threatening diseases before Western medicine. For those who did survive these illnesses and injuries, chronic disease was often a way of life. Practitioners of indigenous medicine were tasked with providing relief from the long-term pain and suffering of their patients. Over hundreds or thousands of years, they learned how to use the plants and herbs around them to improve quality of life. Some of these ancient techniques are being reintroduced as a means of supplementing Western medical treatment plans.

Throughout this book you will learn about animals whose quality and quantity of life was greatly increased through integrative care. The goal is to shine a light on how integrative health care can be successfully used to prevent disease and to treat illness more successfully than any one modality alone.

The Rise of Western Medicine

Through the ages, medicine has evolved just as biological organisms have. The magical aspect of medical practice ultimately gave way to understanding biology and science. With greater scientific understanding came ever more successful health-care options for people with illness and injury. The development of modern anesthesia, surgery, antibiotics, and vaccination has saved countless lives. In 1850, the average life expectancy of an American was less than 40 years. Today that number is almost 80. It is undeniable that many of us would not be alive today without modern medical care.

As modern Western medicine blossomed in the early 20th century, however, there were casualties. Previously well-accepted forms of medical therapy were shunned. This was due, in part, to the development of the modern scientific research paradigm and the evidence-based medicine (EBM) model. The basis of the philosophy for EBM is determining treatment protocols based on proof of efficacy through research trials. It's fairly black-and-white, and it has overwhelmingly been a good thing, leading to more effective and less dangerous health care. Subjecting drugs and medical procedures to rigorous clinical trials means far fewer patients are harmed by the medicine that is supposed to make them better.

Although EBM is positive overall, there are two drawbacks to the rigidity of our current system. The first is the amount of time it takes for a drug to receive final approval to be used in humans or veterinary patients. The painstaking process of ensuring a drug is safe can lead to delays in treatment or even premature death of patients waiting for drug approval.[1] The second issue is the reality that not all forms of medicine lend themselves to a Western clinical trial format.

A perfect example of the shortcomings of the clinical trial–based method is the treatment of arthritis. Western medicine will look at a particular drug to see if it causes a reduction in pain. To be considered "effective," it must demonstrate pain reduction in a statistically significant number of the patients tested and have an acceptable level of side effects.

TCM, however, looks at arthritis differently. Different people (or animals) may share the symptoms of arthritis pain but may have a different Chinese medical diagnosis based on what time of day they have pain, the nature of the pain, and other factors about their body as a whole. Thus, five patients with arthritis may receive five different therapies. These therapies may be equally (or more) successful than the drug tested in the trial above. The entire philosophy does not lend itself well to a conventional research trial; therefore, it may be more difficult to prove efficacy on paper.

The double-blind, randomized clinical research trial has become the litmus test for medical legitimacy. However, many traditional forms of medicine do not fit into the box very well and thus are excluded from what the modern doctor considers to be legitimate. The discussion of the scientific basis for the inclusion or exclusion of various types of medicine has become a matter of debate in medical circles. Specifically, there is reason to believe the playing field is not level when it comes to how the medical community views alternative care. The Western medical and pharmaceutical industry's desire to be the sole purveyor of medical therapy is based on financial as well as humanitarian goals. Like it or not, health care is big business, and medical research requires big money. Funding to prove the efficacy of complementary and alternative medicine is often difficult to come by.

The medical profession's recent, blossoming interest in alternative forms of medicine is simply a matter of demand from the public. The democratization of information through the Internet has (fortunately) led to a generation of amateur researchers. The public is no longer satisfied to wait for the medical establishment to provide them with answers. Now that medical professionals are no longer in sole possession of medical knowledge, more questions are being asked and more treatment avenues are being explored. Pet owners and human patients are letting doctors know they want more. The establishment is responding with greater interest and a willingness to evaluate and discuss alternatives.[2, 3] The results have been extraordinary.

In recent years, the Western medical establishment has taken another look at traditional and other forms of CAM. The "whys" of the renewed interest in traditional medicine are many. Some are practical, such as the search for alternatives in the fight against more and more antibiotic-resistant bacteria.[4, 5] A perfect example is the "discovery" of a traditional Chinese herb, artemisinin, which is now being used to treat drug-resistant forms of malaria.[6] Other reasons include ongoing discoveries that natural compounds can have powerful medical benefits and that often the combinations of chemicals in naturally occurring plants are more effective than single-agent pharmaceuticals alone.[7]

The Bridge Is Evidence-Based Medicine

Regardless of what medical paradigm you subscribe to, everyone can agree on one thing: All effective medical therapies should be on the table and all ineffective options should be noted and excluded from use. It is a noncontroversial statement. The key word, however, is *effective*. Efficacy through any medical therapy should be able to be demonstrated in a group of patients and have repeatable results. That is why the bridge between Western medicine and CAM lies in EBM.

As we discussed, showing repeatable efficacy is the cornerstone of EBM. As a veterinarian and scientist, I rely on EBM to determine how best to treat patients. This is especially important in the field of integrative medicine, as there are plenty of treatments available that lack scientific basis. One of the biggest parts of my job is to help pet owners separate the fact from the fiction, navigate the thicket of treatment options, and choose the ones with the greatest likelihood of success. These judgments are made through a combination of EBM and years of clinical experience.

In later chapters of this book, we will discuss integrative treatment options for a variety of medical problems dogs and cats may encounter. Whenever possible, I will provide references to support the EBM behind the complementary and alternative options for a given therapy. For those therapies that, as of yet, are not supported by EBM, my recommendations are based on years of successful outcomes and an "above all, do no harm" approach.

Why Isn't Integrative Health Care More Widely Available?

There are many aspects of life where exclusivity is a positive. Many business relationships necessitate exclusive partners and assurances through noncompete agreements. The goal of these business arrangements is to ensure all parties will be profitable and not be undercut by the competition.

Health care is a bad business model, because the business of health care often works to the detriment of the individual patient. Patients may be denied access to treatment options either due to financial shortcomings or medical/personal prejudice on the part of the provider. In other words, a physician or veterinarian may have a motivation to recommend treatment options their organization offers in order to keep the business in-house. That may sound horrible, but it is a reality of health care. Although most health-care providers are truly interested in what is best for their patients, the closer business gets to medicine, the muddier the waters can become.

Beyond financial interests are the issues of prejudice among medical professionals. Like everyone else, health-care professionals have a tendency to stick with what they know. This is why many doctors have personal preferences regarding one medication versus another or one surgical approach over another. When the decisions are more or less between equivalent options, there is no real issue. It's like choosing one brand of ketchup over another. However, when legitimate medical options are excluded, the patient gets cheated.

There are a number of reasons for medical prejudice. The first is undoubtedly ignorance. Veterinary and medical schools for the most part teach exclusively Western medical care. Thus, most medical professionals have had little or no exposure to CAM and its potential benefits. Furthermore, educational institutions may have an underlying bias. Professors often feel that alternative options do not warrant serious discussion and may, in fact, communicate this attitude to their students either overtly or in subtle ways. Such was the case with Sly the horse. No one said it out loud, but clearly the faculty was not interested in Dr. Xie's treatments until after they witnessed the extraordinary results.

Given the indoctrination most veterinarians and physicians receive in school, it is not surprising they often have little or no interest in learning about CAM or recommending alternative methods to their patients. Yet there is no shortage of opportunities for doctors to continue their education throughout their professional careers. So why aren't there more open-minded doctors out there?

In many cases, time is a factor. Like any form of medicine, becoming proficient at CAM takes time and practice. Most doctors are very busy in their professional and personal lives and may not have the time to put into more education. These doctors will often refer cases out for CAM when they believe it is appropriate. That's good, although it means that the patient may not be offered alternatives until after Western medicine has failed.

Another issue is one of introspection. Nearly every doctor I have ever met sincerely wants to do right by his or her patients. For an established doctor to embark on the path toward integrative care, however, there has to be a moment of personal reflection. Specifically, the acknowledgment that the medicine he or she has been providing until that point was incomplete and perhaps was not as effective as it could have been. In other words, they have to admit to themselves they have not been doing the best job they could have. When you care as much as doctors do, that can be a tough pill to swallow (pun intended). Not everyone is able to make the journey.

The "Look" of Integrative Health Care

Picture this: You take your pet (or yourself) to a primary health-care provider. During the visit, you receive a consultation regarding nutrition, exercise, and preventive care. Western medicine is provided as it is needed, but that is only a fraction of the full experience. The greater focus is on how to maintain and/or restore health for the long term. Depending on the specifics of your pet's needs, you may discuss herbal/nutritional supplementation, acupuncture, chiropractic, physical rehabilitation, and training in addition to vaccines and pharmaceuticals.

The visit will be significantly longer than the 15 or 20 minutes you have become accustomed to at the veterinarian's office, and you may see both a veterinarian and other practitioners such as an acupuncturist, chiropractor, nutritionist, etc. The visit may also cost more upfront than a standard office visit with a veterinarian, but the money you save by preventing disease will more than make up for that. When you leave, you have a clear picture of your pet's health status and what you can do to maintain and improve their quality of life in both the short and the long term.

This is what health care should look like. It's not a place for hubris or the guarding of knowledge and turf. Health-care professionals working together to achieve better and longer-lasting results must be our goal. If this vision sounds good, I invite you to learn more about integrative care and seek out integrative medical solutions for your pets (and yourself).

This utopian vision of ideal health care has yet to materialize in most areas. If you are fortunate, your pet may have access to alternative medicine practitioners outside the regular veterinary channels, though truly integrative health care is coming for both animals and humans. In some sectors, such as human cancer care, integration is already happening. Renowned centers such as MD Anderson are utilizing nutrition, acupuncture, and other nonconventional therapies to help patients. Progress has been somewhat slower in areas where lives are not immediately in the balance.

There is no doubt that health is best preserved and restored when all aspects of health are considered. During the course of this book, we will examine traditional medicine from many cultures alongside modern medical techniques. We will compare and contrast both the philosophy and science of what works and why, and ultimately discuss how to combine the ancient and the modern into integrative health care that will achieve greater results than either component alone.

The Blueprint to a Long and Healthy Life for Your Pet

Integrative medicine is defined by its multifaceted approach to health care, the major parts of which are nutrition, complementary and alternative medicine (CAM), and conventional Western veterinary medicine. In the coming sections, each of these approaches will be investigated. Particular emphasis will be placed on nutrition and CAM, as these are what tend to be lacking in the current veterinary health-care system. Once we have established solid footing on each of the three points of the integrative care triangle, we will explore the most successful approaches to preventive care and commonly encountered disease conditions in veterinary medicine.

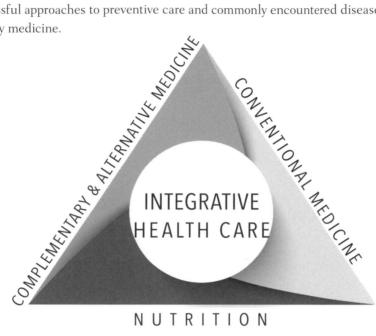

As an integrative veterinarian, my mission is to provide pet owners with the full spectrum of options available to maintain and/or restore the health of their pet(s). The goal of this book is to do the same. Be sure to also check out the accompanying website I've created, www.PetVetExpert.com, for more information and resources to help you achieve a long and healthy life for your pet.

While new medical discoveries may increase the number of alternatives over time, the foundation of an integrative approach will remain constant. By understanding the principles of integrative health care in the upcoming chapters, you will be able to confidently and successfully interact with health-care providers whose common goal it is to provide the highest-quality care.

PART I

NUTRITION IS THE FOUNDATION OF HEALTH

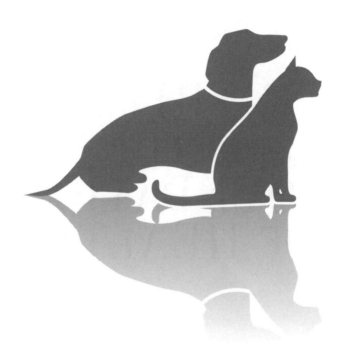

CHAPTER 1

WHY PET NUTRITION MATTERS

The food you eat can either be the safest and most powerful
form of medicine or the slowest form of poison.

— ANN WIGMORE

In 1826, the French physician Jean Anthelme Brillat-Savarin wrote: "Tell me what you eat, and I will tell you what you are." Today we say, "You are what you eat." Nutrition is the foundation of health; without good nutrition, good health is very difficult to come by. As such, the discussion of integrative health care must begin with nutrition.

The human–animal bond dates back millennia. The origins of the domesticated dog began between 16,000 and 32,000 years ago,[1] and scientists debate as to whether humans domesticated dogs or it was the other way around. (Personally, I suspect the answer is "a little of both.") Regardless, our symbiotic relationship with animals has been with us for a very long time. Most of us would agree that what we gain from our relationship with animals is far greater than the food, shelter, and attention we provide them in return.

We obviously love our pets like they are family. (As I write these words, my cat Frieda is nudging my hand away from the keyboard in a ploy for attention.) The mere presence of an animal lifts people's spirits. Bring a cute animal into a hospital ward of sick children and see what happens. Put a purring cat into the lap of a stroke victim who can barely communicate and watch them light up. Bringing comfort to children in need of emotional support as well as veterans with post-traumatic stress disorder (PTSD), pets serve a role in our society that cannot be filled by humans.

The difference between our human family and our fuzzy one is that being the caregiver for animals means you are in total control of your pets' lifestyle, nutrition, and medical care for their entire lives. That's an important responsibility, and the benefits of incorporating integrative care for our pets are exemplified in the story of a black Labrador retriever named Chance.

Success Story: A Second Chance

In late 2013, Chance was brought in to see me by his owner, Walter. Chance, an 11-year-old black Labrador retriever, needed treatment related to a soft-tissue sarcoma (cancer) on his leg, which presented as a large soft growth, or mass, under the skin. While the growth was not painful, it threatened to continue to grow, and ultimately would become painful and infected. Taking no action could eventually cost Chance his leg, or possibly even his life.

Chance and Walter also have an unusually close bond. Walter is a veteran and suffers from chronic, debilitating medical issues related to his military service. Chance is literally the reason Walter gets out of bed in the morning. Although Chance is not officially a service dog, he is Walter's emotional rock and Walter will do whatever he has to do to keep Chance healthy and happy.

Walter can be a little intense, but he knows how to do his homework. When I first met him, he came in with a stack of papers on alternative cancer therapies. Because of his own medical issues, Walter has learned to become a very accomplished researcher. He is one of the few nonmedical people I have met with excellent Internet research skills and the discernment to separate legitimate medical therapies from the endless blind alleys of junk science promising fantastic cures.

Based on the lab reports, Chance's cancer was expected to be difficult to remove completely but was unlikely to spread (metastasize) to distant parts of the body. After weighing the facts, we made the decision to surgically remove as much of the mass as possible and use radiation therapy to treat whatever remained. Chance underwent surgery and radiation, followed by hyperbaric oxygen therapy and herbal support to facilitate his healing.

Chance came through the process with flying colors, but there were bigger issues at hand. Despite having been a very active dog, Chance was markedly overweight due to the cumulative effects of a lifetime of poor nutrition combined with his genetics. His weight limited his mobility, complicated his recovery, and was possibly a contributing factor to his developing cancer in the first place. His condition was already limiting his quality of life; continuing down this path would ultimately limit his *quantity* of life as well.

At the time of that first visit in 2013, Chance was eating a combination of kibble and canned food, resulting in a highly processed, high-carbohydrate diet. The best thing to do for him (and most other pets) was to convert him to a fresh, whole-food–based diet that was lower in carbohydrates, more highly digestible, and rich in micronutrients.

Over the course of five months, Chance lost 20 pounds and is now at his ideal weight. He acts younger now than he did three years ago. The cancer on his leg has not returned, his coat is shinier than it has ever been, and his quality of life has improved immeasurably. Even before the cancer diagnosis, Chance had been slowing down, but after optimizing his diet, he became energetic and now loves to run and play with Walter again.

Chance is a perfect case study in the benefits of integrative health care. While he undoubtedly benefited from surgery, radiation, hyperbaric oxygen, and herbal therapy, there is no way he would have done so well if we had not improved his nutrition.

Pets Eat What We Give Them—They Depend on Us

Don't wait until your pets are sick like Chance to think about their nutrition. I cannot stress enough how many diseases (cancer included) represent the result of a body that has been functioning at suboptimal levels for years, and nutrition is a key component of health.

We are fully in control of exactly what and how much our pets eat. What they eat every day contributes to how efficiently they confront internal and external stresses, prevent disease, and ultimately maintain the "vehicle" they live in. By using nutrition to its greatest advantage in our pets' diets, we can maintain, and often repair, their biological vehicle.

For a moment, let's compare a biological system (you, me, our pets, etc.) to a construction project. Think of nutrients as construction materials. To build a high-quality building, you have to start with the best materials. Unlike a construction project, which requires skilled people to assemble the materials, the DNA in every cell of the body contains the innate programming to build, grow, and heal. Deliver high-quality materials (food), and the body will use them to construct the "building"—and the result is a healthier being. What's more, our bodies are *hardwired* with the innate tendency to be healthy. In other words, given a chance, the building will often repair itself!

While almost any commercial diet will meet our pet's basic nutritional needs, the finer points of nutrition are often overlooked. Your pet may be doing just fine on a day-to-day basis, but consider the longer-term view. Just think of how humans generally fare after years of eating inexpensive and highly processed foods. While eating poorly for one day is not likely to cause major problems, doing so for a lifetime has the tendency to make that lifetime shorter and less enjoyable.

Pets are reflections of us in so many ways. They model our behavior and adopt the lifestyles we choose to give them. Because of their faster metabolism and rate of aging, they show the effects of lifestyle choices more rapidly than we see these effects in ourselves. Many of the diseases of older pets are preventable conditions representing the cumulative effects of years of poor nutrition—metabolic diseases such as diabetes, arthritis, and premature aging. But when it comes to poor nutritional choices, the largest problem among pets today is obesity.

Our Pets' Biggest Nutritional Problem

In 2014, 68.5 percent of Americans were overweight or obese.[2] In 2013, 52.6 percent of dogs in America were overweight or obese (57.6 percent of cats).[3, 4] How's that for the downside of pets imitating their owners? We have become victims of the society of plenty we live in. Overweight pets suffer many of the same maladies as those seen in people; diabetes (mostly cats), arthritis, joint pain, and various chronic inflammatory ailments are all connected to obesity.

It's important to note that when it comes to describing what is a "normal" weight, the general public's perception seems to have undergone a shift. Recently a longtime client, Rodney, told me that he was stopped and chastised by someone on a hiking trail for not feeding his "skinny dog" enough. In reality, his Labrador, Conrad, is the picture of health and fitness— trim, muscular, and very athletic. (Frankly, I wish I had Conrad's body fat percentage!) Yet people have become so accustomed to seeing fat dogs that a healthy animal now appears undernourished.

The great news is that we can solve the obesity problem in pets much more easily than we can with people. This is the upside of being in total control of our pet's nutrition. *We determine what and how much they eat, and their willpower is an insignificant factor in the nutritional equation.*

Think of how healthy we all might be if every bit of food eaten during the day was carefully considered, nutritionally and calorically balanced, and even prepared for us! This is the reality we can achieve for our pets, and creating a sound nutritional plan for them is easy. We need only pay attention to what their needs are and be willing to commit to providing them with ideal nutrition.

Nutrition Is the Problem *and* the Solution

The state of commercial pet food parallels the state of our food today. Prior to the industrial revolution, we were an agriculture-based society and food was typically locally produced. Animals ate scraps left over from their owner's food. As people moved away from farms and into cities, processed and preserved foods became a necessity of urban living. Necessity later evolved into convenience, and a culture of easy, fast food became the new norm.[5]

While modern society has provided us with all kinds of conveniences, it's also left us with highly processed foods with a questionable nutritional profile. Often, processed foods are cooked at very high temperatures to make them more shelf stable in cans or bags. Anyone who has seen a beautiful green vegetable destroyed by overcooking understands that excessive heat makes food less nutritious. This is exactly what happens to ingredients going into most commercial pet foods. Dry pet food is produced in an extruder and processed at almost 400°F. This is definitely not what Mother Nature had in mind.[6]

All living beings evolved to survive and thrive on a certain spectrum of nutrients. When you put the right nutrients in the right proportions into a living system, the result is good health and the prevention or treatment of disease. If you provide the wrong nutrients and/or the wrong amounts, then body systems falter and break down, and disease follows.[7] In other words, poor nutrition causes big problems—good nutrition can solve them.

Preventive nutrition focuses on optimizing all body functions—from the smallest levels of cellular metabolism to regulation of hormonal balance and promoting proper organ function. Once disease becomes apparent, nutrition should be part of a treatment plan and the healing process. For all but the most dire circumstances, it's never too late to improve the health of a pet by changing their diet. The proper balance of vitamins, minerals, and nutrients can slow (and sometimes reverse) the course of various diseases.

It's no secret that a lack of specific nutrients leads to disease. For example, vitamin deficiencies tend to cause a single specific disease process such as scurvy (vitamin C deficiency) or rickets (vitamin D deficiency). Thanks to organizations like the National Research Council, diseases of nutrient deficiencies such as these are rarely seen in the Western world.

These days, overt nutritional diseases in Western society tend to be diseases of excess. Conditions related to excess of particular dietary nutrients and/or energy (calories) result in the slow breakdown of body systems that manifests in any number of ways, ranging from vague signs of malaise all the way to chronic pain and cancer. The diseases that develop in many cases are the result of a poorly functioning endocrine system (diabetes), inefficient organ function (heart disease, kidney failure), and/or chronic inflammation (arthritis). There is little doubt that diet plays a role in many of these life-threatening ailments.

For example, diets with high levels of carbohydrates can lead to insulin resistance and diabetes in cats (and people). Insulin is a hormone the body produces that allows blood sugar to be transported into the cells of the body, where it is used as fuel. Excessive dietary carbohydrates mean excessive energy consumption, which leads to weight gain. The resulting increased body fat releases inflammatory chemicals that alter how cells respond to insulin, making them resistant. Insulin resistance then leads to an inability to transport sugar from the blood into the tissues, which is the definition of type 2 diabetes.[8, 9]

Success Story: Sam, the Cat with Diabetes

When Carol noticed her seven-year-old orange tabby, Sam, was drinking enormous amounts of water, she knew she had to bring him in to be looked at. Sam is a lovable soul who just wants to sit in your lap and purr. He also has an unusual personality trait that I find really endearing in cats: He will lick you like a dog. When we ran blood work and a urinalysis, the diagnosis was clear: Sam was diabetic.

Not surprisingly, Carol was upset to hear of Sam's condition. She loves Sam, and it truly pained her to hear he was sick. As I explained how obesity and a diet high in carbohydrates are contributing factors to diabetes, Carol said she felt responsible. At a little over 20 pounds, Sam was very overweight, and Carol fed him exclusively dry cat food, which is very high in carbohydrates. I explained that none of it mattered at this point. The only thing worth focusing on was how to get him feeling better. Sam would never dwell in the past—why should Carol?

Managing a diabetic cat is tricky. It's a time-consuming and costly process that involves giving insulin injections twice daily and frequent visits to the veterinarian (see Chapter 16 for integrative approaches to diabetic care). In addition to insulin, I helped Carol shift Sam's diet to one that is low in carbohydrates. The goal for him was to slowly lose weight in order to decrease his insulin resistance and hopefully be able to stop the insulin injections.

Sam is lucky in that Carol is very dedicated. Even though we are still in the early stages of his treatment, he is clearly feeling better. He has lost a couple of pounds, and he is more active than he has been in quite some time. Two pounds down was apparently what it took for him to be able to jump onto the kitchen counter again!

Despite the resurgence of the cat's kitchen counter surfing, Sam's owner is over the moon at his progress. Not all cats are so lucky, though. Most veterinarians have, on occasion, euthanized diabetic cats because their owners do not have the means to care for them. Both the treatment and routine monitoring are expensive and time-consuming. Not surprisingly, it's tough to find a new home for a diabetic cat. One of the most difficult things to do as a veterinarian is to take the life of an animal that, under the right circumstances, can be treated. There really are no words to describe what it takes to do this. It's heartbreaking to see a pet euthanized due to a disease that in many cases is both treatable and preventable.

Where Pet Owners Learn About Nutrition

Pet owners rely on their veterinarian to provide them with medical care and guidance regarding what is best for their pet. Yet most routine veterinary visits are for a checkup or medical problems. Generally, appointments last about 20 minutes, barely enough time to address the most pressing issues, let alone basic education on pet care and nutrition.

When it comes to food and nutritional guidance, a lack of time—and perhaps a lack of understanding of the importance of the topic—on the part of veterinarians leads to nutritional advice often being left in the hands of people with less (or no) formal nutritional education such as pet-store employees. Within that realm, advertising and marketing in an ever more competitive marketplace cloud the truths about pet nutrition. Deceptive label claims, buzzwords, and misinformation often influence the decisions people make regarding what to feed their pet. Pictures of "fresh" ingredients and terms such as *grain-free* do not necessarily mean a pet food is high quality. (I'll go into more detail about all of these labels in Chapter 2.) Furthermore, there is no one-size-fits-all diet, regardless of what claims are made by manufacturers.

Our pets can't make the choice for themselves; they have to rely on us.

The Future of Integrative Care

So here we are in the 21st century with all the power that comes from knowledge, and the state of medical care for animals has never been better. Much like the fresh-food "revolution," veterinarians and pet owners are exploring ways to integrate complementary and holistic approaches into cutting-edge Western medical care. The ultimate goal is the creation of a system focusing on prevention as much as on the treatment of disease; the cornerstone of this new paradigm is nutrition. We have the ability to make a huge impact on the quality and quantity of life of our pets. All we need to do is give our pets the building supplies they need and allow them to be healthy.

The upcoming chapters will explore what we do and do not know about the nutritional requirements of dogs and cats and how the pet-food industry approaches nutrition (the good and the bad). We will also evaluate scientific advances regarding how to determine the best foods for your pet as an individual and strategies for how to feed your pet to promote a long and healthy life. We will provide a list of food and treat recipes for our canine and feline family members. The end result will be a greater understanding of the importance of good nutrition and the knowledge of how to either shop for or make food that will optimize your pet's health.

THE BASICS OF NUTRITIONAL REQUIREMENTS FOR DOGS AND CATS

He who takes medicine and neglects diet wastes the skill of his doctors.

– CHINESE PROVERB

A recurring theme throughout the branches of natural medicine is the importance of nutrition. Ancient forms such as traditional Chinese medicine (TCM) and ayurvedic medicine learned long ago about the preventive and therapeutic benefits of food. On some level, we all know that eating right is important for our health; we just don't always act on those instincts. We often choose behaviors we know are unhealthy, taking the short-term benefits while ignoring the long-term effects—like satisfying a cigarette craving.

Contrast this with our natural instincts toward self-preservation. The brain is programmed to avoid situations that are likely to cause us bodily harm. Most of us don't have to actively consider the reasons why we look before crossing the street. We are biologically programmed to quickly process and react to immediate physical danger. Our ancestors evolved this way so they didn't die when a tiger jumped out of the bushes. We have a means of self-preservation and, in a larger sense, species preservation.

Evolution, however, doesn't care whether we live long and healthy lives, only that we live long enough to pass along our genetic material. Evolution never planned on organized civilization, technology, and purposeful living beyond the reproductive age. In our new modern era, we often find ourselves at odds with those very same instincts that helped us survive over thousands of years. In other words, evolution was no better at long-term planning than we are.

The good news is that we (and our pets) are much more than our evolutionary programming. We are able to transcend our natural tendencies when they are not beneficial to us. Accomplishing this feat requires first understanding the innate programming within the body.

Evolution of Food Needs

For now, let's think of food in its most basic sense: food = energy. Eons ago, when food (energy) was scarce, the most successful species were the ones who were the best at finding foods that provided the greatest amounts of energy. Food energy is most dense in the form of fat, carbohydrates (sugars), and protein.[1] For this reason, we are evolutionarily *programmed* to crave these foods.

The conundrum in modern times is that although food is now plentiful, animals (including us) are still biologically programmed with the same cravings and instincts we had when food was scarce. Intellectually, we know that overconsumption is not good for us, but our short-term brain keeps getting in the way and telling us that high-fat and high-carbohydrate foods are highly desirable and delicious—so we crave them.

Animals, especially cats, are creatures of habit and routine. The foods they eat as youngsters shape their preferences as adults. (It's similar to how humans might prefer comfort foods we remember from our childhood.) It is not uncommon for a cat raised on dry food to refuse any other type of food such as canned or fresh, despite its being healthier, because it's just not what they consider to be acceptable. They have been habituated to nutrition that is not ideal; for all intents and purposes, they are "addicted" to dry food in the psychological sense. Changes can still be made, although transitions often take time.

Success Story: Teaching an Old Cat New Things

When James brought his 10-year-old cat, Popeye, into my clinic years ago, he was hoping for a solution for Popeye's chronic skin allergies. The poor cat's skin was red, dry, and itchy all the time. When I suggested to James that we switch Popeye to a fresh, whole-food diet, James literally laughed at me. He explained that the cat was a very picky eater, and he'd never been able to get Popeye to even try another brand of dry food, much less something that wasn't kibble. Still, James agreed to give it a shot.

I told James to slightly decrease the amount of kibble Popeye received each day and put a plate of the fresh food next to his bowl. Popeye resisted the diet change at first, but once we got to about a one-third reduction in his kibble, he relented and began to eat some of the fresh food. After several months, Popeye was eating half kibble and half fresh food, and his skin began to improve.

Today Popeye eats about three-quarters fresh food and one-quarter dry, and his skin problems have fully resolved. James still feeds him some dry food, because he worries Popeye will not eat enough of the fresh food—and frankly, James is a "food is love" person. Although it wasn't easy, making the leap to a fresh-food diet resulted in a happier and healthier cat.

Nutritional Requirements for Cats and Dogs

To optimize health and well-being through nutrition, we need to understand the purpose and function of the major components of nutrition: water, protein, fats, carbohydrates, and vitamins and minerals. Once you have an understanding of nutritional requirements, you'll be able to tailor a routine for your cat or dog based on body weight, size, and age to get their diet on track. The rest of this chapter is a detailed, sometimes very technical, discussion of how to do this. However, for easy reference, I summarize the main points of each section in a "cheat sheet" at the end.

The take-home message is this: What our pets' bodies require to function at optimal levels for the long term is related to, but is not necessarily the same as, what their evolutionary brains are telling them they want to eat at any given moment. Because we live in an environment of plenty and our brains evolved to survive in an environment of scarcity, we must use our intellect to actively choose optimal nutrition for our pets. Mother Nature got us this far; we have to take the reins the rest of the way.

Water

On a day-to-day basis, nothing is as important to maintain optimal body function as adequate amounts of water. Water plays a vital role in nearly every metabolic and physiologic function in the body. The prestigious Mayo Clinic lists the primary functions of water as:

- Protects body organs and tissues
- Lubricates joints
- Regulates body temperature
- Aids the liver and kidneys by flushing out waste products
- Carries nutrients and oxygen to cells

- Dissolves minerals and other nutrients to make them accessible to cells within the body

- Helps maintain appropriate digestion and prevents constipation

- Moistens tissues in the mouth, eyes, and nose

Animals risk permanent physical harm or death by going without water for even a few days. Although we don't generally worry about death through dehydration these days, chronic low-level dehydration can be a real problem for our pets.

Cats in particular are susceptible to dehydration because they tend not to drink a lot of water under normal circumstances. This is because most cats in the wild fulfill much of their daily water needs from the food they eat. Even mild dehydration will result in their kidneys working harder to retain body fluids, which can drive up their urine concentration and cause the formation of crystals in the urinary tract, leading to inflammation and even kidney or bladder stones. This potentially painful condition can be damaging to the kidneys and lead to an inability to urinate due to a urethral obstruction. Obstruction of the urethra caused by crystals and inflammation is almost exclusively seen in male cats and is a life-threatening condition. All of this can be caused by a short-term reduction in water consumption. The prevention of this condition (discussed in Chapter 13) hinges largely on increasing water intake.

The daily water requirement for pets varies based on activity level, environmental temperature and humidity, the amount of food being consumed, and overall health status. In general, however, dogs and cats require between 45 and 65 milliliters per kilogram of body weight per day.

Before you start calculating how much water is in Fluffy's bowl, remember that the amount of water consumed per day is a combination of what animals drink *and* the water content in the food they are eating. Dry foods are usually 6 to 10 percent moisture, while canned and raw foods are around 75 percent. As a result, animals eating high-moisture-content foods will drink less, as much of the water they need is contained within their food.[2]

The question is: Are your pets getting enough water? There are several steps you can take to be sure the answer to this question is yes.

- **Always have a bowl of water available:** Pets should have access to fresh, clean water throughout the day. During puppy training it may be necessary to take up the water a couple of hours before bedtime to limit overnight accidents. In general, however, free access to water at all times is the rule.

- **Change water frequently:** Many animals will instinctively look for clean water to drink. They may be reluctant to dip into a dirty bowl or one with water that has been sitting there for a long time.

- **Make sure the bowl is big enough:** Cats enjoy a roomy bowl. If kitty's whiskers touch the sides, they may be less likely to drink. Whiskers are sensitive organs, and apparently they don't like the sensation of brushing up against the bowl (they are so fussy!). Try a wider, shallow bowl.

- **Consider running water:** Have you noticed how much your pet loves drinking out of the toilet or faucet? That's because animals, especially cats, have a natural preference to seek moving water. In the wild, standing water may be contaminated. Consider getting a circulating water fountain. They're less expensive than you think, and easily available at specialty pet stores or online.

- **Change to food with a higher moisture content:** Throughout history and in the wild, much of the water that animals get is in the food they eat. This is particularly true for cats. The result of dogs and cats eating kibble, which is much lower in moisture content than foods they would naturally eat, can lead to an overall underconsumption of water. While animals on dry food will tend to drink more from the bowl than those on wet food, they may not be drinking enough to make up the difference. This may be the single biggest reason to get pets off of dry food.[3]

In addition to the amount of water consumed, consider the quality of the water your pet is drinking. The issue of water quality has been pushed to the forefront once again due to crises such as lead contamination in the water supply of cities such as Flint, Michigan, and the widespread use of hydraulic fracturing (fracking), which can lead to contamination of surrounding groundwater. Recent studies have shown that drinking water in many areas of the U.S. contains pharmaceuticals including birth control, thyroid supplements, and other hormonal drugs.[4] Many of these potentially harmful compounds are not routinely tested for and thus not reported.

To be clear, most municipal water supplies are relatively safe. Remember, though, this discussion is about *optimal* nutrition. As one of the most vital nutrients both you and your pet are consuming, water quality is a vital consideration for optimizing health.

The most prudent approach is to provide pets (and people) with the cleanest water possible. Using filtered bottled water or installing a water filter at home is often a good idea. A water-quality test may have some bearing on what type of filtration is best for your home. While there are many types of filtration systems, one of the most effective is reverse osmosis, which removes pathogens, heavy metals, and some (hopefully most) drug residues.

Once you've ensured your pet is getting enough clean water, then you can start really assessing nutrition. The best place to begin is evaluating the amount and quality of the protein your dog or cat is consuming.

Protein

The functions of proteins are wide and varied. They are responsible for both body and cellular structure and function. Some of the functions of proteins as described by the National Institutes of Health (NIH) are:

- Proteins form antibodies that bind to foreign particles such as viruses and bacteria and play a vital role in immune system function.

- Proteins form enzymes that carry out chemical reactions in the body. These reactions are responsible for almost all aspects of bodily function.

- Proteins function as messengers such as hormones that signal biological processes to regulate cells and organs within the body.

- Proteins make up many of the structural components that give the body its shape and ability to move.

- Transportation of nutrients and molecules within the body is often facilitated through their binding with proteins.

Proteins are constructed of 22 smaller building blocks called amino acids. Some of these amino acids can be manufactured within the body and some must be obtained through the diet. (Dogs can synthesize 12 amino acids on their own, while cats can synthesize 11.) The amino acids that cannot be synthesized are known as essential amino acids: histidine, methionine, phenylalanine, isoleucine, leucine, tryptophan, arginine, valine, lysine, threonine, and taurine (cats only).

The Association of American Feed Control Officials (AAFCO) gives the following protein requirements for dogs and cats on a dry matter basis. (We will discuss AAFCO and dry matter analysis further in Chapter 4.)

- Dogs (adult): 18 percent minimum

- Dogs (for growth and reproduction): 22 percent minimum

- Cats (adult): 26 percent minimum

- Cats (for growth and reproduction): 30 percent minimum

Remember these are the *minimum* values required to prevent disease caused by a lack of dietary protein. To reiterate, we have a much loftier goal than the prevention of disease by nutritional deficiency. Most animals reach optimal health with higher levels of protein. Many raw or fresh dog food diets have upwards of 40 percent protein, while many raw or fresh cat food diets are in the neighborhood of 50 percent.

While oftentimes higher protein levels are beneficial, there are conditions in which dietary protein should be kept toward the lower end, such as with cats with significant kidney disease (see Chapter 19). Regardless, elevated protein levels in any pet can lead to weight gain if the protein contributes to excess calorie consumption.

Cats are very clear in their requirements. They are obligate carnivores through and through, which means that they *must* have meat to survive. Cats will occasionally eat non-meat items such as grass or even cantaloupe. (Some say that cats are attracted by the scent of cantaloupe because the aroma is caused by amino acids that to cats smell like meat![5, 6]) The vast majority of a feline diet should be meat based, and *all* the protein should be sourced from meat.

However, when we consider what is best to feed our dogs, we must evaluate whether dogs are omnivores or carnivores. Certainly wild canids (wolves, wild dogs, etc.) will eat nonmeat foods, but they do have a strong inclination toward eating meat. That's not the full story, though, as the modern dog is not a wolf. During the past 16,000 to 32,000 years, as dogs were domesticated and became more dependent on humans for food, they were also (inadvertently) being selected for their ability to adapt to a more omnivorous diet.[7] Essentially, dogs evolved away from wolves in order to better live with humans. While dogs have a greater ability to survive on a higher-starch diet than their ancestors, the ideal protein for dogs is *meat*. Dogs who are fed meat-based diets maintain a larger percentage of lean muscle and a lower percentage of fat than dogs who are fed diets containing plant-based protein sources. This in turn leads to a dog who is less likely to be overweight or obese, which decreases the chances of chronic disease.

To be clear, I am not saying that your pet should be fed 100 percent meat. I am advocating for diets in which the *protein sources are 100 percent meat* rather than any vegetarian sources such as soy or gluten.

However, not all animal-based protein sources are created equal. In principle, from a nutritional perspective, there is no "bad" animal protein. But the real world tends to throw us a few curveballs. Animal protein ingredients to be cautious with are *fish, meat by-products*, and *meat meal*.

While the protein and amino acid content of fish may be nutritionally sound, our oceans are not as clean as we would like them to be, and so the fish living in them are often contaminated with heavy metals and other dangerous chemicals. Larger predatory fish such as salmon eat smaller, contaminated fish, increasing the amount of pollutants in their own body. (Small fish that are lower on the food chain, such as sardines, may be a better choice.) Farm-raised fish are often fed antibiotics to grow faster, and grains that alter their nutritional profile. Additionally, some seafood-based pet foods are preserved with the potentially dangerous preservative ethoxyquin.

To be clear, not all seafood-based pet foods are bad; some pets do very well on diets that include fish. Ultimately, you must consider the needs of the animal when you are working out the considerations of ideal nutrition. Remember, however, that companies will often seek out the least expensive, lower-quality ingredients, so it's probably best to stick with mammals and birds as main protein sources.

When looking at land-based protein sources, we must consider the manner in which the animals were raised. Even conventional meat production for human consumption involves feeding animals large quantities of high-energy grains, antibiotics, and hormones, which change the nutritional composition of the resulting meat. Grass-fed cattle is preferable to conventionally raised, grain-fed cattle. Compared to grain-fed cattle, beef from grass-fed animals has a lower overall fat content, and the fat contained has a spectrum of fatty acids that are much more beneficial to overall health. What's more, grass-fed meat is higher in vitamins A and E as well as cancer-fighting antioxidants.[8]

Meat by-products and meat meal (chicken meal, lamb meal, fish meal, etc.) are commonly found ingredients in pet foods because they are such an inexpensive source of meat protein. However, they may not be "meat" in the way we traditionally think of it. By-products and meal can be made up of scraps of meat, organs, collagen, and/or connective tissue—essentially, the leftovers from meat processing.

Although the description may sound a little gross, these ingredients are not, by definition, bad in a nutritional sense. The catch is in the *quality* of the material being added to the food. Where did the material come from? What, exactly, was in the batch of by-product or meal put in the food? How was it handled and stored before making its way to the pet food manufacturer? We as consumers have no way of answering any of these questions, and the answers are likely to be different for every batch brought into the processing facility. Increased amounts of collagen and cartilage in these products can lead to lower quality and less digestible protein. Lamb meal, for example, may be contaminated with *wool*, which also affects overall quality.

Although the pet food regulations consider meat by-products and meal to be appropriate ingredients, I would argue that the unknown quality and digestibility of these products makes them highly undesirable for pets to consume. I strongly advise against purchasing commercial pet foods with by-products or meat meal listed in the ingredients.

Another issue comes up when animals eat the same thing over and over for long periods of time. This may cause them to develop food sensitivities or allergies. Therefore, one of the best things to do when it comes to feeding dogs and cats is to rotate the protein source in their food. This helps lessen the chance of your pet developing food intolerance due to prolonged exposure and ensures that you are providing a varied spectrum of nutrients and amino acids. With a little luck, you are also keeping things interesting for them.

When an animal is "sensitive" to food, it is due to a protein component within the food. Even in cases of grain sensitivity, it is the protein fraction of the grain (usually wheat gluten) that causes the response. The most common allergens in pet foods are beef, dairy, chicken, lamb, fish, eggs, corn, wheat, and soy.[9] The reason these ingredients are on the list is not because they are inherently allergenic; it is because they are the most commonly found ingredients in pet food. While some proteins can be slightly more reactive than others with regard to food sensitivities and allergies, no particular protein is "highly allergenic" in pets.

With an understanding of proteins, we can move on to fats, carbohydrates, and vitamins. Each has an important role to play in how food either positively or negatively affects our pets' health. Just as with water and protein, the source and amount present in food is crucial to optimizing nutrition.

Dietary Fats

Apart from being a not-so-complimentary adjective, fat is an essential part of the diet. In the body, fat serves a number of roles, including being an energy source and a necessary part of the absorption of the fat-soluble vitamins A, D, E, and K. In recent years, researchers have discovered that fat plays a vital role in mediating inflammation and in the body's ability to regulate hormones. We also now know that fat is a major reservoir within the body for stem cells, which promote repair and healing. As you can see, there's a lot more to fat than meets the eye.

Although there are many types of fats, the most important ones to consider from a dietary perspective are the omega-3 and omega-6 fatty acids. These are known as essential fatty acids (EFAs) because the body cannot make them and they must be obtained through the diet.

Omega-6 fatty acids are found in a wide variety of foods and are readily available in most diets. The essential omega-6 fatty acids are linoleic acid (LA), arachidonic acid (AA), and gamma linolenic acid (GLA).

Omega-3 fatty acids are not as widespread in foods as omega-6s, so we must be careful to be sure our pets are getting adequate amounts. The essential omega-3 fatty acids are eicosapentaenoic acid (EPA), docosahexaenoic acid (DHA), and alpha-linolenic acid (ALA). Each of the omega-3 fatty acids serves a vital purpose, ranging from mediating inflammation to regulating hormone balance and protecting the body from disease.

Evolutionarily speaking, many animals were not able to get optimal levels of EPA and DHA in their diets. In this event, the body is able to convert the more commonly found ALA into EPA and DHA. But the process is inefficient, which is why supplementation with EPA and DHA can be so beneficial to health. Additional supplementation of essential fatty acids is discussed in Chapter 6.

Dietary fats come from both plant and animal sources. Plant fats include plant oils such as corn, soybean, canola, etc. Animal fat is the fatty portion of the food animal in question—chicken, beef, lamb, fish, etc. As with protein, the sourcing of the ingredient is as important as the ingredient itself.

Of the omega-3 fatty acids, ALA is the easiest of the three to come by in that it occurs naturally in plant oils, nuts, etc. The richest sources of EPA and DHA come from marine lipids (fats).[10] EPA is found in high quantities in marine animal products such as fish oil, mussel oil, krill oil, etc. DHA is also present in these products, but marine algal oil is the richest source of DHA.[11] (The body is able to convert the more commonly found ALA into EPA and DHA, but the process is inefficient. For this reason, supplementation with EPA and DHA is beneficial to good health.[12])

In addition to the type and source of dietary fat, varying levels of saturation and amounts and ratios of omega-3s to omega-6s play a part in the nutritional advantages (or disadvantages) of a given fat. Fortunately, saturated fats are not as big of an issue in pets as they are in people. Dogs and cats do not get coronary artery disease and thus don't have heart attacks. There are, however, a couple of matters to consider when choosing fat sources for pet diets.

It's important to avoid oils made from genetically modified organisms (GMOs). GMO plants are engineered by scientists to provide greater yields per acre of crop grown. When you say it like that, it sounds pretty good, right? More food produced on fewer acres of farmland. Yet the method by which these plants are made to be more productive seems a little less wholesome.

Plants are genetically modified to become resistant to herbicides and pesticides so the crops can be heavily sprayed with materials that would kill normal crops. Not surprisingly, many of the herbicides and pesticides used are toxic, carcinogenic, and environmentally harmful.[13, 14] When we use GMO plants or plant oils in our pets' food, we are potentially exposing them to toxic chemicals whose long-term effects are not fully understood.

When sourcing fats from animals, try to avoid animals raised on a grain diet, which is common with conventional meat and farmed fish. (As we discussed, there are significant differences in the nutritional composition of grass-fed beef as compared to corn-fed beef.[15]) Farm-raised fish are fed grains to make them grow faster and get to market quicker, but this leads to a food product that is lower in omega-3 fatty acids and thus less healthful to eat.

Toxins are also a particular concern for fats coming from fish because, as we discussed, ocean fish absorb toxins in the water they live in as well as from the other fish they eat, and these toxins are often concentrated in their fatty tissues.[16] Therefore, when sourcing fish oil, find a company that does independent testing for heavy metals and other contaminants. If a company is testing for contaminants, it will talk about it in its literature and on its website. A few minutes of extra research here will really pay off. By using safe supplements from reputable companies, you are in control of the quality and quantity of the essential nutrients your pet is consuming.

When it comes to nutritional amounts of fat in food, it's best to look at amounts of fat in two ways. The first is the total amount of fat in the food. The total amount is a source of dietary energy and also serves as a substrate for fat-soluble vitamin absorption and production of tissues within the body that require fat.

AAFCO guidelines for crude (total) fat content* in dog and cat food are as follows:

- Canine growth/reproduction: 8.5 percent minimum
- Canine adult maintenance: 5.5 percent minimum
- Feline growth/reproduction: 9 percent minimum
- Feline adult maintenance: 9 percent minimum

The second consideration is the level of essential fatty acids contained within a diet. As we will discuss later, pet food manufacturing is a business, and as such manufacturers will seek out the most cost-effective way to construct a diet. Omega-6 fatty acids are far more plentiful in most foods than omega-3s, and thus there is a tendency to use more omega-6s. In addition, when it comes to dry food, fats present a challenge when it comes to spoilage. The National Research Council (NRC) has determined that 2,800 milligrams per 1,000 kilocalories of combined EPA and DHA is the safe upper limit for canine diets.[17] That translates to about 950 milligrams of EPA and DHA daily for a 10-pound dog. Although the NRC has not made a statement about feline diets, the numbers are very likely to be similar. If we work within these "safe upper limits," essential fatty acids can be safely used in the treatment of specific diseases and conditions (see Chapter 6).

Given the complexities of fats in commercial diets, giving your pets a high-quality fish oil or marine algal oil supplement is the best way to ensure they are getting the appropriate levels of the omega-3s EPA and DHA. Supplementing with omega-6 fatty acids is unnecessary, as they are plentiful in food. Research shows that a ratio of omega-6 to omega-3 between 5:1 and 10:1 is ideal for optimal health.

Like all the other nutrient groups, fat should be fed in appropriate amounts and proportions relative to the rest of the diet.[18] Too much can lead to gastrointestinal upset and/or cause pets to put on weight. (In many cases, however, carbohydrates are equally, if not more, responsible for the extra pounds.[19]) Very high-fat diets may also lead to gastrointestinal upset and a potentially serious condition called pancreatitis.[20] The ideal amount of fat in a diet varies based on species, age, and underlying medical conditions.

The Conundrum of Carbohydrates

Carbohydrates consist of a large group of compounds of plant origin that make up sugars, starches, and celluloses. Most of us recognize carbohydrates in the form of grains, fruits, sugars, and vegetables.

---

*Percentages expressed on a dry matter basis (see Chapter 4).

Although water, protein, and fat are essential nutrients that dogs and cats cannot live without, carbohydrates are a different story. For the most part, dogs and cats do not need to eat carbohydrates, though they do serve a physiologic purpose. Digestible carbohydrates are a quick energy source that the body converts to blood sugar for short-term use and to fat for energy storage. Indigestible carbs (fiber) aid in digestion.

As we have discussed, dogs and cats evolved to consume a high-protein, high-fat diet. High carbohydrate loads are foreign to them in the metabolic sense. Excessive dietary carbohydrates can lead to obesity, a variety of inflammatory conditions, and a shortened life span. While it is unclear whether excessive dietary carbohydrates contribute to diabetes in cats, they are certainly detrimental to those cats that are already diabetic. When it comes to carbohydrates and pets, less is more.[21]

While dogs and cats are able to use carbohydrates as an energy source, the question is: Is this an optimal part of their diet? Can we justify the carbohydrate load of the modern commercial diet of dogs and cats?

The diet of a dog's wild ancestors was around 6 percent carbohydrates, consumed in the form of grasses, berries, nuts, and other vegetation.[22] Modern dry dog food averages between 45 and 75 percent carbohydrates.[23, 24] Although modern canines digest carbohydrates more efficiently than their wild ancestors, that's quite a leap!

The disparity between a cat's "wild" diet and commercial food is even more drastic. Wild cats do not generally consume carbohydrates directly, and the only carbohydrates they do get are from whatever is present in the gut of their prey. A natural carbohydrate load for a cat would be 5 percent or less, yet commercial dry cat foods have similar levels of carbohydrates to dry dog foods (45 to 75 percent).

If there is a boogeyman of ill health hiding in pet foods, it is carbohydrates—a "starch in sheep's clothing," if you will. As people, we know what happens if we eat lots of pasta, rice, bread, potatoes, etc.: We gain weight. To be specific, we gain fat. (It's one of life's little ironies that we gain more fat from eating carbs than we do from eating fat.) The same is largely true for dogs and cats, particularly if they are consuming excess calories.

While animals may not need carbohydrates as a nutritional absolute, they will eat them. (We humans are not the only ones who will eat things our bodies don't necessarily need!) With our goal of optimal nutrition, however, we should keep carbohydrate levels in both dog and cat foods to a minimum.

So why are carbohydrates—which are nutritionally unnecessary and can potentially lead to health problems in dogs and cats—the predominant energy source in many commercial pet foods? It comes down to convenience and profit.

Carbohydrates are cheap and thus keep manufacturing costs down. High-protein and high-fat ingredients cost much more to obtain and process. In addition, carbohydrates are necessary in conventional dry food. Kibble is basically a baked good like a small cookie or a biscuit. In order for the baked good to hold together, manufacturers have to add carbohydrates.[25]

Before you let your righteous indignation loose on the pet food industry, remember that pet food companies are only creating what the consumer is buying. Yes, there is misinformation in marketing, but ultimately consumers control the market. The same goes for every other unhealthful, cancer-causing, or dangerous product that exists. If no one were buying it, no one would sell it.

In recent years, food companies have been developing "grain-free" and "low-carb" dry foods. While these foods may be lower in carbohydrates than traditional kibble, don't be fooled. Dry food is by necessity high in carbohydrates, and even the grain-free and low-carb varieties generally still contain 30 to 70 percent carbohydrates. By contrast, canned and fresh foods tend to have much lower levels of carbohydrates (more on comparisons of food formats in Chapter 4).

When it comes to carbohydrates, less is more, and the format of the food (dry versus fresh) you are feeding your pets has everything to do with it.[26] Comparisons of carbohydrate and other nutrient levels between dry and canned or fresh foods can be tricky because of the need to account for the different water content of the diets. We will discuss how to accurately make these comparisons in Chapter 4.

Vitamins and Minerals

The last nutritional requirement for cats and dogs is vitamins and minerals.

Vitamins are organic compounds that are required for normal growth and nutrition. Vitamins such as A, B, C, D, E, and K are vital nutrients in that they cannot be synthesized within the body.

Minerals, on the other hand, are inorganic compounds such as calcium, phosphorus, potassium, and iron. Minerals play a wide range of roles and are part of almost every aspect of the body's functions.[27]

In our analogy of the body as a building, vitamins are the engineers, cleaning personnel, repairmen, and landscapers—they are active participants who keep the building in good order. Vitamins protect the body from damage, help repair damage, and take part in cellular functions. Minerals are much more simple and take a more passive role. Minerals are part of the building blocks of large structures: The smaller, simpler minerals are needed to create the larger, more complex vitamins, cells, and organs.

These nutrients are vital and can lead to ill health and/or disease when they are deficient *or* in excess. Appropriately balancing vitamins and minerals in a home-prepared diet is a complicated task that is beyond the ability of most people. Diet formulation requires advanced education and software for diet analysis. That is why an animal nutritionist is invaluable when feeding your pet a fresh-food diet, and why it is so important to carefully follow supplementation instructions when using a balanced recipe for pet food.

While there are guidelines in place to ensure that commercial pet foods do not cause disease through over- or underdoses of vitamins and minerals (see Chapter 3), by necessity they are blanket recommendations for dogs and cats within specific life stages. I am frequently asked the question, "How do I supplement the diet if my pet is eating a store-bought food?" There is not an easy answer to this, and recommendations must be made on an individual basis. What a specific animal needs to stay healthy depends on age and lifestyle, the quality of the food and its ingredients, and any underlying medical conditions.

As is the case with people, supplementing when it is not necessary is a waste of money, and it is possible to oversupplement and cause problems. Chapter 6 offers the basics about supplements, but ultimately the decision of what to supplement your pets with should be a conversation with your veterinarian and/or a nutritionist.

NUTRITION
QUICK-REFERENCE GUIDE

WATER

- **Access to clean water is vital to good nutrition.** Always have fresh, clean water available. Consider a circulating water fountain for cats.

- **Clean water is relative.** Consider having your water tested and getting a filtration system to address your specific water quality.

- **Switch to food with a higher moisture content.** Remember that animals get water from their food as well as from drinking. Canned or fresh, whole-food diets have a much higher moisture content than dry kibble.

PROTEIN

- **Protein in dog and cat food should be from meat sources.** Foods containing soy, gluten, or other grain-based proteins are not optimal nutrition.

- **Keep it real.** Meat by-products and meat meals are inconsistent in their nutrient availability and digestibility. Pet food manufacturers use them because they are inexpensive. Stick to foods that use actual whole-meat products.

- **Aim for higher levels of protein.** All foods balanced by a nutritionist have adequate levels of protein, but higher-quality foods and fresh foods tend to have higher levels. Somewhat higher levels of protein provide good nutrition and pose no harm to most animals, provided the diet is properly balanced by a nutritionist.

- **Calculate protein on a dry matter basis.** Comparing and evaluating amounts of protein as listed on pet food labels can be tricky, so please review Chapter 4 for instructions on how to calculate protein on a dry matter basis.

FATS

- **Remember your essential fatty acids (EFAs).** EFAs are fats the body cannot make and must be included in the diet: omega-3 and omega-6 fatty acids. Omega-6 is mostly found in plant sources, while omega-3s are mostly from animal sources (primarily fish).

- **Supplement your pet's diet with a fish or marine algal oil supplement.** This is the best way to ensure they're getting enough omega-3s. (Omega-6 is plentiful in food, so supplementing is unnecessary.)

- **Research your supplement companies to avoid toxins.** Find a company that does independent testing for metals and other contaminants in their fish oils. Avoid oils and supplements made from genetically modified organisms (GMOs); farmed, grain-fed fish; and conventionally raised farm animals.

- **Feed fat in appropriate amounts.** Too much fat can lead to weight gain and/or gastrointestinal upset.

CARBOHYDRATES

- **Carbohydrates can be a useful part of your pet's diet.** Carbohydrates can be found in plant material, fruit, and grains. Digestible carbs are a quick energy source for the body, while fiber aids the digestive process.

- **Less is more.** Dogs and cats evolved to thrive on low amounts of carbohydrates. Excessive amounts of carbs can lead to weight gain, inflammation, and potentially disease. Keep carbohydrate levels low for diabetic cats in particular.

- **Commercial kibble contains far more carbohydrates than your pet needs.** Even "grain-free" and "low-carb" dry foods contain several times the optimal amount of carbohydrates. Carbohydrates are primarily used in pet foods because they are an inexpensive source of energy and are necessary in the manufacture of extruded dry food. This, if for no other reason, is justification to move away from kibble.

Vitamins and Minerals

- **Always use foods and recipes balanced by a qualified nutritionist.** Do not attempt to create a nutrition plan yourself; having the correct level of vitamins and minerals is essential to your pet's health. Oversupplementing can be as unhealthful as undersupplementing.

- **Don't make your own substitutions in recipes.** When purchasing supplements to utilize in a home-prepared diet, be certain to get exactly what is recommended. It is very easy to inadvertently over- or underdose by getting the wrong product.

- **Additional supplementation is not needed when your pet has a nutritionally balanced diet.** However, there are occasions when additional supplementation can be healthful. Always consult with your veterinarian or a veterinary nutritionist to determine what may be the most beneficial for your pet.

CHAPTER 3

UNDERSTANDING THE REGULATIONS

> The greatness of a nation can be judged by the way
> its animals are treated.
>
> – Mahatma Gandhi

When most people purchase pet food (or any food, for that matter), they often don't give too much thought to how the food is created or what regulations exist to ensure the food is safe and healthy. The underlying assumption from the public's perspective is that there *are* regulations—but how many people really know what they are?

In this chapter, we'll explore the regulations involved in the pet food industry, and what you need to know so you can pick the right food for your pet, from reading labels to choosing the best food format.

How We Got Here: The History of Pet Food

How did we move from feeding our pets table scraps to buying them their own special food? The history of commercially prepared pet foods dates back to the turn of the 20th century, coinciding with the industrial revolution and the translocation of our population from agrarian to urban lifestyles. Fresh, whole-food diets were no longer the norm, because the necessity of providing food to population-dense cities led to the production of processed and preserved foods. Table scraps were still on the menu for many city pets, but consumer demand was asking for other alternatives (with convenience being the driving force).

The logical solution was canned foods. Canned goods were affordable and had a long shelf life. The industrial technology and infrastructure were already in place, and pet owners were eating out of cans, so why not feed the dog the same way? When metal was rationed during World War II, however, the cans had to go, and dry food (kibble) was born.

The next big innovation came in the 1950s, when Ralston Purina (now known simply as Purina) developed a process of making dry food called extrusion. In this process, ingredients were mixed to form a kind of dough and then heated and forced through a small opening (extruded). The product expanded and cooled as it came out of the extruder, and kibble was born.[1] This revolutionary new process created a uniform product that was less dense than previous forms of dry food. Less density meant the bag looked fuller and created a perception of greater value.[2]

That was great news for business, but not so great for pets. The process of extrusion requires very high temperatures, which causes degradation of nutrients.[3] Extrusion also requires a mixture high in carbohydrates in order to make a successful kibble. This advent led to the unnecessarily high levels of carbohydrates in pet foods we discussed in Chapter 2. Between ingredients and the process necessary to successfully make extruded food, palatability became an issue and food companies found they had to spray flavorings and fats onto the kibble after it cooled in order for pets to eat it.[4, 5]

By mid-century, commercial pet food was big business and was looking to get bigger. In the 1960s, a newly formed organization called the Pet Food Institute (which still exists) began a campaign warning consumers of the dangers of feeding table scraps to pets. The campaign recommended pet owners only feed their pets "complete" foods and avoid the dangerous remnants from their own dinner table. On its surface, it sounds like a good thing.

Logically, one would assume the Pet Food Institute was formed as a grassroots humanitarian organization whose mission was to ensure the good health and nutrition of all pets, right? Think again. The Pet Food Institute represents the manufacturers of 97 percent of the commercially prepared dog and cat food in the United States, and its purpose is to promote the industry. The pet food industry was responsible for an estimated $58 billion in consumer spending on pet food in 2014.[6] As with every for-profit business, decisions must be made, at least in part, with profits in mind.

Who Sets Pet Food Guidelines?

In the U.S., there are multiple state, federal, and nongovernmental agencies that have a hand in ensuring the safety of pet foods as well as the legitimacy of their labeling, marketing, and advertising. The framework surrounding pet food manufacture is complex, and the following information is intended to serve as an overview of the state of the regulatory landscape.

Government Regulations: The FTC, USDA, and FDA

Pet food regulations are set by the Federal Trade Commission (FTC), the United States Department of Agriculture (USDA), the Food and Drug Administration (FDA), and agencies at the state level.[7] Each regulatory agency has its own jurisdiction as it applies to pet foods, although there is some overlap.

- **Federal Trade Commission:** The FTC guards against false and misleading practices in labeling and advertising.[8] For example, if a company produces a pet food that claims to be "naturally preserved" and turns out to contain ethoxyquin (an artificial preservative), this would be a violation of FTC regulations.

- **United States Department of Agriculture:** The USDA's primary concern is the origin and safety of ingredients. All meat products, including pet foods, sold commercially within the U.S. must be processed within a USDA-inspected facility. Imported products are also subjected to USDA scrutiny. The goal is to ensure that ingredients in human and animal food are free from contaminants and do not pose a health threat. When there is a food recall because of safety concerns, the USDA is in charge.

- **Food and Drug Administration:** The FDA is concerned with the ingredient list rather than the individual ingredients.[9] In particular, the FDA regulates what ingredients can be labeled as "food" versus a "drug." (Unlike labeling for people, there is no classification for nutritional supplementation in animals. Legally speaking, something is either a food or a drug.)

  The FDA is very particular about what ingredients can go into pet food. It has a published list of approved animal food ingredients. Anything not on the list is not supposed to be put into food for animals. Since there is no legal definition for supplements, putting them in commercial pet food is technically illegal.[10]

The Nutritional Guidelines: NRC and AAFCO

- **National Research Council:** The NRC is part of the National Academy of Sciences and has been providing nutritional guidelines for feeding dogs, cats, and rabbits since the 1940s. When the NRC releases guidelines for animal nutrition, it should theoretically offer objective recommendations based on scientific research and calculations that use optimal ingredients. In other words, there is an assumption made by the NRC that the ingredients going into your pet's food are high quality, with easily absorbed and assimilated nutrients. However, that assumption does not always bear out, which explains the shortcomings in some commercial pet foods.

- **Association of American Feed Control Officials:** AAFCO is an independent organization that publishes pet food standards based on NRC research. AAFCO has no regulatory authority, but its guidelines are used by regulatory agencies. While the NRC generates recommendations about *optimal* nutrition for animals, AAFCO analyzes pet foods and provides *minimum* nutritional parameters for pet foods to meet in order to be considered "complete and balanced." The term *complete and balanced* is actually a legally protected term and can only be used by foods meeting AAFCO standards. State and federal regulatory agencies utilize AAFCO standards to determine their pet food regulations.

The Business of Pet Food

Like any other business, the pet food industry is a for-profit venture. With the ultimate goal of making money, companies often seek out the least expensive ingredients, which are usually not the optimally digestible and bioavailable ingredients the NRC had in mind when it made its recommendations. This is why AAFCO developed guidelines that take into account ingredients that may be less than perfect. Although AAFCO guidelines are based on NRC data, they diverge in places where AAFCO deemed the NRC guidelines to be impractical.[11]

AAFCO evaluates foods in two categories: adult maintenance; and growth, reproduction, and lactation. AAFCO labels foods as "complete and balanced" for one or both of these categories based on either a biochemical analysis of the food or a successful feeding trial. Pet food does not need to be certified by AAFCO in order to be on the market. As mentioned previously, however, a food cannot make the claim "complete and balanced" without the AAFCO seal of approval.

The entire regulatory framework is designed to monitor safety of ingredients and adequacy of nutrient profiles, as well as to prevent deceptive claims and labeling, but it's important to note that setting *minimum* standards is as far as the government and AAFCO will go. For a food to be considered "complete and balanced" according to AAFCO guidelines, it needs only to not get your pet sick from a nutritional deficiency and not have too much of anything that could cause illness from excess. It's a pretty low bar to clear.

The waters get even more murky when you consider who is funding the research. The Pet Food Institute indirectly provides funding to the NRC, whose research forms the basis of AAFCO feeding guidelines and ultimately influences pet food regulation.[12] Conflicts of interest, to say the least!

Demanding More Than the Minimum

While everything stated about the pet food industry is 100 percent accurate, don't let that leave you with the impression that all commercial pets foods or pet food companies are inherently bad. Truly they are not. Smart, sincere people work for big companies such as Hills, Royal Canin, and Purina, not to mention dozens (if not hundreds) of smaller companies. These people are dedicating their professional lives to improving the health of pets through nutrition. I've met a lot of them, and trust me when I say their sincerity is genuine.

If the people behind the curtain at the large pet food corporations are sincere, then what is standing between our pets and the perfect commercially prepared pet food? In the end, it has a lot to do with profits, consumer demand, and convenience. As long as there is demand for something cheap and easy, pet food companies will fill the shelves. Convenience is everything in our society, and healthful food is generally less convenient than unhealthful food.

Intuitively, everyone can agree that a fresh, whole-food–based diet is better for humans and animals alike. These diets, however, are often perishable, require refrigeration, and are much more costly to produce than kibble or cans. Not everyone has the time and/or resources to purchase or make fresh, whole foods for their pet(s), never mind the education to understand the importance.

The good news is that if we feed our pets foods that meet USDA, FDA, FTC, and AAFCO regulations, our furry friends will not die from vitamin and mineral deficiencies or other nutritional imbalances. While that's a great baseline to start with, what about ingredients and nutrient profiles that are optimal to promote ideal physical health? How do we up the ante from averting death by malnutrition to helping our pets live stronger, healthier, and longer? That's the focus of the next chapter.

CHAPTER 4

INGREDIENTS AND PREPARATION

The part can never be well unless the whole is well.

– PLATO

Our goal is for our pets to thrive rather than merely survive—an impossibility unless we begin with a foundation of optimal nutrition. Luckily, pet foods have come a long way in recent years. The larger companies are starting to add more meat-based proteins to their recipes and use fewer plant fillers. Perhaps even more exciting is the upswell of smaller companies offering higher-quality products, such as freeze-dried and frozen raw meals for pets. Make no mistake, the change is consumer driven. Companies are responding to the demands of their customer base.

In this chapter, we begin to transcend pet food regulations and "adequacy" in our quest for the ideal diet. With this in mind, there are two primary considerations in evaluating diets: food ingredients and food format (method of preparation).

Ingredients

When evaluating the quality of pet food ingredients, we are using a different scale than you would for gourmet dining. High-quality ingredients do not necessarily mean filet mignon or heirloom potatoes. What we're looking for are ingredients that are predictably highly nutritious and easily digestible. Any number of meats, organs, vegetables, fruits, and even whole grains can fit in this category. By contrast, lower-quality diets may contain fillers such as corn or wheat that bulk up the food at a lower cost.

Exotic Protein Sources

There seem to be new and ever more exotic ingredients being used in our pet food all the time. The protein options in ingredient lists now read like a list of attractions at a wild animal park, with bison, kangaroo, and even opossum as options. All of these exotic ingredients are ostensibly there to help animals with dietary sensitivities to standard pet food proteins. While there is no doubt some animals do have these sensitivities, marketing would have us believe they are of epidemic proportions.

Most pets do just fine on more "mundane" proteins such as beef, chicken, and lamb. The important thing is that your pet food's main protein source is *real meat*, not meat by-products or meal, or a vegetarian source such as soy, corn, gluten, or grains.

Meat By-products, Meat Meal, and Gluten

Inferior proteins in pet foods can be found as meat by-products, by-product meal, or gluten. By-products are generally organs, fat, and/or leftover scraps. As stated in Chapter 2, by-products are not by definition poor nutrition, but the vagueness of the term allows manufacturers far too much leeway in what they are actually putting in the food. Always avoid foods listing meat by-products or meat meal as ingredients.[1, 2]

The Truth about Grains

A recent trend in pet foods is the "grain-free" movement. Pet food companies producing these diets aren't overtly saying it, but the implication is that grains are inherently bad for animals. This is only partially accurate. Many "grain-free" pet foods are, in fact, good-quality diets; the term, however, is a marketing tactic.

Grains encompass a wide swath of agricultural products ranging from corn and rice to barley and amaranth. Making a blanket judgment about grains is a bit like saying all pizza is bad because you don't like anchovies. The appropriateness of a given grain in pet foods hinges on the species being fed, the amount of grain being used, and the nutritional purpose of the grain in the diet.

On the negative side, grains are sometimes used as cheap fillers in pet foods. Corn and/or wheat can be utilized to bulk up pet food and to provide an inexpensive protein in the form of gluten. Furthermore, gluten and soy are also likely genetically modified.

On the upside, grains can be used as a source of complex carbohydrate and fiber, particularly in canine diets. These diets should still utilize meat for protein, but high-quality grains can add to the nutrient profile. Grains such as millet, barley, and oats are generally not genetically modified and have excellent nutritional value in canine diets. Proper use of these ingredients (like all others) is why we rely on our highly trained nutritionists to create ideal diet recipes.

Comparing Methods of Preparation

Equally as critical as ingredients within the ideal diet is the method of preparation. Preparation methods affect both palatability and nutritional value of food. In this section, we will evaluate the most common methods of preparing pet foods and compare what they have to offer our pets.

Pet food manufacturers create and market many pet foods based on cost and convenience rather than ideal nutrition. It is up to you, the consumer, to determine which products meet the standards you believe are important. For the purposes of comparison, food formats must be normalized to allow evaluation on an even playing field. Accomplishing this is going to take a bit of math.

Compare Different Foods by Calculating Dry Matter (DM)

The relative moisture (water) content of a food has an enormous impact on nutrient content when expressed as a percentage. Therefore, pet food labels express nutritional analysis on an *as-fed* or *dry matter (DM)* basis. The term *as-fed* means that the percentage of a given nutrient includes the water content of the food, while DM indicates the percentages with the water removed.

Consider this: If I have 100 grams of pure protein in a bowl, the bowl contains 100 percent protein. If I add 100 grams of water, the same 100 grams of protein are there, but the bowl now contains 50 percent protein. Nothing changed but the water.

Using our example above of 100 grams of protein and 100 grams of water in the bowl, we would express the amount of protein in two ways:

- 50 percent protein on an as-fed basis
- 100 percent protein on a DM basis

This concept is critical if you are going to try to compare pet foods that have different moisture contents. If you don't account for water, you are metaphorically comparing apples and oranges. Even foods of the same format (two different brands of canned food, for example) may contain different moisture content.

If you can find the ingredients of two diets expressed on a DM basis, then comparison is easy. Dry matter analysis of one food is directly comparable to dry matter analysis of another; apples and apples, so to speak. Go ahead and make your comparison.

However, if DM is not available, it can be easily calculated with the following formula:

$$\text{DM percent} =$$
$$\text{percentage of a given nutrient} \div (100 - \text{percentage of moisture content}) \times 100$$

For example, say you want to find the protein content of a food on a DM basis. The package label states the protein content of the food is 15 percent, and the moisture content is 50 percent. Plug in those values in the above equation thus:

$$\text{DM percent of protein content} = 15 \div (100 - 50) \times 100 = 15 \div 50 \times 100 = 30$$

In this example, the protein content of the diet is 30 percent on a DM basis.

Using the formula, you can easily take any nutrient (protein, fat, fiber, etc.) and convert it to DM. Without comparing dry matter nutrients, there is really no way to make a meaningful comparison of nutritional content.[3]

Accounting for Toxins:
MRPs and AGEs in Pet Food

Most commercially prepared dog and cat foods are cooked in some way. Not surprisingly, cooking methods affect nutritional value. Less intuitively obvious, however, is that cooking methods can lead to the formation of potentially harmful chemicals within the food itself.

Maillard reaction products (MRPs) and advanced glycation end products (AGEs) form as a result of browning proteins and carbohydrates during the cooking process. The brown color that develops on the outside of food during cooking is due to the Maillard reaction. (Think of when you've cooked meat or baked bread.) The Maillard reaction changes the bioavailability of certain amino acids in food and can cause disease in humans. MRPs and AGEs are associated with causing oxidative damage to our bodies and may either cause or complicate diseases such as cancer, diabetes, and chronic kidney failure.

When researchers evaluated the presence of MRPs and AGEs in dogs and cats that consumed kibble or canned diets, it was found that dogs and cats consume 122 and 38 times more MRPs per day, respectively, than the average adult human.[4, 5, 6] By utilizing a homemade, fresh-food diet, we can largely avoid these toxins altogether.

Raw Feeding

I have been an advocate of raw feeding for many years and have seen overwhelmingly positive results in my patients with regard to allergies, digestive issues, and overall well-being. However, raw feeding is not right for every individual or every household.

Dogs and cats tend to be more resistant to food-borne illness than people, and clinical disease from bacteria such as salmonella, E. coli, and campylobacter is exceedingly rare. That said, there is the potential for problems in sick animals as well as for possible cross-contamination to humans in the house. In other words, your dog or cat may eat food containing bacteria and be fine, but if they eat that food and then give you a big, wet kiss, they could potentially transfer the bacteria to you. Before beginning raw feeding, educate yourself regarding potential risks and how to take the appropriate, commonsense precautions outlined in Appendix C in the section discussing raw versus cooked food preparation.[7, 8]

Comparing Pet Food Formats

Now that we have taken both quality of ingredients and some of the pitfalls of preparation into account, we can compare the different pet food formats.

Dry Food (Kibble)

Kibble is by far the most popular format of food. Most kibble is manufactured through the process of extrusion.

- You can't beat the convenience. Just open the bag and pour into the bowl.

- It is inexpensive.

- The food has a long shelf life.

- It's made in a high-temperature process, which may affect the nutrient profile.

- This method of production leads to the presence of MRPs and AGEs.

- The level and type of preservatives used in dry food vary. Some foods use natural preservatives such as mixed tocopherols and rosemary extract. Others use artificial (and potentially harmful) preservatives such as ethoxyquin.

- Kibble is by definition high in carbohydrates, even the "low-carb" and "grain-free" varieties. High-carbohydrate diets can lead to weight gain and chronic inflammation. Note: Some smaller companies have begun to introduce baked (rather than extruded) kibble that is lower in carbohydrates.

- The low moisture content in kibble may also lead to pets (particularly cats) having chronic mild dehydration, which can affect health in both the short and long term.

Canned Diets

There is a range of canned diets from super premium to very low quality. It is important to read ingredient labels and know what you are buying.

- Canned foods are convenient and have a long shelf life.

- The high moisture content helps provide extra water in the diet (which is a benefit over dry foods).

- Canned foods are lower in carbohydrates than kibble. (Note: Canned foods containing grains such as rice will have higher levels of carbohydrates.)

- Canned foods are by necessity processed at very high temperatures, which leads to the presence of MRPs and AGEs. The process may also result in the loss of micronutrients and enzymes that are beneficial for your pet.

- Metals or plastics (from the can or the can liner) can potentially leach into the food.[9, 10]

Low-Temperature Processed Foods

These diets are generally freeze-dried or dehydrated versions of fresh, whole-food diets. Many pet stores carry them.

- Freeze-dried diets retain many of the benefits of the fresh, raw diets. The low-temperature processing preserves micronutrients that might be lost in higher temperature methods. (Note that dehydration is a somewhat higher-temperature process than freeze-drying but is still preferable to kibble or cans.)

- Since water is added to the diet before feeding, moisture content is controlled, which helps make sure pets are getting enough water.

- As with the fresh-food diets, these diets tend to be made with high-quality ingredients.

- These diets have a long shelf life at room temperature.

- Several freeze-dried pet foods are certified pathogen-free when packaged. (This means they are tested and found free of bacterial contamination.)

- Freeze-dried raw products carry the risk of cross-contamination. Be careful in households with small children or immune-compromised people. (Cross-contamination refers to exposure to bacteria from secondary contact. In other words, if the dog eats his raw food and then licks someone in the face or someone touches the plate the food was on and then puts their finger in their mouth.)

- These products tend to be more costly than kibble and cans, which can sometimes present a financial challenge for people with a large dog or multiple pets.

Fresh-Food Diets

These diets include either raw or lightly cooked foods purchased fresh or frozen or made at home using a balanced recipe.

- A balanced, fresh, whole-food diet contains excellent nutrition and high moisture content while minimizing exposure to artificial ingredients and preservatives.

- The lack of high-temperature processing preserves micronutrients and enzymes that may be lost in other food formats. Many pets with chronic inflammatory conditions, such as allergies or inflammatory bowel disease (IBD), fare better on fresh-food diets.

- These diets tend to be made with high-quality ingredients.

- Several raw pet foods are certified pathogen-free when packaged. This means they are tested and found free of bacterial contamination.

- When made at home, fresh-food diets can be reasonably cost effective.

- Fresh food is perishable and requires frequent preparation and/or significant freezer space for storage.

- Appropriate precautions should be taken when handling and feeding raw meat regardless of prior testing for bacteria. Potential cross-contamination to humans should be considered.

- Homemade fresh-food diets can be cost-effective but time-consuming to prepare.

- When purchased premade in stores, these diets can be expensive for larger dogs or in multiple-pet households.

The Bottom Line: Good vs. Optimal

Most good-quality pet foods, regardless of format, provide good nutrition. The "super premium" brands of food use excellent ingredients. Once they are processed into cans or kibble, though, some of the nutrition is lost. *Optimal* nutrition can only be achieved through fresh, whole-food diets. While the particular ingredients and nutrient profiles of optimal diets will vary with species, age, and medical conditions, the future is leaving kibble and canned diets behind in the distance.

In our quest for optimal nutrition, practicality must play a role. (This is the real world, after all.) No doubt we would all be healthier if we had a private chef preparing all of our meals with the best and freshest ingredients. Sadly (for me, at least), this is not reality. When it comes to our pets, store-bought foods are practical. In these cases, frozen raw, freeze-dried, or dehydrated foods that are readily available provide excellent options that are far superior to kibble and cans.

For those with the time and interest, well-constructed, home-prepared diets are usually the best way to feed a dog or cat. Preparing food at home means you are in control of the quality and freshness of ingredients and the food can be custom-tailored to your pet's needs. Recipes must, however, be properly nutritionally balanced by a trained nutritionist. The road to poor nutrition is often paved with the good intentions of loving pet owners. Long-term feeding of an unbalanced diet can lead to serious medical consequences. Thus, creating a home-prepared diet is absolutely not the time to wing it.

CHAPTER 5

GUIDE TO CREATING A BALANCED DIET FOR YOUR PET

Let food be thy medicine and medicine be thy food.

— HIPPOCRATES

The sage words of Hippocrates are as true today as they were more than 2,000 years ago. Back in his day, there were no synthetic pesticides, fertilizers, and antibiotics. All food was by definition organic. Food was medicine, and medicine was food by necessity.

Since Hippocrates's time, we have strayed from letting "medicine be thy food" into letting medicine be *in* thy food. Industrialized farming has led to food that is contaminated with antibiotics, hormones, pesticides, etc.[1] Furthermore, our food is not as nutritious as it used to be. In 2004, a researcher from the University of Texas analyzed USDA data on common fruits and vegetables and determined that 6 of the 13 nutrients evaluated had declined between 1950 and 1999.[2]

How did this happen? Decades of research into how to increase crop yield per acre has led to soil depletion as farmers selected for crops that grow faster but have fewer nutrients.[3] It is more efficient (and profitable) to have cows graze on high-energy grains such as corn rather than grasses as they naturally would. Compared to grain-fed cattle, beef from grass-fed animals has a lower overall fat content, and the fat contained has a spectrum of fatty acids that are much more beneficial to overall health. What's more, grass-fed meat is higher in vitamins A and E as well as cancer-fighting antioxidants.

Industrialization of farming has led to increased toxins and decreased nutritional content in food. As consumers, our best option is to buy locally grown, organic produce that is as "clean" and nutritious as possible. The more food is processed, the greater the loss of nutrients. Given that we are already somewhat behind the eight ball with regard to declining nutritional value of foods available to us, the best dietary option for our pets is fresh, whole foods with minimal processing and the appropriate combination of water, protein, fat, energy, vitamins, and minerals. It bears repeating that the market is consumer driven. What we buy governs what the food industry produces.

While Hippocrates's food may have been more nutritious than ours, we do have an advantage over him today: We have a much greater understanding of the science of nutrition. Many of the shortfalls in the nutrient profiles of our food can be overcome by using a variety of ingredients and appropriate supplementation. And what's more, nutritional supplementation (see Chapters 6 and 7) can be used to create food that is closer to "medicine" than perhaps even Hippocrates could have dreamed.

What Makes Up Optimal Diets

We have now successfully laid the foundation regarding how and why dog and cat diets are what they are and, in the broader sense, what they need to be. We know that not all food ingredients are created equal; how crops are grown or how livestock is fed has a significant bearing on their nutritional value. In many cases, we literally cannot compare apples to apples. It's also important to know that when a pet food company designs a diet, it is not enough to rely on published tables. To ensure accurate nutrient composition, the company should have individual ingredients and/or the entire diet analyzed for its nutrient content—and even then variability occurs, as different ingredients are sourced over time. In a home setting, it is not realistic to submit ingredients for analysis. This is why utilizing a diet created by a nutritionist is critical. It takes a highly trained eye to navigate these murky waters and come out with an ideal diet on the other side.

As we begin our discussion of optimal diets, we will evaluate the levels of protein, fat, carbohydrates, vitamins, and minerals required by the individual needs of the dog we are feeding. These needs vary based on age, breed, lifestyle, and reproductive status.

Both AAFCO and NRC publish data regarding nutritional requirements for animals in various life stages, such as growth, maintenance, reproduction, lactation, etc. As discussed in Chapter 2, NRC calculations are made using ingredients assumed to provide optimal nutrition with regard to digestibility and bioavailability. AAFCO guidelines adjust the NRC recommendations, taking pet food manufacturing concerns into account. When developing home-prepared diets, nutritionists can choose to use AAFCO, NRC, or a combination of both to calculate nutritional analysis.

Ultimately, the nutrient value of a diet is the sum of its parts. The relative nutritional analyses of individual ingredients are combined and compared to the dietary needs of the animal in question. Nutrient value of an ingredient is best determined by analyzing each one separately. The USDA's data regarding the nutritional analysis of food ingredients can be used to determine the overall nutrient content of a diet—just understand that there is going to be a certain degree of variation in nutrition relative to how given ingredients are produced.

Dietary Energy and Basal Metabolic Rate (BMR): Discover Your Pet's Daily Energy Requirements

Food comes down to energy: Energy is needed to support all body functions, from the lowest levels of cellular metabolism through organ function and body movement. Dietary energy is found in fat, protein, and carbohydrates and is measured as kilocalories (kcals). (When we humans talk about calories in our food, we are really talking about kcals. The term has been abbreviated to "calories" for convenience.) The number of calories (energy) required by an individual is based on factors such as age, breed, lifestyle, and overall health status.

Basal metabolic rate (BMR) is the measurement of how much energy is required to support and maintain the basic functions of the body. BMR is a fairly static number, as it is a measure of the minimal amount of energy the body needs for maintenance.

In reality, however, bodies have lots of other things to do than just exist. Pets move, digest food, chase a ball, etc., and all of these additional actions consume energy. The number of calories needed to power an individual's daily activities, combined with their BMR, makes up the daily energy requirement (DER).

The amount of food consumed, however, does not match up with the amount of energy the body can extract from that food. In other words, just knowing your DER is not enough. You need to know about the digestible energy of a food as well.

Digestible Energy (DE) of Food

Not every kcal consumed is a kcal absorbed. Unfortunately, nobody's digestive tract is 100 percent efficient, and thus a certain number of calories are "wasted." You know all that poop you are picking up on walks or out of the litter box? That is, in part, undigested kcals. Assuming we are not feeding a gross excess of kcals that are just passing through, what we are witnessing here is the difference between kcals fed and kcals left undigested. That difference is a function of digestible energy (DE).

DE is the percentage of food that can be absorbed by an animal. The level of digestive efficiency is a function of the relative digestibility of the food and the efficiency of their gastrointestinal (GI) tract. The great news is, we have at least partial control of both variables.

The relative digestibility of food is within our control. It is up to us as pet owners to make the choice to feed optimal diets with highly digestible ingredients. As a veterinarian, one of the consistent reports I receive after a client has switched their pet from kibble to a whole-food diet is that the pet's stool has become markedly smaller and has very little odor. This is a function of relative digestibility; when the body can digest most of the food, there is very little left to pass into the stools. Additionally, fewer undigested kcals are passing into the colon, where they would become food for our bacterial friends down there. Less bacterial activity translates to less smell.

Smaller poops that don't stink! Maybe I should just stop writing now. Does anyone need a better motivation to switch to a fresh, whole-food diet?

Digestible energy as a function of GI tract health is something we have control over as well, although less directly than manipulating food ingredients. Poor digestion has many potential origins that we will discuss in more detail in the coming section on gastrointestinal issues. For now, suffice it to say that underlying inflammation is the cause of many gastrointestinal problems and leads to poor nutrient absorption. Through the feeding of correct proteins to sensitive individuals and using appropriate supplementation, very often we can improve the health and efficiency of the GI tract.

Armed with this new information regarding the various functions and activities an animal needs energy for, the energy content of food ingredients, and factors involved with digestibility, it's time we looked at determining resting energy requirements (RER). (For our purposes, you can think of RER as very similar to BMR.)

Resting Energy Requirements (RER)
for Ideal Body Weight

RER can be calculated using the following formula[4]:

$$\text{RER in kcal/day} = 70 \times (\text{body weight in kilograms})^{0.75}$$

Then again, why bother with math? The table below is an extrapolation of RER calculations for dogs and cats by body weight. (Note that 1 kilogram = 2.2 pounds.)

Body weight (pounds)	Body weight (kilograms)	RER in kcal/day
2	0.91	65
4	1.82	110
6	2.73	149
8	3.64	184
10	4.55	218
15	6.82	295
20	9.09	366
25	11.36	433
30	13.64	497
35	15.91	558
40	18.18	616
50	22.73	729
60	27.27	835
70	31.82	938
80	36.36	1,037
90	40.91	1,132
100	45.45	1,225
110	50.00	1,316
120	54.55	1,405
130	59.09	1,492
140	63.64	1,577
150	68.18	1,661

Now we have the resting energy requirements for an animal based on its body weight or body surface area and we are one step closer to determining the daily energy requirements for your individual pet. You can use RER as a baseline to extrapolate the energy needs of an individual animal using multipliers to account for specifics such as activity level, age, breed, reproductive status, etc. The table below shows the calculation for daily energy requirements (DER) for dogs and cats.[5]

Determining DER by RER

Activity	Dog DER	Cat DER
Weight loss	1.0 × RER	1.0 × RER
Neutered adult (normal activity)	1.6 × RER	1.2 × RER
Intact adult	1.8 × RER	1.4 × RER
Light activity	2.0 × RER	N/A
Moderate activity	3.0 × RER	1.6 × RER
Heavy activity	4–8 × RER	N/A
Pregnancy (0–42 days)	1.8 × RER	1.6 × RER (free feed)
Pregnancy (42+ days)	3.0 × RER	2 × RER (free feed)
Lactation	4–8 × RER	2–6 × RER (free feed)
Puppy/kitten (weaning to 4 months)	3.0 × RER	2.5 × RER
Puppy/kitten (4 months to adult size)	2.0 × RER	2.5 × RER

The Variability of DER by Age and Breed

Keep in mind that all of these numbers and calculations are approximations based on large populations of dogs and cats. Variability among individuals is guaranteed. In addition, DER changes over time. Dogs who are younger than 2 years old may have a DER that is up to 20 percent higher than an adult dog between the ages of 3 and 7. Dogs who are older than 7 may require 20 percent less energy.

Similarly breed can make a difference, particularly with dogs. Smaller dogs have a higher energy requirement per pound of body weight than larger dogs. Even within dogs of the same size, there are going to be breed-related differences. Take a 15-pound shih tzu who is relatively sedentary and compare it to a very active Jack Russell terrier of the same size. Metabolism and breed-related differences with regard to activity level are significant factors. There is data regarding breed differences out there if you care to take the time to research it.

Large-breed puppies do have specific nutritional requirements that go beyond what we have discussed so far. Because proper nutrition of large-breed puppies has such a profound effect for the life of the dog, I've addressed this specifically in Appendix C.

Monitor Your Pet's Weight with the Body Condition Score (BCS)

A numerical system called the body condition score (BCS) is a simple way of tracking whether your pet is at an ideal weight, too fat, or too thin. Veterinarians use this tool to assess the body weight and overall condition of a dog or cat based on fat deposits and how prominent the animal's bones are.

There are two types of BCS charts. One is a 5-point scale in which a BCS 2.5 is average body weight, while the other is a 9-point scale in which a BCS 5 is average. Veterinarians commonly hand out a copy of the BCS chart with pictures so dog and cat owners have a visual reference for comparison.

Body Condition Score (BCS) Chart for Cats
Score: 1–4 = underweight, 5 = ideal, 6–9 = overweight

1	Can't feel any fat when touching cat's body. Ribs clearly observable by sight alone on short-haired cats. Upper hip bone and lower vertebrae (lumbar) easily felt by hand. Extreme abdominal tuck.
2	Can't feel any fat when touching cat's body. Ribs clearly observable by sight alone on short-haired cats. Lumbar vertebrae are easily felt and contain only a slight bit of muscle around them. Prominent abdominal tuck.
3	Small amounts of fat can be felt when touching cat's stomach. Ribs easily felt by touch with only slight layer of fat. Waist prominently tapers and stands out below ribs. Lumbar vertebrae are easily felt.
4	Lack of a distinct and palpable abdominal fat pad. Ribs can be felt by touch under a slight layer of fat. Waist visibly tapers and stands out below ribs. Moderate abdominal tuck visible.
5	Slight palpable abdominal fat pad. Ribs can be felt under a small layer of fat. Visible waist below ribs, but without a sharp taper into body.
6	Ribs can be felt under a minimal amount of extra fat. No visible abdominal tuck. Abdominal fat layer and waist are both discernible but not prominent.
7	Waist is difficult to see. Ribs have a noticeable fat covering and are not easily felt. Noticeable abdominal fat pad. Stomach is beginning to become bulbous.
8	No discernible waist. Ribs cannot be felt due to large amount of fat. Fat pockets developing around lower back (lumbar vertebrae). Stomach is clearly bulbous and has pronounced fat pad.
9	No waist whatsoever, with a stomach that is bulbous and hangs beneath the body. Many abdominal fat pockets as well as excess fat around limbs, face, and lumbar spine area. Ribs cannot be felt, covered with significant layer of fat.

Body Condition Score (BCS) Chart for Dogs
Score: 1-4 = underweight, 5 = ideal, 6-9 = overweight

1	No visible body fat. Bones visibly protrude from body. Easy to see the pelvis, ribs, and lumbar vertebrae. Emaciated and with clear signs of decreased muscle mass.
2	No tangible body fat when touched. Pelvis, ribs, and lumbar vertebrae all easy to see; other bones slightly visible. Small loss of muscle.
3	Pelvis is beginning to stand out. Tops of lumbar vertebrae are showing. Ribs can be easily felt, with no tangible body fat around them. Prominent abdominal tuck. Prominent waist.
4	Abdominal tuck and waist both easy to see. Ribs can be felt easily, with a small layer of fat covering them.
5	When looking down on a dog, easy to see waist as distinct from ribs. When viewed from side, abdominal tuck is evident. Ribs can be felt even though there is some fat–fat layer is not too thick.
6	When looking down on a dog, waist is visible with some difficulty. Can see abdominal tuck. Ribs can be felt underneath a moderate layer of extra fat.
7	Abdominal tuck may or may not be present, but can no longer see waist when looking down on dog from above. Visible fat buildup where tail meets body, as well as around lumbar area. Ribs can be felt with difficulty under significant amounts of fat.
8	Waist and abdominal tuck are not visible. Stomach and abdomen may be hanging out from the body and look distended. Large fat buildups around lumbar and tail area. Ribs either cannot be felt when touched or are able to be felt only when pressed forcefully. Significant fat covering the ribs.
9	Abdomen is clearly distended. Abdominal tuck and waist are completely missing. Ribs cannot be felt. Huge pockets of fat over the base of the tail, spine, and chest. Fat buildup on individual limbs and the neck.

Practical Use of This Information

Optimal nutrition is achieved through careful consideration of ingredients, digestibility, nutritional profile, and the amount fed. What you now have in your arsenal is an understanding of what nutrients and energy levels should be present in the ideal dog and cat diet. Your basic options at this point are to buy it or make it.

If you choose to make your own pet food, remember that balancing diets is highly complex and cannot be done by eye. After 10 years of college and nearly 20 as a veterinarian, I defer to veterinary nutritionists when I need a custom diet formulation. The stakes are too high to do it any other way. A dog or cat can be eating the freshest organic ingredients and still get into nutritional trouble if the diet is not properly balanced.

You now also have the information you need to compare the different types of commercial foods available. Many of the raw and freeze-dried diets available on the market today are far superior to the cans and bags of kibble that used to be our only options. The drawbacks of buying commercially prepared raw or freeze-dried diets are cost (particularly for large dogs) and a lack of flexibility with ingredients in the case of a pet that has specific dietary requirements.

My advice is to start by determining DER via calculation or the chart and use it as a starting point. After that, monitor your pet's BCS and employ good old common sense when determining how many kcals your dog or cat requires in a day. What's the worst that can happen? If you feed him too much, he'll gain weight, so you cut him back. Vice versa if you feed him too little. Biology is forgiving.

CHAPTER 6

THE LOWDOWN ON SUPPLEMENTS

The best doctor gives the least medicine.

– BENJAMIN FRANKLIN

In the preceding chapters, we have discussed nutrition in the context of an ideal diet for dogs and cats based on their evolutionary biology. However, we can do even better than that. By understanding how our pets' bodies work, we have the potential to achieve a far loftier goal than ideal nutrition. We can utilize nutrition, nutritional supplementation, and herbal therapy to prevent and cure disease.

In the world of medicine, there is often more than one way to get from A to B. For example, a pet with allergies can often be relieved of their itching through the use of steroids (prednisone) or through dietary changes and natural anti-inflammatory supplements such as omega fatty acids. Both are effective at relieving symptoms, but long-term use of steroids can have profound negative effects on the body such as muscle atrophy and liver damage, whereas the fatty acids do not.

The unfortunate reality is that Western medical care frequently favors short-term benefits over long-term consequences. If you doubt this, listen to the list of potential side effects for any prescription medicine advertised on television. Undeniably, we live in an instant-gratification society, and this plays a part in the tendency of doctors and pet owners to look for the quick fix.

Natural medicine, on the other hand, is often, but not always, about the long view. Admittedly, there are times when instant relief is needed and potent short-term conventional therapy is a blessing. This is the very nature of integrative care: utilizing the best of both worlds to achieve the greatest result while minimizing negative side effects.

Walking hand in hand with the desire for instant gratification tends to be a lack of consideration for recognizing factors that contribute to disease. In other words, preventive medicine is not a big part of the Western medical paradigm. With the exception of vaccinations, there is not a lot of preventive care in conventional medicine, although that is starting to change. (See Appendix B for more information on vaccinations.) Holistic and integrative doctors view illness as a late stage of the disease process. By the time a disease is detectable, often it has been brewing beneath the surface for quite some time. These things really don't come out of nowhere. When viewed through this lens, the importance of prevention and treatment of disease before it is a visible entity becomes crystal clear.

Supplements to Support General Health and for Specific Conditions

Fresh, whole-food diets should form the basis of your pet's nutrition, while nutritional supplementation fills in the gaps. Consider the fresh-food platform as the foundation of our health-care structure, which we continue to build upon with concentrated nutritional supplementation that we direct toward general health and specific body systems.

Dogs and cats in good health that are eating a balanced, fresh, whole-food diet may require few, if any, additional vitamins and minerals. If your pet is eating a commercially prepared or a homemade diet with a balanced recipe, then they have their basic nutrient needs covered—no need for a multivitamin. Remember, in order for a food to gain AAFCO certification, it must contain levels of specific nutrients to prevent diseases caused by nutritional deficiency or excess. That's more than a lot of people can claim with their current eating habits!

It's important to note, however, that some smaller pet food manufacturers may not be evaluating their foods according to AAFCO standards. (AAFCO certification is not a *legal* requirement.) In such instances, do your due diligence and find out what veterinary nutritionist the company is using and how the nutrient profiles of the diet in question are being evaluated.

Our quest is to move *beyond* the prevention of diseases caused by deficient (or excess) nutrition and into *optimal* health. How do we determine what supplements are needed by our dogs and cats? The answer depends on criteria such as age, lifestyle, underlying medical conditions, and the quality of their diet. How much supplementation and of what type is clearly the question at hand.

There are so many examples of nutritional supplementation improving the quality of life for animals. In many cases, nutritional supplements can improve or resolve medical conditions that have plagued pets for months or years. For example, severe arthritis is a debilitating disease that significantly affects quality of life. It is not that uncommon in veterinary medicine to euthanize large dogs because of intractable arthritis pain and an inability to move. These pets with arthritis often benefit from glucosamine and chondroitin supplements to support their damaged cartilage. Taking it one step further and controlling the pain and inflammation by adding Boswellia, turmeric, fish oil, gotu kola, etc., can often decrease a pet's need for prescription pain medications.

Nutritional and herbal supplementation can (and should) be thought of in the same light as conventional drug therapy. These compounds have documented biological activity just like drugs do. Just because they are natural does not mean they are less effective than drugs. It also does not mean they are completely harmless. The key to safe, successful therapy is to know how specific supplements work and what their potential interactions may be within the body or with pharmaceuticals. We will discuss many nutritional supplements and herbs, their uses, and necessary precautions in Part III, in the sections discussing specific medical conditions.

A Caution about Supplementation

The requirements for all essential nutrients varies based on the life stage of a pet. During periods of rapid growth or reproduction, dogs and cats also have an increased demand for nutrition. Similar increased requirements occur in geriatric animals as immune function and the bioavailability of these nutrients tend to wane with aging.

Indiscriminate supplementation, however, is not the answer. Excessive supplementation can lead to significant clinical problems, many of which are similar to the respective deficiency states of these ingredients.

The solution is to feed a diet that is balanced optimally for your pet, taking into account its age, lifestyle, and underlying medical conditions (if any). Frequently, this can be accomplished through a commercially prepared high-quality, fresh, whole-food diet or homemade food using a balanced recipe. For those pets with complicating medical issues or nutritional needs that fall outside the norm, a veterinarian and/or nutritionist is an invaluable resource.

How to Determine Supplement Quality

Quality in nutritional supplementation can be summed up in one statement: There is no government oversight regarding labeling claims on nutritional supplements. When you buy a bottle of vitamins, supplements, fish oil, etc., there is no one policing the contents of the bottle.[1, 2] It may or may not contain exactly what is on the label. The name of the game is caveat emptor—let the buyer beware.

Sales of nutritional supplements in the United States were estimated at $36.7 billion in 2014.[3] With this kind of money being spent, you can be sure that being an educated consumer is vital to getting the best-quality products available. You can also be sure that someone is out there looking to make money by selling mislabeled, ineffective, and potentially harmful products. When shopping for the highest-quality supplements, keep the following in mind:

- **Where you buy matters:** Get supplements from a reputable health-care provider or vitamin store, people whose business it is to carry high-quality products. Although convenience stores, drug stores, and discount stores tend to have lower prices, they also may have lower quality.

- **Brand matters:** Choose either reputable brands that come recommended by someone knowledgeable or brands that can demonstrate a guaranteed analysis of their product through independent laboratories. This way you will know you are buying what is printed on the label.

- **Buy only what is on the label:** Look for brands that can show independent analysis to guarantee the product is free of contaminants such as heavy metals or other toxins.

- **Look For GMP:** Many high-quality supplements will bear the Good Manufacturing Processes (GMP) seal on the label. This claim can only be made by facilities inspected by the FDA and found to be upholding the highest standards of cleanliness and quality in manufacturing.

- **Look for NASC:** The National Animal Supplement Council is a private organization that evaluates veterinary supplements for safety and accuracy of label claims. You can feel good about the quality of supplements with the NASC seal on the label. There are certainly excellent animal supplements out there that are not NASC-approved, but keeping to the guidelines above will ensure quality.

Bioavailability refers to the level to which the body is able to absorb and use the nutrient in question. Bioavailability is one of those topics that fill textbooks and doctoral dissertations. Let's not get too deep into the weeds, though. Generally speaking, high-quality supplements made by reputable companies factor in bioavailability when they formulate a supplement. This is yet another reason to use only high-quality supplements.

Vitamins and minerals that naturally occur in food are, not surprisingly, highly bioavailable. In an ideal world, this is how we would provide our pets (and ourselves) with all necessary nutrition. Hence the push toward a whole-food diet. The reality, of course, is that in most cases this is difficult to achieve—which is particularly true in regard to therapeutic levels of nutrients to treat a disease condition. In such cases, a pet often needs much higher levels of nutrients than those in food.

Supplementation can balance a diet deficient in certain nutrients and make it safe for long-term consumption. This is particularly useful with pets that have dietary sensitivities and can only tolerate very limited ingredients. Take, for example, a pet whose dietary sensitivities allow them to eat only chicken and rice. Anything else seems to cause severe gastrointestinal upset. The combination of chicken and rice alone is not nutritionally balanced, so supplements are critical.

In addition, higher, therapeutic doses of certain nutrients can be helpful in the treatment of disease. For example, omega fatty acids are sometimes used in the treatment of cancer (more on this in Chapter 20). While certain levels of omega-3 and omega-6 fatty acids are present in food, diet alone cannot achieve the therapeutic levels required.

For the most part, we will discuss specific supplements and herbs and their usage in the sections addressing specific medical conditions. That said, there are a few that warrant discussion here. Despite variability among individuals, a few supplements are almost universally beneficial in maintaining good health and preventing disease while having few (if any) side effects.

The Importance of Probiotics and Prebiotics

The term *probiotic* means a supplement containing live bacteria intended to be ingested for the benefit of the GI tract and, by association, the body as a whole. When most people think of bacteria, they think of infections and contamination. While bacteria is sometimes responsible for such things, it can get a bad rap. Under the right circumstances, bacteria can:

- Help with digestion and nutrient absorption
- Prevent diarrhea and constipation
- Support optimal immune system function
- Prevent inflammation

Supplementing the diet with the right kind of bacteria can accomplish all the things listed above and more. Probiotics are possibly the most benign *and* most beneficial supplement almost all animals can benefit from.

The secret to beneficial bacteria lies in understanding how the body works. The GI tract begins at the mouth and ends with the anus; it includes the mouth, esophagus, stomach, pancreas, gallbladder, duodenum, jejunum, ileum, cecum, colon, rectum, and anus. That's a lot of stuff! This amazing collection of tissues and organs is responsible for the body's ability to absorb and assimilate nutrients and get rid of toxic waste products; it's an integral part of the immune system.

The fascinating part of all of this is that the gut is filled with bacteria! If you don't generally think of bacteria as a particularly good thing, consider that you have 10 times more bacteria in your gut than you have cells in your entire body.[4] Did that give you the creeps a little? Believe me, you do not want to live without these little buggers. As symbiotic organisms, we rely on trillions of bacteria to keep us healthy.[5]

Along with countless bacteria, the GI tract is also home to approximately 70 percent of the immune cells in the body.[6] The balance of the bacterial population (flora) in the gut is crucial for proper function of the immune system. Imbalances of the GI flora can lead not only to vomiting and diarrhea, but also to more widespread issues affecting all aspects of body function. Bacterial imbalance (dysbiosis) can lead to immune system dysfunction, which leads to ill health. If you have ever known someone with irritable bowel syndrome or Crohn's disease, you may have seen the toll GI dysfunction can take on total health.[7, 8, 9]

Probiotics support the body through enhancing the barrier of the intestinal wall, which in turn supports the immune system. This, in turn, aids in the tolerance of food antigens and protects against pathogens (harmful organisms) in the gut. Thus, probiotics are useful to prevent and treat diarrhea and many other manifestations of GI upset.

Keeping the GI flora happy and balanced leads to a more optimally functioning body as a whole. When bacterial imbalance and/or GI inflammation occurs, the results can range from vomiting and diarrhea to constipation, gas, and systemic disease. Overall, there are a lot of great reasons to pay attention to probiotics and GI tract health.

Probiotic supplements are either mixed in with food or given directly orally. They often contain a number of bacteria such as lactobacillus, bifidobacterium, and enterococcus. High-quality probiotic supplements should contain billions of cells, or colony forming units (CFUs), per dose. Look on the label; it should guarantee CFUs in the billions (not merely millions). Probiotics generally need to be refrigerated once opened, as the product is live.[10]

Good probiotic supplements are often combined with prebiotics. Prebiotics are nondigestible food ingredients that selectively stimulate the growth and/or activity of one or a limited number of bacteria in the colon, thus improving host health. In short, prebiotics are food for the beneficial bacteria of the gut—the colon in particular. Generally, these can be found in the form of fructooligosaccharides (FOS). You will find these listed on product labels in several ways including FOS, oligofructose, inulin, and oligosaccharides.

The benefits are positive with few, if any, potential side effects. Every dog and cat can benefit from probiotics.

Essential Fatty Acids

Much like probiotics, supplementation with essential fatty acids (EFAs) is almost universally beneficial. Adding these fats to the diet benefits the body in the following ways:

- Supports normal digestion and nutrient absorption

- Supports a healthy immune system

- Improves skin and coat quality

- Decreases allergic response

- Provides nutrients to every cell in the body

Recall from Chapter 2 the importance of omega-3 and omega-6 fatty acids, also known as essential fatty acids. These are fats that the body cannot synthesize from other dietary components, so their inclusion is essential for a complete and balanced diet. Omega-6 fatty acids are found in a wide variety of foods. Most diets have plenty of omega-6 and do not require supplementation, with the exception of the feline requirement for arachidonic acid. Omega-3s are not as common, so I recommend supplementation.

Omega-3 fatty acids can be broken down into three major types: eicosapentaenoic acid (EPA), docosahexaenoic acid (DHA), and alpha-linolenic acid (ALA). ALA is by far the easiest of the three omega-3s to come by in food. ALA is present in plant and nut oils. EPA and DHA are primarily found in marine sources such as fish oil, krill oil, and mussel oil.[11] EPA and DHA can also be synthesized from ALA in the diet. The process is highly inefficient, however (although dogs do it better than cats), and should not take the place of directly supplementing EPA and DHA.[12]

Now that we have extolled the virtues of EPA and DHA, how much are you supposed to give? The answer to that depends somewhat on whether you are using them to support general health or to treat a pet with a particular condition.

On the whole, the dosing recommendation for general health in dogs and cats is 220 to 330 milligrams of combined EPA and DHA per 10 kilograms (22 pounds) of body weight. Remember that we are talking about 220 to 330 milligrams of EPA and DHA, not the milligram weight of the full dose of fish oil. You will have to read the label to see how much EPA and DHA is in any particular product.[13]

Therapeutic use of EPA and DHA is a bit of a different story, and I often recommend using higher doses to support pets with specific conditions. The following doses of combined EPA and DHA are recommended in therapeutic applications in dogs.[14]

Disorder	Combined EPA + DHA daily dosage for a 10-kg (20-lb) dog
Hyperlipidemia	675 milligrams
Chronic kidney disease	790 milligrams
Cardiovascular disease	645 milligrams
Osteoarthritis	1,745 milligrams
Inflammatory or immunologic disorder	700 milligrams
General health	220–330 milligrams
NRC recommended	170 milligrams
NRC safe upper limit	2,080 milligrams

As you can see, these numbers are quite a bit higher than the NRC-recommended level, but still significantly lower than the published safe upper limits. While the chart above was published based on canine data only, the numbers likely hold true for cats as well. Just remember that the doses listed are combined EPA and DHA for a 10-kilogram (22-pound) animal.

Medium-Chain Triglycerides

Medium-chain triglycerides (MCTs) are a beneficial fat in much the same way as EFAs. While not essential in the sense that they must be added to the diet, MCTs have widespread health benefits. Many of these benefits arise from the unique way MCTs are digested and utilized by the body. Compared to other ingested fats, MCTs are absorbed more quickly and are much more likely to be accessed as an energy source rather than being stored as fat. Among other things, this rapid utilization as energy makes MCTs an excellent food source for the brain. Because of this, MCTs have been found to be effective in enhancing cognitive function in older dogs and humans.[15, 16]

In addition to being brain food, MCTs have widespread effects on the body. Research has shown MCTs to be an effective therapy for weight loss, in the treatment of seizure disorders, and reduction of GI inflammation, as well as being an effective antibacterial and antiviral therapy.[17, 18, 19, 20] There is also evidence that MCTs may be beneficial in cancer therapy as well.[21] In short, medium-chain triglycerides are an excellent nutrient that supports multiple body systems.

MCTs occur naturally in palm oil and dairy products, although the most readily available and highest concentrations are found in coconut oil. Regular coconut oil contains four different types of MCTs, which vary in molecular size and bioavailability. The most biologically active of these, caprylic acid, makes up about 6 percent of coconut oil. Caprylic acid is very quickly metabolized compared to other MCTs and other fats.

When it comes to supplementing pets with MCTs, cats can be tricky. They usually don't like the taste and thus are reluctant to eat it (even mixed in with food). There is also concern that MCT supplementation could predispose cats to a liver condition called hepatic lipidosis (see Chapter 18). It is unclear if the condition is a direct effect of the MCT or if it is secondary to cats going off their food due to palatability issues. If you do wish to try MCT supplementation in cats, use one-eighth (small cats) to a quarter (larger cats) teaspoon of organic coconut oil in food per day.

Supplementing your dog with MCTs is easily done by mixing organic coconut oil into their food. Give between a half and one teaspoon per 10 pounds of dog per day. If MCTs are being used to treat a specific condition or you just want to increase the potency of the supplementation, consider using a refined coconut oil instead. Products like Brain Octane, made by Bulletproof, contain 10 times more caprylic acid than regular coconut oil. The higher dose of highly bioavailable caprylic acid is formulated to have greater efficacy.

Practical Use of This Information

The takeaway from this chapter is understanding the benefits of nutritional supplementation for home-prepared diets and realizing that not all supplements are created equal. Read labels. Ask questions. Know what you are buying. Lastly, the use of probiotics, prebiotics, EFAs, and MCTs will benefit almost any pet.

When it comes to supplementation of healthy pets and those dealing with illness, I recommend essential fatty acids and a supplement with probiotics and prebiotics nearly across the board. MCTs are a great idea for most dogs. The only exception would be in animals that are sensitive to them, which is uncommon. For all other supplements, be sure to consult with a veterinarian or veterinary nutritionist.

Modern medicine continues to improve its ability to put out medical fires and save patients' lives. However, many of those fires were started by years of poor nutrition and detrimental lifestyle choices. Nutrition (good or bad) forms the foundation of the body's health.

In Part II of this book, we'll build on the base of knowledge you learned in these first chapters. With this understanding, we discuss the next steps to take after you've established your pet's nutritional foundation for health: preventing and treating disease through the use of nutrition, nutritional supplementation, and herbal therapy. You'll use the rest of this book to help you shape your nutritional and health-care decisions for your pets.

If the answers to all of your questions are not illuminated, do not despair. Although one book cannot cover *every* treatment option for every disease process and their inevitable variants, in the information age your goal should not be to know everything. Instead, it is far more important to know how to ask the right questions and access the information you seek.

I hope that you will take what you have learned here and use that knowledge to open a dialogue with a veterinarian you feel comfortable with. Successful medical outcomes require a hands-on approach and a collaborative effort between pet owners and medical professionals. And as you read success stories of animals who have been helped through natural and integrative medicine, please keep this critical thing in mind: All patients respond differently to therapy as a result of their genetics and the specifics of their condition, and so all good medical treatment plans are customized to the individual. The information contained is offered to you as an inspiration in your own personal journey.

PART II

INTEGRATIVE MEDICINE: MAINTAINING AND RESTORING GOOD HEALTH

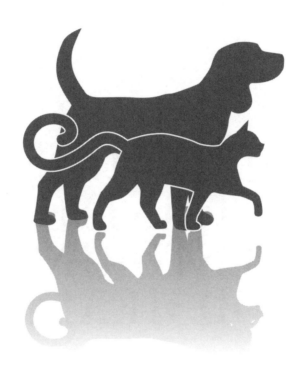

CHAPTER 7

BEYOND BASIC NUTRITION

Using Food as a Medicine

The doctor of the future will no longer treat the human frame with drugs, but rather will cure and prevent disease with nutrition.

— THOMAS EDISON

Up to now, our discussion of nutrition has been largely centered on how to provide the body with optimal amounts of water, protein, fat, fiber, vitamins, and minerals to allow biology to work at its most efficient. However, evolutionary biology is a miracle, and the power to positively affect health does not start and end with simply providing the body with all of its nutritional needs.

Beyond the basics of nutrition lies the potential to use food as medicine and change the ways a body reacts to its environment. We have the power to transcend merely "building the house" that is programmed by genetics and create something better. We can "hack" nutrition to directly manipulate gene expression—in other words, turn genes on and off like flipping a switch—and change the landscape of how the body builds and repairs itself. Through glandular therapy, whole-food medicine, oral tolerance therapy, and the new science of nutrigenomics, we are going to exchange some old-school hammers and saws for power tools.

Glandular Therapy

Glandular therapy is the use of tissues and extracts from animals to treat disease. The two most readily recognized examples of this kind of treatment are the use of thyroid and pancreatic tissue to treat hypothyroidism and exocrine pancreatic insufficiency. These two conditions are defined by the body's inability to produce hormones and enzymes necessary to maintain normal body functions. Feeding your pet tissues containing these compounds balances the body's deficiency. (Hypothyroidism and pancreatic insufficiency are discussed in detail in Chapters 21 and 15, respectively.)

Using glandular therapy in this way is well accepted and completely noncontroversial even for the most dedicated Western medical practitioner. However, glandular therapy goes further than this, illuminating how foods can have very direct and profound medical effects beyond their empirical nutrient value.

Beyond glands such as the thyroid that contain active hormones, the makeup of specific foods can make them medically beneficial. Whole tissues contain proteins, enzymes, and other nutrients that are often specific to those glands and organs. Medical reports from the 1600s describe the treatment of "night blindness" through the feeding of liver. The liver is very high in vitamin A, which can be beneficial for vision.

The easiest way to think of the broader use of glandular therapy is through the lens of "like supports like."[1] In other words, the best way to provide nutrition for the purpose of treating a medical condition is to provide the body with the building blocks it needs to repair the tissues in question. For example, what food contains all the components that make up heart muscle? Clearly the answer is the heart. Feeding heart to a patient with heart disease provides them with the precise nutrient profile they need to help maintain their heart muscle. It's a fairly intuitive concept that seems to have been forgotten in many medical circles.

Glandular Therapy through Whole Foods and Supplements

Treating disease through glandular therapy can be accomplished by including specific dietary ingredients—heart, liver, etc. By adding them to an already nutritious diet, damaged or at-risk organs are supported. This frequently involves feeding a home-prepared diet with recipes that include glands. However, whole-food supplements utilizing these same principles are also available.

The goal of glandular therapy is to increase the amount of specific nutrients fed to a patient. Through the use of specific supplements, we are able to do so for nutrients and ingredients that can be difficult to source otherwise. When you read the ingredient lists of these supplements, you'll generally find the organs that the supplement is designed to target. In other words, liver supplement contains liver and (generally) other organs that support liver function within the body.

Look for supplements that are derived from whole-food ingredients. I recommend those by companies like Standard Process, which designs and manufactures an extensive line of supplements. (Standard Process was founded nearly a century ago on the principle that food was becoming less nutritious and disease would result. It is now common knowledge that food is becoming less nutritious as a result of soil depletion, GMOs, and agribusiness pushing for increased yield at the expense of nutritional quality.)

Success Story: Roscoe's Biceps Battle

Roscoe, a beautiful Brittany spaniel, is a good example of the power of whole foods and glandular therapy. At only 20 months old, Roscoe began limping and favoring his right front leg. Concerned, his owners brought him to their family veterinarian, who recommended that they restrict his activity level and start him on Rimadyl (a nonsteroidal anti-inflammatory) and Traumeel (a homeopathic remedy for muscle soreness).

Unfortunately, four weeks into his period of rest and treatment, Roscoe was no better and continued to limp severely. His owners were referred to an orthopedic specialist, who diagnosed Roscoe with biceps tenosynovitis. This condition involves inflammation of the biceps tendon and can be a long-term, nagging injury that may never completely resolve.

Roscoe's owners were given the option of surgery to cut the biceps tendon, which would relieve the pain but leave Roscoe with decreased range of motion and strength. Not surprisingly, they elected not to perform the surgery and instead tried a cortisone injection in hopes of relieving the inflammation and pain. Sadly, four weeks later, Roscoe was still in pain and limping.

At this point, Roscoe's veterinarian started him on a glandular therapy regimen, which included Calcifood and Ligaplex by Standard Process. Both supplements contain highly bioavailable nutrients derived from bones, organs, and plants. Within one week, Roscoe's owners were seeing improvements. Eight weeks into treatment, his limp resolved and his activity level slowly returned to normal without complications.

In this case, Western medicine simply masked the pain without treating the underlying cause, while surgery was considered too high a risk for too little reward. The answer lay in whole-food products that provided Roscoe's body with the nutrients he needed to repair his injured tendon.

How You Can Use Glandular Therapy as Part of Your Pet's Treatment Plan

While glandular therapy can be used as a primary treatment for conditions like hypothyroidism and pancreatic insufficiency, most commonly it is used as preventive or complementary therapy.

I would never suggest that you forgo conventional treatments or pharmaceutical support in favor of stand-alone glandular therapy unless recommended and supervised by your veterinarian. In many pets, prescription medications are necessary and lifesaving. That said, adding glandular therapy into the regimen for these patients could improve their quality and quantity of life by providing needed nutrition to their damaged organ(s).

Following are suggestions on how to utilize glandular therapy to benefit your dog or cat:

- If your pet has a known condition such as organ disease, chronic inflammation, or cancer, consult a veterinarian or holistic practitioner who is familiar with the use of glandular therapy. Some glandulars, such as natural desiccated thyroid or pancreas, are available by prescription only. A good resource to find veterinarians trained in holistic medicine is the website of the American Holistic Veterinary Medical Association: www.ahvma.org. (Click the "Find a Vet" tab.)

- Provide your pet with a fresh, whole-food diet containing organ meats such as heart, liver, and kidney. These ingredients will help support your pet's vital organs. Diets can be purchased or made at home using a balanced recipe.

- Purchase supplements that are made with whole-food ingredients by reputable companies, such as Standard Process. Check the ingredient list to make sure it contains the organs that you wish to support.

Oral Tolerance Therapy

While glandular therapy is a strategy to affect specific organs through feeding your pet specific tissues and extracts, oral tolerance therapy is a strategy to directly access the immune system through feeding your pet small amounts of an allergen. This ability to affect immune function brings a whole new level to using food as medicine—it is advanced nutrition. Before explaining oral tolerance, however, we must first explain how and why we would *want* to affect the immune system.

How and Why We Affect the Immune System

Imbalances in the immune system can lead to devastating health effects. Underfunctioning immunity leads to infections or cancer, while even a mildly overactive immune response can lead to hypersensitivities and allergies. A severely overactive immune response leads to massive inflammation and tissue destruction that can sometimes be fatal.

A familiar way that we affect, or modulate, immune function is through allergy treatments. I used to get allergy shots when I was a kid. When a person or animal is regularly injected with a very small amount of the material they are allergic to, over time the body reduces, or downregulates, its response to the allergen through the mechanism of *immune tolerance.*

A crucial function of the immune system is its ability to recognize self from nonself, which is how the body defends itself against bacteria, viruses, cancer cells, and other foreign materials. When a body recognizes something perceived as foreign, the immune system attacks in an effort to eliminate it. However, it is critical for the body to be able to differentiate what is normal from what is abnormal. Immune tolerance describes the immune system's ability to not respond to certain substances it might otherwise react to, allowing normal body processes to continue without interference. In other words, it's how the immune system knows what not to react to.[2]

The immune reaction is a vital immunological function that is crucial for healthy living, but it also has a dark side. When the immune system overreacts to certain foreign material—dust, pollen, food, etc.—the result is a hypersensitivity or allergic response. When the immune system overreacts to a normal component within the body such as blood cells or connective tissues, the result is autoimmune disease.[3] (Immune response to allergies and autoimmune conditions is discussed in detail in Chapters 11 and 23, respectively.)

While there are many factors affecting immune system status, nutrition and nutritional supplementation can have a profoundly positive effect. This brings us to the subject of oral tolerance.

Modulating the Immune System through Oral Tolerance

Oral tolerance is a subset of immune tolerance that can be used as therapy for allergic or sensitive pets. Feeding a very small amount of something your pet normally would react to can "train" their immune system to leave it alone.

Inducing oral tolerance is the same process as allergy shots, but using oral or sublingual administration—no shot necessary![4] As antigens (foreign material such as allergens) are administered orally and pass through the GI tract, they are exposed to immune cells. Seventy percent of the immune system lives within the GI tract, and this exposure stimulates an immune response.

When we regularly expose immune cells to a given antigen, they tend to downregulate the natural inflammatory response. Through oral tolerance, the immune system is being trained to not react to what your pet has eaten or to the normal bacterial flora residing within the GI tract. While these bacteria are highly beneficial for both digestion and in the prevention of invasion by pathogenic (bad) bacteria, without oral tolerance even these "good" bacteria could lead to severe inflammation and clinical disease.[5, 6]

Oral Tolerance and Food Sensitivities

Oral tolerance also prevents hypersensitivity to food proteins. Of course, all animals routinely eat foods containing proteins and other compounds that could be described as "foreign," but the immune system accepts these nutrients without complaint through the process of oral tolerance.[7] Without oral tolerance, the immune system would constantly be reacting with inflammation, and food sensitivity would be the norm rather than the exception.

Although food sensitivity does occur (see Chapter 14), it is relatively uncommon. In some cases, it appears to be due to the feeding of the same protein for several years. The constant presentation of one particular protein to the immune cells of the GI tract overwhelms oral tolerance and leads to an inflammatory response, or sensitivity, to that protein. This is why many holistic practitioners recommend rotating through ingredients in a pet's diets over time.

Oral Tolerance and Allergies

We can use the principles of oral tolerance to improve immune system responses even when allergens are inhaled or absorbed by the skin rather than ingested. Environmental allergies, known as atopic dermatitis, or atopy, are extremely common. Atopy is the most common cause (besides fleas) for dogs to be itchy. It's very common for animals to be sensitive to a variety of environmental factors, which can be determined through testing. Allergy testing performed by a veterinarian often reveals reactions to a myriad of weeds, grasses, trees, molds, and fungi. Preventing exposure to all environmental allergens is generally impossible, so treatment options focus on reducing the allergic response.

To relieve allergy symptoms, we can use omega fatty acids, natural anti-inflammatories, antihistamines, and even steroids in severe cases. More ideal, however, is desensitization therapy, which modulates the immune response through oral or immune tolerance. (A more detailed description of allergy testing and treatment can be found in Chapter 11.) While oral or immune tolerance therapy often takes months to achieve desensitization, it can be very effective. It also limits the need for stronger medications like steroids, which can have serious long-term side effects.

Allergy desensitization therapy is an excellent example of holistic therapy that is commonplace in Western medicine. The administration of a benign substance that stimulates the animal's own body to adjust and become healthier is exactly the kind of care we are looking for.

Holistic practitioners sometimes administer other antigens to control allergies. Bee pollen is the one most commonly recommended to treat allergies. The idea is that the pollen contains allergens from the many different plants visited by the bees, packaged into convenient little balls, so this will help desensitize a pet through oral tolerance. However, there is limited scientific evidence to support this, and individual response varies.[8] If you choose to supplement your pet's diet with bee pollen, it is important to use *local* bee pollen, as it will contain antigens from plants in your geographic area. For safety's sake, never use bee pollen and honey in patients with a known severe allergy to bee stings.

Success Story: Duffy, the Itchy Westie

Treating allergic pets is an everyday activity for most veterinarians. It also can be one of the more challenging aspects of our jobs. Allergies are nagging problems that make pets itchy and their owners frustrated and unhappy. One such pet that sticks out in my mind is Duffy.

Duffy was a nine-year-old West Highland white terrier, or Westie. These are adorable stocky little dogs with a big personality. They also happen to be well known for their skin issues and allergies. In Duffy's case, he was a chronic foot licker. Duffy was a regular at my office, as he often developed sore, red, infected feet due to his allergies and incessant licking. We tried all the conventional therapies and a spectrum of herbs and supplements. The only thing that gave him relief was prednisone. Since long-term steroid use was not an option, we needed an alternative.

Although they were initially reluctant, Duffy's owners, Scott and Pam, finally agreed to do some allergy testing. We submitted a blood allergy test to the lab, and a week later the results were in. Duffy was highly allergic to many of the grasses and trees in our area, as well as to dust mites. The severity of his allergies made it clear why Duffy had been largely unresponsive to most of our previous efforts to make him comfortable.

Based on the results of the allergy testing, we had the lab make a custom formulation of allergy drops that were given to Duffy orally every day.

By the end of the first month, Scott and Pam thought maybe there was a little less foot licking. Two months in, there was no doubt he was improving. By month three, Duffy's foot licking and chewing had decreased by 75 percent, and Scott and Pam were thrilled. We used the principle of oral tolerance to control his symptoms. Duffy is always going to have allergies and the occasional flare-up. These are much easier to control now with antihistamines.

How You Can Use Oral Tolerance Therapy
as Part of Your Pet's Treatment Plan

Oral tolerance therapy is most useful for pets with allergies or chronic GI issues. (More detailed recommendations can be found in Chapters 11 and 14.)

- Ask your veterinarian about allergy testing for your pet and recommendations for using oral tolerance to relieve your pet's symptoms. There are many laboratories offering testing, and your veterinarian likely has a lab they use regularly.

- The results of allergy testing may be used as a guideline for creating oral drops or injections to desensitize the pet to specific allergens. Note that the drops are custom-designed based on test results and can only be obtained through your veterinarian.

- Bee pollen may be beneficial in limiting the effects of environmental allergies in dogs and cats. Feed one ball of bee pollen per day for the first month. (It is best to administer this directly orally rather than mixing it in with food.) Add one additional ball to the dosage monthly, for four to six months; large dogs may require a little more. If the pollen is effective, results should be seen within four to six months.

  Remember to use local bee pollen, as it will contain the pollen present in your immediate area. Watch for worsening signs of allergies, which may indicate the pollen exposure is causing symptoms. If this occurs, decrease the dose and start again. If allergy signs are severe, discontinue use immediately and consult with your veterinarian.

- Rotate food ingredients periodically (two to three times yearly) to prevent the development of food sensitivities. (This will also provide a broader spectrum of nutrition over the long term.)

Nutrigenomics

Now you know how glandular therapy can replace deficient hormones and support damaged organs, and you understand how oral tolerance can help access the immune system. The next step on the food-as-medicine continuum is to access the genetic code. We can dramatically impact health by affecting gene expression through nutrition.

Dr. Jean Dodds, one of the foremost researchers in the field of nutrigenomics in animals, describes nutrigenomics as "the emerging science that studies the molecular relationships between nutrition and the response of genes in promoting health." While we certainly understand that vitamins, minerals, phytonutrients (beneficial plant chemicals), and other natural compounds often have profound health benefits, the specifics of how these nutrients work, interact with one another, and show variable effects between individuals are still being studied. When certain nutritional ingredients are ingested, they send signals to the body to stimulate healthy expression of genes and/or protect the genome from damage.[9] This is perhaps the best application of the term *functional foods*, and the study of how foods elicit varied responses due to individuals' different genes is at the heart of nutrigenomics.

One good example of nutrigenomic research was an evaluation of broccoli. Researchers determined that broccoli reduces acute liver injury and toxicity through stimulating gene expression. In other words, broccoli induces the expression of a gene that leads to the production of compounds that naturally protect the liver.[10] A food (broccoli) is directly affecting the behavior of DNA!

There is great variation among individuals when it comes to their genetic makeup and, thus, their optimal nutritional profile. Consider how it is that some people (or animals) can eat all the "wrong" foods and still live long, healthy lives, while others can do all the "right" things and still end up with heart disease—it has a lot to do with individual genetic makeup. Perhaps this is best illustrated through an interview with the famous comedian George Burns, who died at 100 years old:

"Is it true that you smoke eight to ten cigars a day?"
"That's true."
"Is it true that you drink five martinis a day?"
"That's true."
"Is it true that you still surround yourself with beautiful young women?"
"That's true."
"What does your doctor say about all of this?"
"My doctor is dead."

While genetic programming certainly has a big impact on longevity, understanding how and why genes do what they do will help more and more pets and people live a long life like George Burns (minus the cigars and martinis). Nutrigenomics is one pathway to get us there.

Unlocking all the benefits of nutrigenomics is going to hinge on our ability to evaluate an individual's genome. In 1990, the Human Genome Project began its quest to map the entire human genetic code. It took 13 years and $2.7 billon to complete.[11, 12] Today you can have your genome analyzed 30 times (to ensure accuracy) for around $1,000.[13, 14]

As the field of nutrigenomics progresses, customized nutritional profiles will be developed based on an analysis of an individual's genetics. Consider it: Your pet's genome will be analyzed and a list of optimal nutrients will be generated so as to access the greatest power of their genes. It is the pinnacle of optimal nutrition. It's in the future, but not as far off as you think.

How You Can Use Nutrigenomics as Part of Your Pet's Treatment Plan

- Remember that nutrigenomics is a scientific field in its infancy. How we may be able to utilize the information coded in the DNA to individualize nutrition for both humans and animals is just now being evaluated.

- There is a test available through Dr. Jean Dodds's lab called NutriScan (www .nutriscan.org). The test evaluates a pet's immune response to a wide variety of foods in order to screen for dietary sensitivity. In other words, the test looks for which foods cause inflammation within an individual animal. The test provides a way to quantitatively measure which foods are best for a given individual.

- Consider other DNA and gene testing that is currently available for pets. Although not specifically for the purposes of nutrigenomics, DNA analysis can be used to determine the breed makeup of an individual dog, which may provide some insight into sensitivities to certain drugs or susceptibility to certain diseases. Different kits can be ordered online, at pet shops, or at your veterinarian's office.

If you come away from this chapter with anything, I hope it is the understanding that nutrition is more than raw materials. What we feed our pets frequently has direct effects on the immune system. Feeding the right ingredients can treat disease, decrease inflammation, and support health through healthy immune function.

CHAPTER 8

COMPLEMENTARY AND ALTERNATIVE MEDICINE

The healing comes from nature and not from the physician. Therefore the physician must start from nature with an open mind.

— PARACELSUS

Before there was a pharmaceutical industry, all medicine was natural medicine. Healers used remedies derived from plants and animals to treat every manner of malady. Every indigenous culture across the globe has a form of traditional medicine. As the world has modernized, some forms of traditional medical knowledge have been lost to the ages. Other forms, however, have survived and even found a foothold outside of their countries and cultures of origin. We'll be exploring some of these modalities in this chapter, including traditional Chinese medicine (TCM), chiropractic, homeopathy, physical therapy, and herbal medicine.

Proficiency with any form of medicine requires years of study. Most lifelong medical practitioners (regardless of their field) will say after 30, 40, or even 50 years of study, they are still learning. As such, the goal of this section is to familiarize you, the reader, with key concepts and definitions of traditional and herbal medicine and how they relate to integrative care. In other words, you want to be an educated consumer of integrative health-care services rather than an expert in all fields. In this way, when you need to seek out a veterinarian for your pet, you will know what to look for and what questions to ask when you get there.

Alternative Care at Its Finest: Anka the Cat

Among the most rewarding things about practicing complementary and alternative medicine are those times when a pet comes in and a medical "miracle" happens. Anka the cat is one of those patients.

As a kitten, Anka seemed to have some kind of death wish. After being hit by a car at a young age, he lost his left eye and suffered nerve damage to the left side of his face. Years later, another car accident lost him his tail and caused a loss of neurologic function to his urinary bladder. Despite it all, he continued to be an inquisitive and affectionate cat.

Anka came into my clinic about one year after the second accident. (He walked in on a leash—no carrier necessary!) His owners explained that ever since the accident, Anka had not urinated on his own. Five times a day, every day, his owners had to manually express (physically squeeze) his bladder or else it would overfill and cause severe kidney damage.

I explained that his old neurologic injury would be difficult to overcome, and it was unclear how much we could do or how long it might take to see results. It might be months before we'd know if anything would be possible. Still, we got started right away, and Anka received acupuncture during his first appointment.

While Anka and the couple were in the reception area scheduling their next visit, the cat squatted and peed on the floor. Seeing such results after a single acupuncture treatment was nothing short of miraculous!

Anka continues to receive acupuncture, and he is now urinating multiple times per day. Although his owners still need to manually express his bladder, they need do so only twice daily. Time will tell how much he will continue to improve.

How Western Medicine Differs from Complementary and Alternative Care

The Western medical paradigm is a uniform landscape. By and large, the entire conventional medical community subscribes to the same set of principles, knowledge, and therapeutic options for patients. The bar for what is considered effective treatment is set very high and requires rigorous and extensive testing and trials before a new therapy can be brought into the fold.

The benefit to this uniformity is that everyone practicing Western medicine is speaking the same language, and there is generally a high degree of certainty regarding the potential effects (and side effects) of any given medical therapy. A patient can go from one doctor to the next anywhere in the world (assuming quality of care is good) and experience consistency.

Complementary and alternative medicine, however, is a different story. There are literally dozens of medical philosophies that can be found within the scope of complementary and alternative medicine. Some therapies, such as TCM, have foundations in thousands of years of medical practice and teachings. Others, like homeopathy and chiropractic, have more recent roots. While some forms of alternative medicine are intended as stand-alone therapies, most are frequently interwoven with multiple forms of traditional and modern medicine.

Although the combination of several medical disciplines may prove challenging for the uninitiated, the benefits can be overwhelming. Introducing additional medical perspectives into treatment strategies is akin to bringing a new voice to a stale conversation dominated by a single opinion. Many solutions are uncovered when a new and different light is shined upon a nagging problem.

Be an Educated Consumer

It goes without saying that we want the best medical care for our pets. Choosing the types of medical care they receive is a big part of achieving this goal. Western medical care offers rigorous standards and consistency throughout the field, but the path may be less clear when it comes to navigating the various forms of complementary and alternative care.

So how does one determine the ideal complementary and alternative treatment plan when Western medical research standards are often not present and there is a lack of consensus among medical professionals? The marketplace can be challenging. There are bad actors selling supplements and cures on the Internet using buzzwords and unfounded claims. More commonly, however, well-intentioned people attempt to treat pets despite inadequate or nonexistent veterinary training. The result can be ineffective treatment, and sometimes harm to the pet.

Despite intentions to the contrary, pets treated by sincere and talented nonveterinarian holistic practitioners can be harmed by treatments that are dangerous to animals. A pet may suffer from adverse effects of the treatment or due to the practitioner's inability to recognize symptoms that require immediate Western medical care. For this reason, direct veterinary supervision is legally required in many states for an animal to receive treatment by a nonveterinarian. It is never a good idea to allow an acupuncturist, chiropractor, or any other practitioner trained only in the treatment of humans to treat your pet without the knowledge and supervision of a veterinarian.

This is not to say that nonveterinarian health-care practitioners don't have a lot to contribute. In my office, we employ a human-trained chiropractor and a human-trained acupuncturist.

They work under my supervision, and we monitor the patient's progress and together decide how to best integrate Western and alternative therapies.

As a veterinarian trained in both chiropractic and acupuncture, I know what these highly skilled practitioners can do, and I am not shy to admit they can do things I cannot. The story of Anka as told above is a prime example. An incredibly talented acupuncturist named Kaylah Sterling is administering the kitty's acupuncture. She is helping him in ways that are beyond my abilities. There is no room for pride in medicine and I am happy to coordinate medical care with talented nonveterinarians. If someone can provide more than I can, I am quick to get out of the way.

So how does one make the right decisions regarding medical care to integrate with, or use as an alternative to, conventional medicine? One option is to exercise due diligence, to research multiple therapies extensively and make decisions based on your findings. While effective, that path is time-consuming. The much easier alternative is to find a veterinarian who has already done this for you and consult with him or her regarding the best treatment alternatives. I strongly recommend the latter. While you can make yourself better informed, it is unrealistic for most people to become experts in multiple medical disciplines.

Strategies to Find Safe and Effective Complementary and Alternative Care for Your Pet

- Locate a veterinarian experienced with integrative and complementary care. Start with www.ahvma.org to find one in your area.

- Do your own research and tap into your own personal experiences with alternative care. Begin by investigating what resonates with you on a personal level and determine (with your veterinarian) the most promising treatment options.

- Always keep your veterinarian in the loop regarding what care your pet is receiving. Never keep secrets from your veterinarian regarding herbs, supplements, or hands-on therapy; it benefits no one and is potentially dangerous.

Traditional Chinese Veterinary Medicine

Just about everyone has either had an experience or knows someone who has had an experience with acupuncture or traditional Chinese herbs. TCM is one of the most widely accepted forms of nonconventional medical therapy, and its use in animals (often referred to as traditional Chinese veterinary medicine, or TCVM) has become increasingly popular over the last 20 years.

The medical philosophy of TCM is many thousands of years old. It utilizes acupuncture, herbal therapy, medical massage (tui na), exercise (qigong), and dietary therapy to prevent and treat illness in humans. TCVM developed out of necessity in much the same way treatment for humans did. At that time, animals were not only a source of food, they were beasts of burden and war. Animal health and well-being was fundamental to the health of society as a whole, and thus TCVM developed somewhat in parallel with treatment for humans.

Like many forms of traditional medicine, TCVM is about balance. The origins of this balance are described in the form of yin and yang. Yin represents darkness, coolness, night, femininity; yang represents light, heat, day, masculinity. All living beings are a combination of yin and yang. One does not exist without the other, and health is achieved when the two are in balance. In the well-known yin-yang symbol, we can see how the yin (black) and yang (white) shapes combine to form a perfect circle. (See figure to the right.) In addition, there are circles within the circle. A small amount of yin exists in yang and vice versa.

Terminology in TCM and TCVM

The language used in TCM is highly metaphorical—almost poetic. This is because when this system of medicine was developed, there was little or no knowledge of physiology as we now understand it. Doctors dissected bodies and made assumptions about how things worked. Some organs such as the heart were fairly obvious in their function (it is quite visibly a pump). Others, however, such as solid organs like the liver and spleen were less clear in their purpose. This lack of understanding and the belief that internal and external forces affect the flow of energy throughout the body led to descriptions that sound strange to the Western ear.

Chinese medical practitioners often use terms like *stagnation*, *phlegm*, *wind*, *heat*, and *cold* to describe a patient's condition. Understanding these terms allows for translation to Western terminology. The ability to move back and forth between various terminologies is a key factor in integrating Western medicine with more traditional methods.

According to TCM, there is a life force within the body called qi. Qi flows through the body along specific pathways called meridians. The meridians are circular and qi constantly moves through the body in this way. Qi can be lost though injury, illness, age, etc. Qi is gained and/or maintained through nutrition and healthy living. The goal of TCVM is to maintain both the amount and regular flow of qi throughout the body. When a body runs out of qi, life comes to an end.

When the flow of qi is interrupted, a patient is said to have stagnation, or phlegm. TCVM phlegm is not what we Westerners think of when we say *phlegm*. Phlegm can be a swelling or a mass (such as a tumor), but sometimes it is a metaphorical description of the interruption of qi within a meridian. For example, a patient with chronic inflammatory bowel disease could be described as having a "spleen qi deficiency with phlegm."

Descriptions of Chinese herbs are complements to the TCVM diagnosis. They are often described as "qi tonics," "blood tonics," "yin supportive," etc. To use the example above, a practitioner may reach for an herbal formula that is a "spleen tonic" and a "blood mover" as a means of supporting the deficiency in the spleen and breaking up phlegm. The herbs, acupuncture, etc., correct the imbalance in order to restore health through the balancing of energy, yin, and yang.

Chinese Medicine in Clinical Usage

TCM is now commonly practiced in the Western world and is often integrated with other forms of natural medicine and even conventional medical care. It encompasses a variety of treatment modalities, including nutrition, herbal medicine, and medical massage. However, the most well known by far is acupuncture.

Several veterinary schools are now integrating acupuncture and herbal therapy into their curriculum and teaching hospitals, and veterinarians have the opportunity to become trained in TCVM through one of three international accreditation programs. While the majority of veterinarians are not trained Chinese medical practitioners, most are open to the potential benefits of acupuncture and herbal therapy in pets.

In my own practice, we treat many patients with a combination of TCVM and other methodologies. Commonly, pets are treated with acupuncture and herbs (Chinese and others), as well as Western medical care. When it comes to patients with cancer, it is common practice for me to provide the holistic side of a pet's care while they are receiving some combination of surgery, chemotherapy, and/or radiation. Acupuncture and herbs can help pets cope with the stresses of the Western end of their care, mitigate chemotherapy side effects, support appetite, and fight cancer.

Acupuncture

Although everyone knows about acupuncture as a treatment, how it works is a mystery to most people. From the Chinese medical perspective, acupuncture needles are used to normalize the flow of qi through the body.

In a normal, healthy state, qi travels along specific circular pathways (meridians) traversing the body. At certain points, the meridians are internal, and at other points they are on the body surface. By placing needles (acupuncture) or pressing/massaging the points (acupressure), we affect the flow of qi. Different meridians affect specific areas of the body or specific organs, and organs can be affected by multiple meridians.

Even within TCM, there are multiple philosophies regarding how best to improve the flow of qi. If all of this sounds complicated, that's because it is. In some ways, TCM is more complex than modern conventional care.

One of the fascinating things about acupuncture is how placing a needle can have an effect on an organ or body part that is nowhere near the needle itself. TCM explains this through the meridian pathways. For example: The large intestine meridian courses through the large intestine internally and also travels outside the body along the arm and hand. Large Intestine 4 (LI 4) is a point between your thumb and forefinger. Placing a needle in LI 4 can have effects on digestion and abdominal discomfort despite the needle being quite far from the area affected. Although this effect is counterintuitive to our Western minds, it is perfectly logical from a Chinese medical perspective.

All this talk of qi and meridians is perfectly fine for those who subscribe to the paradigm of TCM. On the other hand, how can the effects of acupuncture be explained through the lens of Western medicine? The answers lie in the complex neurochemical networks within the body. The current understanding of the mechanisms of action of acupuncture include the following:

- Acupuncture needles stimulate nerves that can have both local and distant effects on the body by causing the release of chemicals and neurotransmitters that relieve pain and inflammation.

- Microtrauma from the needles causes the release of chemicals in the body that promote healing.

- Acupuncture improves blood flow.

- Acupuncture causes muscle spasms to relax in the same way as trigger point therapy.

Whether your perspective is through Chinese or Western medicine, the efficacy of acupuncture is beyond question. Combined with Chinese herbal and/or nutritional therapy, TCVM is a powerful tool to keep your pets healthy.

Some of the ways in which acupuncture can be a beneficial part of your pet's treatment plan include:

- Relieving chronic pain, such as arthritis and back pain

- Maintaining appetite and energy level in pets with cancer and chronic illness

- Mitigating the side effects of chemotherapy, anesthesia, and Western medications

- Facilitating recovery for pets with neurologic disorders such as spinal trauma

How You Can Use TCVM
as Part of Your Pet's Treatment Plan

- Locate a veterinarian certified in TCVM or an acupuncturist working under the direct supervision of a veterinarian. You can search for certified veterinarians on the following websites:

  - American Holistic Veterinary Medical Association (www.ahvma.org)

  - International Veterinary Acupuncture Society (www.ivas.org)

  - Chi Institute (www.tcvm.com)

- TCVM can be used as both a preventive to maintain good health and for the treatment of medical conditions. Prevention is always easier than treatment, so ask a practitioner how to use TCVM to keep your pet healthy.

- Don't let your needle phobia prevent your pet from benefiting from TCVM. The vast majority of dogs and cats do great with acupuncture.

- Be patient. Like many forms of natural medicine, the effects of TCVM are cumulative and may take time. While immediate results sometimes happen, pets with chronic conditions such as arthritis may take weeks or even months to realize the full benefits of therapy.

While TCVM can be used as a stand-alone treatment, integrating it with other alternative or Western therapies is often more effective than TCVM alone. There are many complementary and alternative care therapies that are highly beneficial for both people and animals, including chiropractic, homeopathy, essential oils, physical rehabilitation, and massage therapy.

Chiropractic Medicine

Originating in the late 1800s, chiropractic medicine is the practice of manipulating joints within the body to improve health. A chiropractic adjustment can improve range of motion of joints, relieve pain, and improve posture.

However, chiropractic is much more than moving bones. Despite the perception of chiropractic care being primarily orthopedic in nature, it is better to think of it in terms of neurology.

Literally thousands of nerves traverse into and out of the spine. When the spine is adjusted, energy is put into these nerves and transmits signals to the rest of the body. Since the entire body is controlled by the nervous system, any organ or body system can be affected by a chiropractic adjustment.

Conditions Commonly Treated
with Chiropractic Care

- Back/neck pain
- Arthritis
- Gastrointestinal disease
- Reproductive issues

Homeopathy

Dating back to the 1700s, homeopathy works on the principle that disease-causing compounds, when given in very small doses, can actually prevent disease. On its face, there is plenty of modern science to validate this hypothesis. Vaccinations started this way. A very small quantity of an organism that causes disease can be used to prevent the same disease. Homeopathy takes things a little further.

In homeopathic medicine, the material being given (called a remedy) is diluted in water. In many cases, the remedy is diluted to the point where there is no detectable trace of the original material left in the water. From a homeopathic perspective, only the "energy" of the substance remains. These remedies are then used to treat patients with a variety of diseases.

A good example of a commonly used homeopathic remedy is nux vomica. The seed of the strychnine tree (*Strychnos nux-vomica*) is loaded with toxins. When diluted as a homeopathic remedy, however, nux vomica is commonly used for gastrointestinal upset and as a hangover cure.

The part of my brain that holds its ground as a Western-trained veterinarian has a hard time with homeopathy. By the logic of modern medicine, homeopathic remedies are literally sugar pills and nothing more; they should have no medical effect other than placebo. That said, homeopathy does sometimes work, and I have very intelligent and critical-thinking colleagues who successfully use homeopathy in their practices. Personally, I file homeopathy in the part of my brain that houses the "things that I can't fully explain but are legit."

Although some medical practitioners dabble in homeopathy, a true homeopathic education requires years of study. Classical homeopathic practitioners evaluate their patients and develop a "constitutional analysis." This analysis is then referenced within a large volume called the *materia medica*, and a remedy is recommended.

True homeopathy is intended to be practiced as a stand-alone therapy, although many practitioners will use other therapies alongside homeopathic remedies. Homeopathy is only effective in treating an existing condition; it cannot be used as a preventive.

Never use homeopathy as a substitute for vaccination. This is ineffective and may leave a pet susceptible to deadly diseases. Homeopathy can, however, be used to treat vaccination side effects, as discussed in Chapter 23.

Conditions Commonly Treated with Homeopathy

Homeopathy can theoretically be used to treat any acute or chronic medical condition. It cannot, however, be used as a preventive. Common uses include treatment for the following conditions:

- Arthritis
- Muscle soreness
- Gastrointestinal distress
- Anxiety
- Respiratory diseases

Essential Oils

Many plants contain compounds called volatile oils, which are the chemicals that make up the aroma. When extracted from plants and concentrated, they are known as essential oils.

Prior to the advent of modern medicine, essential oils were used as a means of primary care for the sick. Today essential oils are more commonly utilized for relaxation and to support patients who are undergoing other forms of medical therapy.

Essential oils can be applied topically, or their scent can be inhaled. They are rapidly absorbed into the bloodstream and body tissues. Various oils have differing affinities for specific body systems or tissues.

Parameters for Safe Use of Essential Oils

A note of caution: Pets are very sensitive to essential oils, and toxicity is possible. Essential oil protocols and dosages for pets cannot be extrapolated from those used in humans. In other words, a safe dose for a human could be lethal for your pet. Always consult with a veterinarian regarding the types and dosages of essential oils that can be used for your pet's conditions.

Some essential oils contain contaminants, which are potentially harmful. Only the purest products are safe for pets. I recommend the brand Young Living, which makes very high-quality products that have been used safely on animals.

Some animals are more sensitive than others. When using essential oils either for your pet or in your house, provide the pet an escape to get away from the scent if they need to. Topical application should be done sparingly and under direct veterinary supervision.

Pure essential oils are too strong to use full strength. They must be diluted in a neutral oil, such as coconut or grapeseed, before being used on pets. Dilution guidelines are as follows:

- Dogs up to 10 pounds: one part essential oil in four parts neutral oil
- Dogs 11–25 pounds: one part essential oil in three parts neutral oil
- Dogs 26–45 pounds: one part essential oil in two parts neutral oil
- Dogs 46–75 pounds: one part essential oil in one part neutral oil
- Dogs 75–100 pounds: two parts essential oil in one part neutral oil
- Dogs over 100 pounds: three parts essential oil in one part neutral oil
- Cats: one part essential oil in 10 parts neutral oil

Some essential oils are too strong for safe use in pets. Do not use the following oils around pets unless specifically instructed by a veterinarian:

- Melaleuca (tea tree)
- Pennyroyal
- Camphor
- Wintergreen
- Citrus oils
- Cinnamon
- Oregano
- Thyme
- Clove
- Birch

Comprehensive information on the use of essential oils for animals can be found in *The Animal Desk Reference: Essential Oils for Animals*, by Melissa Shelton, D.V.M.

Conditions Commonly Treated with Essential Oils

- Anxiety and stress (consider lavender)
- Skin problems (consider myrrh, melrose, frankincense, or lavender)

- Skin growths or tumors (under veterinary supervision, consider frankincense, lavender, sandalwood, and myrrh)

Physical Rehabilitation and Massage Therapy

It is arguable whether these therapies are truly "alternative." However, as they are not truly mainstream in the veterinary field, they are included here.

Physical rehabilitation (rehab) in the veterinary field is what is known as physical therapy for humans. (*Physical therapy* is a legally protected term.) The uses for rehab and massage are exactly the same as for humans: they improve circulation, range of motion, strength, and coordination. The big differences with pets are the strategies employed to encourage patient participation.

In humans undergoing physical therapy, the patient is told to push through the pain because it is good for them in the long term. That strategy is a nonstarter with pets. Rehab has to be a game for them. In addition to various forms of exercise therapy, specialized equipment such as underwater treadmills, therapeutic ultrasounds, and cold laser therapy are utilized.

In my clinic, we set up fun obstacle courses, bribe them with treats, and give them lots of love and encouragement. We burn through bags of treats and order peanut butter by the case.

Conditions Commonly Treated with Physical Rehab and Massage Therapy

- Post-orthopedic surgery
- Back/disc problems with or without surgery
- Neurologic disorders
- Arthritis
- Strength and athletic training
- Maintaining good health and having fun!

Herbal Medicine

The term *herbal medicine* is broad and encompasses natural remedies derived from natural sources. All traditional forms of health care had a pharmacopoeia derived from what was available to people in their geographic region. Some of the most extensive uses of herbal medicine can be found in traditional Chinese medicine, ayurvedic (Indian) medicine, and the indigenous cultures of North and South America.

Derived from plants, animals, and minerals, these medicines formed the cornerstone of health care for ancient cultures. Many of these are still in use today in traditional medical practice. Some have even been co-opted and adapted for use in conventional Western care. The following are some examples of herbs commonly used in conjunction with Western veterinary care:

- Valerian: used for anxiety; may also help with seizures

- Marshmallow root: used to treat respiratory disorders, urinary tract irritation, and gastrointestinal upset

- Slippery elm: used to treat gastrointestinal upset

- Milk thistle: provides support and protection to the liver

- Chamomile: used for anxiety

- Ginger: helpful with nausea; can be used for muscle pain/soreness

- Yunnan Baiyao: a Chinese herbal formula that can help stop bleeding

The specific applications of herbal therapy in dogs and cats will be discussed in much greater detail in Part III. In that section, we will explore the use of herbal medicine in health and wellness care and in the treatment of a wide range of medical conditions in dogs and cats.

Adverse Reactions of Supplements and Herbal Medicine

While herbal medicines tend to be very safe, something being natural does not mean it is harmless. Regardless of their origins, effective medicines work because they are pharmaceutically active. This means they have a direct effect on body processes. Without this effect, these compounds would be useless as medicine.

Any medicine that has an effect can also have side effects. All medicines, natural or otherwise, must be treated with respect. Admittedly, side effects are uncommon with natural medicines, but their relative "uncommonness" means little to those who suffer from an unexpected reaction.

Any medication (natural or pharmaceutical) has the potential to cause vomiting and/or diarrhea. Gastrointestinal upset, while uncommon, is the most frequently seen side effect with herbal medications. Sometimes gastrointestinal upset can be mitigated by giving the medication with food or by lowering the dose. In other circumstances, an individual animal may not be able to tolerate certain herbs. In such cases, alternatives are usually available.

There are no specific herbs commonly used in veterinary medicine that regularly cause gastrointestinal upset. When it happens, it is usually an individual animal's specific response.

There are a few herbs and supplements that are worth discussing with regard to side effects. Some herbs have the potential to negatively impact the liver, cause excessive sedation, and even affect blood clotting.

Any medication or supplement affecting blood clotting is of particular concern for patients that may be undergoing surgery. While I have never seen a patient experience spontaneous bleeding attributed to supplements, I have seen cases in which there was excessive bleeding during surgery because certain supplements were not discontinued.

Some commonly used herbs and supplements in pets have the potential to cause real medical problems:

Ginger	May alter blood clotting time[1]
American ginseng	GI upset, changes in blood pressure and heart rate, lowers blood sugar, may cause liver damage[2]
Licorice root	Lowers blood potassium, increases blood pressure, may cause abnormal heart rhythm[3]
Fish Oil	May affect blood clotting time[4]
Glucosamine and chondroitin	May affect blood clotting time[5]
Ginkgo	May affect blood clotting time[6]
Hawthorn	Potentiates the effects of the cardiac drug digitalis[7]
Valerian	May cause drowsiness
Cannabis	Potential for toxicity requiring medical treatment (see Chapter 9)

Outside of a few rare exceptions when a pet's life is in immediate danger, starting herbs and supplements is not an emergency. Just as with a diet change, any regimen should be started slowly. Don't give multiple new supplements to your pet at the same time. Space out the administration of new supplements by several weeks, so that in the event of an adverse reaction, you can know what caused the problem and make appropriate adjustments. As always, inform your veterinarian about any and all supplements and herbs your pet is receiving.

Warning about Manufacturers' Standards for Herbs and Supplements

Remember that there is no government oversight regarding inaccurate or misleading product claims when it comes to herbal remedies and supplements. However you may feel about the pharmaceutical industry, at least they maintain rigorous standards to prevent unwanted materials in the drugs they produce. Unfortunately, the same cannot be said for some herbal manufacturers. Therefore, if a product makes claims that sound too good to be true, they probably are. Be wary of cheap products and unknown manufacturers, as toxins such as heavy metals have been found in some herbal supplements.[8] The best recommendation I can give is to only buy products from reputable companies recommended by a trained health-care practitioner.

How You Can Use Herbal Therapy and Supplements as Part of Your Pet's Treatment Plan

- Find a veterinarian with experience using herbal medicine. The American Holistic Veterinary Medical Association (www.ahvma.org) is a good resource.

- Be certain to use herbal medicine only from reputable companies and use formulas made for pets unless instructed otherwise by your veterinarian.

- If your pet is prone to gastrointestinal upset, start any new herb or supplement slowly. Give a half dose for a few days and see how he responds before giving the full measure.

CHAPTER 9

MEDICAL CANNABIS

The evidence is overwhelming that marijuana can relieve certain types of pain, nausea, vomiting and other symptoms caused by such illnesses as multiple sclerosis, cancer and AIDS or by the harsh drugs sometimes used to treat them. And it can do so with remarkable safety. Indeed, marijuana is less toxic than many of the drugs that physicians prescribe every day.

— JOYCELYN ELDERS, M.D.

Cannabis? Really?

Legitimate uses of medical marijuana and hemp (both forms of cannabis) are swathed in undeserved controversy. Thanks, in large part, to the government and the medical establishment, misconceptions about the perceived dangers of medical cannabis have become ingrained in much of society. Only in the past few years has medical and public opinion, and subsequently legislation, begun to swing the other way.

Some physicians and veterinarians (including myself) use marijuana and hemp in much the same way we would utilize any other pharmaceutical. In my own professional experience, I have seen pain relieved, seizures abate, chronic gastrointestinal problems resolve, and anxiety lessen through the use of this powerful medicine. Cannabis, in my opinion, is perhaps the *most powerful and effective* medicine that is not embraced by the medical community at large.

The extent of the medical potential of this amazing herb has not even been fully realized. As state and federal restrictions ease, medical cannabis will move into the mainstream. Given the importance of this powerful medicinal herb in veterinary medicine and the controversy that surrounds it, now is the perfect time to dispel the myths and look at its medical application in pets.

Success Story: Ella the Cat and Cannabis Oil

Jen brought her six-year-old cat, Ella, into my clinic and explained that the kitty's sensitive stomach had gotten worse in the last 12 months. Ella had begun having consistent liquid diarrhea with gas. After visiting a regular veterinarian several times, they were referred to an internal medicine specialist who diagnosed Ella with inflammatory bowel disease (IBD).

Ella was started on appropriate Western medical therapy, including prednisone (a steroid) and metronidazole (an antibiotic). Ella got a little bit better, but her stools were still very soft. When the specialist recommended starting cyclosporine (an immunosuppressive) or chlorambucil (chemotherapy), Jen decided to look for alternative therapies.

After a thorough evaluation of Ella and a long discussion with Jen, my treatment recommendations were to begin a probiotic and clay powder to support normal gastrointestinal flora and decrease bacterial toxins within the gastrointestinal tract (more on this in Part III). In addition, we discussed starting Ella on cannabis oil.

Within two weeks of beginning therapy, Ella's stools were normal. Over the next six weeks, Jen successfully weaned Ella away from the steroid and antibiotic, with no ill effects. Ella is now eating normally and having perfect digestion without any conventional pharmaceutical intervention.

Ella is a perfect example of how an animal who might otherwise end up on long-term immunosuppressive therapy can have their life turned around through natural medicine including cannabis.

The Facts

Marijuana and hemp both come from the same plant, *Cannabis sativa* L. Compounds naturally occurring in cannabis affect the endocannabinoid system (ECS) within the body. The ECS is a group of receptors within the central and peripheral nervous systems that are found throughout the body.

The development of the ECS is very old on an evolutionary scale, as evidenced by its presence in primitive invertebrates as well as more complex animals like dogs, cats, and people. The function of these receptors is to modulate physiologic processes such as pain, appetite, and mood.[1] While study is ongoing, it appears that the overarching purpose of the ECS is to normalize body functions. Medically, this is called "supporting homeostasis." The ECS receptors and their associated neurotransmitters help to keep the body on an even keel when there are emotional or physical stresses such as trauma, injury, inflammation, etc.

The concept of plant-based compounds affecting neurotransmitters is not unique to cannabis. This is exactly how opiates (derived from poppies) work. Appropriate medical use of opiates relieves pain and improves the quality of life for countless humans and animals by affecting opioid receptors in the body. The ECS is affected in much the same way through the use of the cannabinoid compounds found in cannabis. While there are many compounds in cannabis (with more being described all the time), the big players are tetrahydrocannabinol (THC) and cannabidiol (CBD). Most research of medical cannabis focuses on these two cannabinoids.

Safety Considerations

There are many factors to consider regarding the medical use of cannabis in pets, and like any other form of medical care, veterinary supervision is critical to success and safety. The risk of giving an ineffective product or one that leads to toxicity and a trip to the emergency room is very real. The following parameters should always be adhered to when considering the safe use of medical cannabis in pets:

- Always consult with your veterinarian before administering any cannabis product to your pet.
- Know the dose of THC; this is critical to avoid toxicity. (THC, not CBD, is the psychoactive substance that gets people and animals stoned.)
- Don't dose your pet without veterinary supervision. Different diseases respond to differing ratios of THC and CBD, and not every preparation is appropriate for every condition.
- Use only products designed for animal use, unless otherwise directed by a veterinarian. Most cannabis products on the market are made for humans and are not applicable for safe use in pets.
- Be cautious when it comes to doses and labeling. Although states with legal commercial dispensaries may have prepared medical cannabis products, inaccurate or incomplete labeling can make accurate dosing impossible. Don't just make an educated guess; this is an invitation to the emergency clinic.
- In states where marijuana is illegal, hemp is a great alternative. Hemp products are legally available over the counter countrywide, and can be effectively used to treat many conditions. Hemp products contain high levels of CBD and very little THC (less than 0.3 percent).

History and the Legal Issue

Marijuana and hemp plants have been used for literally thousands of years for a myriad of purposes, including fiber, food, oil, and medicine. Many indigenous cultures were aware of the power of this herb to relieve pain and ease the sick. Writings extolling the virtues of cannabis are found in many cultures, including the ancient Chinese and Greeks.[2, 3, 4] Throughout the 1800s and early 1900s, cannabis and hemp were widely used in the U.S. for medicinal and industrial purposes. All of that changed in the 1930s when a series of laws ultimately made cannabis illegal.[5, 6]

Since then, marijuana has been criminalized and classified in the U.S. as a Schedule I controlled substance, a substance the FDA considers to have no medicinal application as well as "some potential for abuse sufficient to warrant control under the CSA [Controlled Substances Act]."[7] In other words, as far as the FDA is concerned, marijuana has no medical value and is no different from heroin and cocaine.

Setting the FDA and apoplectic legislators aside for a moment, let us shift the focus to the actual science of medical cannabis. Even a casual appraisal of the literally thousands of published research papers makes it clear cannabis does, in fact, have many medical applications. As with any drug, determining how we can utilize medical cannabis in pets hinges on an evaluation of its safety and efficacy.

Dosing

When researchers evaluate drugs for use in humans or animals, one of the cornerstone parameters for safety used is LD_{50} (lethal dose 50 percent). In other words, LD_{50} is the dose of a medication that causes death in 50 percent of a research population. While the concept may seem draconian, it is critical in the determination of the margin of safety for a medication. For example: If it takes 50 milligrams of a drug to have a desired effect and the LD_{50} is 60 milligrams, the drug has a very narrow margin of safety, and the FDA must decide if the drug can be approved for safe use. The narrower the margin of safety, the more carefully the medication must be used in order to prevent serious complications. Every over-the-counter and prescription drug available for humans and animals has been researched to determine its LD_{50}.

Orally ingested cannabis has no known LD_{50} in dogs.[8] Despite some pretty concerted efforts, researchers have not been able to find a lethal dose of cannabis in dogs. This is not to say there is not an issue with toxicity. Certainly animals can get stoned just as easily as we humans, and sometimes emergency medical intervention is required. In nearly all cases, however, the effects are transient (hours to days) and leave no lasting damage. While the research has not been done on cats, the same is likely to be true. For all of the hubbub about the dangers of cannabis and its FDA Schedule I status, there are almost no other Western medications that can make this kind of safety claim.

Notes Regarding Safe Cannabis Use in Pets

- Although the cannabis itself does not have an LD_{50}, deaths have been reported from pets eating "edibles" made for people. These often contain chocolate, raisins, coffee, or other compounds that are toxic to animals.

- Dogs have a higher number of endocannabinoid receptors in their cerebellum and brain stem.[9] These parts of the brain control coordination, heart rate, respiratory rate, etc. This makes dogs particularly susceptible to toxicity from too much THC.

- Dogs intoxicated with THC may show signs of static ataxia. These dogs will seem rigid and have difficulty standing. This condition is unique to dogs and, while not fatal, often requires supportive medical therapy.

Efficacy

Medical researchers are publishing reports detailing the benefits of cannabis at an amazing rate. One needs only to look at the National Institutes of Health database (just do an Internet search for "PubMed") and search for the word *cannabis*. You will find literally thousands of research studies, many evaluating the benefits of cannabis for conditions such as arthritis, pain, inflammation, gastrointestinal disease, epilepsy, cancer, etc.[10, 11, 12]

However, when it comes to pets and disease treatment, there is not as much published data available. That said, we know all mammals have an endocannabinoid system, and there is no evidence to suggest medical cannabis works differently in animals than it does in humans. Additionally, anecdotal reports and my own professional experience with medical cannabis in dogs and cats lead me to be 100 percent certain that it is safe in appropriate doses and, in many cases, effective in the treatment of disease and in relieving pain.

In veterinary medicine, we commonly use "human" drugs that are not specifically approved for use in animals. This is because it is not financially worthwhile for a pharmaceutical company to spend millions of dollars to get a drug specifically approved for dogs and cats. This standard of practice is known as extra-label usage. Thus, extrapolating the benefits of medical cannabis in pets based on research in humans is a completely acceptable platform upon which to base treatment recommendations.

Guidelines for Safe and Accurate Dosing of Medical Cannabis

Like all botanical medicines, cannabis is not made up of a single compound. There are dozens (more likely hundreds) of cannabinoids and other active components present within the plant. It is theorized that there is a synergistic effect between these chemicals that ultimately is greater than the sum of the plant's parts. This phenomenon, known as the entourage effect, is one of many reasons why utilizing a whole plant as medicine is often better than attempting to isolate a single compound for pharmaceutical use. That said, it is impractical to calculate the concentration of all the compounds present in a given plant as a means of determining dosage. Since THC and CBD are the most biologically active cannabinoids, medical cannabis dosing is based on these two components.

The following section discussing dosing of cannabis in pets reflects the most up-to-date information available at the time this book was written. As previously stated, medical cannabis is an evolving science, and information may change over time. Based on my professional experience, however, the following information is an excellent guideline that will provide therapeutic benefit while limiting the chance of unwanted side effects.

Medicine Labeling

Like any drug, the most important consideration with cannabis is to know exactly how much active ingredient(s) is in the medication. With conventional pharmaceuticals this is easy, as standardized labeling allows us to know exactly what is contained within every liquid, pill, and capsule on the market.

Because our friends at the FDA have stated that cannabis has no legitimate medical use, they do not regulate or oversee product manufacture or labeling. The upside of this is there are a lot of boutique companies that are making artisan products much like fine wine. A lot of love goes into these products. The downside is inconsistency and/or inaccuracy in labeling. A cannabis preparation needs to be labeled with both the amount of THC and CBD contained in a given quantity, such as milligrams per milliliter (mg/ml), and the ratio of THC to CBD. We must have both pieces of information for safe and successful medical use.

Biphasic Dosing Curve

Medical cannabis displays a phenomenon called the biphasic dosing curve.[13] In short, there is an optimal dose for a given condition and individual. Dosing below *or* above this dose will lead to less-than-optimal results. In other words, giving too much cannabis can result in a decreased effect of the medication in much the same way as underdosing will. There is effectively a sweet spot with cannabis where it works optimally.

Given that there is no way to know exactly what the ideal dose is for any individual, the recommendation is to begin with low dosing and slowly increase on a weekly basis until the optimal response is found. Gradual dosing increases help determine optimal dose and reduce the risk of toxicity by allowing the body to become accustomed to the psychoactive effects of THC.

The biphasic dosing curve proves both the old sayings that "more is not always better" and sometimes "less is more." Step-by-step instructions regarding how to calculate dosing can be found at the end of this chapter.

THC:CBD Ratio

The relative ratio of THC to CBD is as important to successful treatment as is the actual amount of each compound present in a medication. THC and CBD each mimic a different neurotransmitter in the ECS and thus have different effects on the body. The individual amounts of THC and CBD in a formula create a medicine that affects the body relative to the specific ratio used. For example, a formula that is well suited to fight cancer often will have a higher THC content, whereas one designed for seizures will have a higher CBD content. Since formulas can be made with specific ratios, it is possible to create medicines to help a wide variety of conditions.

Even though the research may indicate more successful uses for specifically high-THC or high-CBD formulas for certain conditions, there is usually a benefit to both being present. The entourage effect suggests that the combination of compounds in the medication is partially responsible for its efficacy. In other words, a small amount of THC in a high-CBD formula may potentiate the CBD effects and vice versa.

Product Selection and Dosing Calculation

When choosing a cannabis product for use in pets, it is imperative to know both the concentration of the medicine and the ratio of THC to CBD. The following chart is a guide toward product selection with regard to specific disease conditions and the most appropriate THC-to-CBD ratio. For some conditions and in smaller animals, it may be beneficial to begin with a lower-THC product and work up to a higher-concentration product. This allows for a greater margin of safety and, if needed, acclimation to THC, which helps limit toxicity.

Access to medical marijuana products and/or veterinary guidance may be difficult to come by for some pet owners. In these cases, a safe place to start is with products made from hemp. Hemp contains very little THC, which minimizes negative side effects and toxicity concerns. Hemp-based products also have the advantage of being legal to sell over the counter in all states. Thus, if you live in a state that does not have legal medical or recreational marijuana, you still have options.

Recommended THC:CBD Ratios of Marijuana or Hemp Products for Particular Conditions

High CBD, low THC (THC:CBD ratio between 4:1 and 20:1)	Epilepsy/seizures Pain, inflammation Anticancer effects Neuroprotective effects in cases of stroke, head injury Anxiety, restlessness, as an aid for pets who are not sleeping well
Even THC and CBD (1:1)	Inflammatory bowel disease Pain, inflammation Anticancer effects Possibly beneficial effects for spinal cord injuries
High THC, low CBD (THC:CBD ratio between 4:1 and 20:1)	Severe pain such as advanced arthritis or cancer pain Appetite stimulation Anticancer effects

Guidelines for Product Selection

- Complete and accurate labeling of medical cannabis is critical for safety and success. Select only products with labels that contain both the concentration of THC and CBD (usually expressed in milligrams) and the ratio of THC to CBD.

- Different medical conditions respond better to specific THC-to-CBD ratios. Choose a product that is most appropriate for the condition to be treated.

- Always begin at a very low dose (see dosing information that follows). This will limit the chance of adverse reactions, allow your pet to acclimate to the effects of THC, and optimize efficacy due to the biphasic dosing curve.

- Think of cannabis as a prescription-strength medication. Use it with appropriate caution, and consult your veterinarian every step of the way.

Dosing Calculation

My colleague, Dr. Rob Silver, originally determined much of the following dosing information through available data in human medicine and his own experience with veterinary patients. Rob is a good friend and a highly accomplished herbalist with years of experience formulating natural medicines for pets. His book, *Medical Marijuana and Your Pet*, is available online and is a great read for pet owners who really want to dive into the topic of medical cannabis for pets. The chart below represents a combination of Dr. Silver's data and extrapolation from reports from research in human medicine as well as my own personal experience treating animals.[14]

Note: Dosing calculation for all drugs, including medical cannabis, must be done precisely to ensure safety and efficacy. The following dosing information is included for you to bring to your veterinarian. Unless you are trained in calculating drug dosages, contact your veterinarian for assistance. A simple mathematical error can result in a tenfold overdose and a trip to the emergency room. As they say on TV: "Do not try this at home."

THC*

- Starting dose: 0.1–0.25 milligrams per kilogram of pet's body weight per day

- Calculated dose should be divided for twice- or thrice-daily dosing.

- Start low and slowly increase to allow for tolerance to develop and due to biphasic dose response.

- Reports suggest higher levels of THC may be beneficial, but caution at higher doses must be used in pets due to toxicity concerns.

CBD

- Starting dose: 0.1–0.5 milligrams per kilogram of pet's body weight per day

- Calculated dose should be divided for twice- or thrice-daily dosing.

- Doses up to 5 milligrams per kilogram per day have been reported for difficult seizure cases.

- Start low and slowly increase due to biphasic dose response.

---

*Although the amount of CBD in a given medicine is important, THC is the compound in cannabis that has the potential to be toxic. Thus, THC is always the limiting factor for any product containing THC. To prevent toxicity and a trip to the emergency room, accurate dosing is critical. Consult with a veterinarian and have them calculate dosing whenever using a cannabis product containing moderate to large amounts of THC.

Applying the Dosing Information to Your Pet

Most medical cannabis and hemp products for pets are in liquid form, and calculating the appropriate dosage is easy. All that is required are a few pieces of information and basic math skills. The following steps will walk you through how to calculate a dose of medical cannabis for your pet.

1. Start with accurate information. Specifically, you will need the following:

- Your pet's current body weight in kilograms (kg). To convert your pet's weight from pounds to kg, divide the number of pounds by 2.2. For example, a 50-pound dog is 22.7 kg (50 ÷ 2.2 = 22.7).

- The ratio of the cannabis product you will be using (if you are using a hemp product, the ratio is less important because of the very low levels of THC).

- The dosing range of both THC and CBD (see the previous guidelines).

2. Multiply your pet's body weight in kilograms (kg) by the low and upper ends of the THC dose range: 0.1 to 0.25 mg/kg/day.

- Low dose with a 22.7 kg dog: 22.7 kg × 0.1 mg/kg/day = 2.27 mg/day

- Upper dose with a 22.7 kg dog: 22.7 kg × 0.25 mg/kg/day = 5.67 mg/day

3. Multiply your pet's body weight in kilograms (kg) by the low and upper ends of the CBD dose range: 0.1 to 0.5 mg/kg/day.

- Low dose with a 22.7 kg dog: 22.7 kg × 0.1 mg/kg/day = 2.27 mg/day

- Upper dose with a 22.7 kg dog: 22.7 kg × 0.5 mg/kg/day = 11.35 mg/day

4. Determine how many milligrams of THC and CBD are in a given quantity of medicine by dividing the number of calculated milligrams of THC by the number of milligrams in a given quantity of medicine. (The label may list milligrams per milliliter, per drop, per dropper, etc.)

- The medication you are using has 5 mg per ml of THC. You want to dose your 22.7-kilogram dog between 2.27 and 5.67 mg of THC per day.

    - Low dose of THC = 2.27 mg ÷ 5 mg/ml = 0.45 ml per day

    - Upper dose of THC = 5.67 mg ÷ 5 mg/ml = 1.13 ml per day

- The medication you are using has 5 mg per ml of CBD. You want to dose your 22.7-kg dog 2.27 to 11.35 mg of CBD per day.

- ▫   Low dose of CBD = 2.27 mg ÷ 5 mg/ml = 0.45 ml per day
- ▫   Upper dose of CBD = 11.35 ÷ 5 mg/ml = 2.27 ml per day

5. Most of the time, cannabis and hemp are best administered twice or thrice daily. So be sure to divide the daily calculated doses of THC and CBD by two or three when measuring out your doses.

6. Once the dose range is determined, begin at the low end of the dose range and increase slowly. Increase the dose no more than weekly to allow for your pet to acclimate to the new dose. (This is particularly important when THC is in the mix.) It should take at least three or four weeks to move from the low end to the high end of the dose. Remember to always watch for effect.

Remember that because of the biphasic dosing curve, the most optimal dose may be less than your highest calculated dose. Monitor carefully for any signs of loss of balance, excessive sedation, or abnormal behavior that might be an indication of too much THC. Discontinue the medication and contact your veterinarian immediately if you see anything concerning.

CHAPTER 10

TECHNOLOGY AND HOLISTIC MEDICINE

Two Sides Coming Together

There is no need for fiction in medicine, for the facts will always beat anything you fancy.

– SIR ARTHUR CONAN DOYLE

When most of us think of the term *holistic medicine*, the image conjured up is one of traditional remedies, herbs, acupuncture, etc. Western medicine, on the other hand, is more frequently associated with cutting-edge research and innovation. Overall, the tendency is to view holistic medicine as old and Western medicine as new.

Until recently, this presumption held water pretty effectively. Technological advances over the past few years, however, have created more and more exceptions to the old-versus-new rule. And as we all know, the exceptions to the rule are always the most fascinating things.

One of the defining aspects of holistic medicine is its propensity to facilitate healing. More specifically, holistic therapy stimulates the body to heal itself by providing the patient with the nutrients or energy they need to address the root cause of a problem rather than covering things up by only alleviating symptoms. Well-accepted holistic therapies such as acupuncture, herbal medicine, nutritional and glandular therapy, etc., are effective due to their ability to promote the body's own natural healing abilities.

Technology can also be holistic. By learning some of the secrets of how the body works, researchers have been able to take advantage of healing pathways to create a body-healing hack. In this way, technology *can* be holistic—and the following are some of the most successful options that modern technology has made available. Used in conjunction with more traditional holistic care as well as conventional medicine, they can help us achieve even better outcomes than were previously possible.

Pulsating Electromagnetic Field Therapy (PEMF)

All living things are electrical systems. The nervous system, along with every cell in the body, communicates with its neighbors through the use of minute amounts of electrical current. Just as in every mechanical electric device, biological systems create an electromagnetic field.

The electromagnetic fields created by biological organisms are more than merely by-products of electrical impulses between cells. The fields themselves affect body function. For example: Plant growth and development is influenced by exposure to varying magnetic fields.[1] In addition, concerns regarding human exposure to electromagnetic fields such as cell phones and power lines are commonplace. While there is ongoing debate about whether such exposure will be our undoing, there is no controversy surrounding the fact that exposure to electromagnetic energy has biological effect.[2, 3]

Setting aside concerns of "death by cell phone," there are legitimate medical applications for PEMF, and the positive effects can be quite dramatic. Both veterinary and human patients are routinely treated successfully with PEMF to facilitate healing of bone, cartilage, and chronic wounds. Following are examples of some of the currently available PEMF applications and technologies.

PEMF for Bone Healing

Fractures happen. Dogs and cats may be hit by a car, fall from a height, or get bitten by something larger and stronger than they are. Most fractures in dogs and cats are repaired surgically (they don't tolerate casts) and tend to heal very well. There are occasions, however, when the healing process does not go as planned.

The medical terms for a fracture that doesn't want to heal are *delayed union* or *nonunion*. This can be caused by an inability to effectively immobilize the fracture, such as a pet being too active during the healing process, or sometimes it can occur spontaneously. Regardless of the cause, a delayed or nonunion fracture is a serious complication that often requires additional surgery or, in some cases, amputation.

In 2009, a miniature dachshund named Figaro mysteriously broke his toe. The little guy was one and a half years old and was staying with a friend of the owner. He came home limping, and X-rays revealed a fractured toe on his front foot. Given that the bone was so small, surgical repair was not an option, so Figaro's leg was splinted for six weeks. After that time, follow-up X-rays showed minimal healing of the fracture. He was given another four weeks in the splint, with no significant improvement. The radiologist diagnosed a nonunion fracture and recommended amputating the toe.

It was around that time that I was beginning to build a holistic practice, and we had just installed a new piece of equipment called Pulsed Signal Therapy (PST). PST technology was developed to help stimulate cartilage regrowth and repair of damaged joints in humans.[4, 5] While clearly cartilage and bone are not the same thing, medically speaking, they are close. I had the opportunity to speak with the inventor of PST, Dr. Richard Markoll, and he recommended a protocol to use to stimulate healing of Figaro's broken bone.

Figaro was treated with PST for nine days, and we maintained his splint for an additional six weeks. At the end of the six weeks, the bone was healed! Figaro got to keep his toe, and the new holistic practice had a fantastic success story.

PEMF for Cartilage Healing

As mentioned above, cartilage is close to bone. It is, in fact, attached to bone. Everywhere in the body where two bones come together to form a joint, the ends of the bones are lined with cartilage. It is a very smooth, very tough surface that allows joints to move with minimal friction. Most forms of arthritis are characterized by damage or loss of cartilage due to injury and/or age. When the cartilage is worn, bone rubs on bone and the result is pain.

We can provide our pets with nutrients such as glucosamine and chondroitin to supply building blocks to make new cartilage, but the process is slow and somewhat limited. PEMF puts the system into high gear. The electromagnetic energy literally stimulates the chondrocytes (cartilage-forming cells) to become more metabolically active and repair damaged cartilage.[6]

Treating a pet with PST is completely painless and works by stimulating the body to heal itself. Most animals require a daily series of nine 30-minute treatments. After the course of treatment, it takes between one and three months to see the full effect; cartilage growth takes time. Most pet owners begin to see subtle changes within the first month. Sometimes the results are so subtle, they initially go unnoticed. Oftentimes it begins with a little more stamina and interest in longer walks. Then one day the owner comes home to find the dog has jumped onto the couch or the bed (or the kitchen counter), which they have not done in months or years.

I have used PST successfully for dogs and cats with nonhealing fractures, arthritis, and neck and back pain. Many pets are able to decrease or discontinue the use of prescription anti-inflammatory drugs within several months after treatment. Cartilage growth as a result of treatment lasts anywhere from one to three years. Injuries such as fractures are healed permanently, of course. However, pets with conditions such as arthritis will need further treatment every one to three years as they continue wearing down the new cartilage.

PEMF for Soft-Tissue Healing

PEMF devices are tuned to the waveform of the tissues they are designed to affect. Bone and cartilage (hard tissues) respond to different frequencies than skin, muscle, and nerves (soft tissues). While utilizing different frequencies than PST, the FDA-approved Assisi Loop exerts biological effects on soft tissues leading to reduction in pain and inflammation, and stimulation of healing.[7, 8]

Devices like the Assisi Loop are more widespread than PST because of their relative affordability and availability. Whereas a PST unit is costly and generally owned by a veterinary hospital, loops are affordable for pet owners and allow treatment of pain and inflammation on a daily basis. This can be a real advantage, since multiple acupuncture sessions per week can become logistically (and financially) challenging for many pet owners. In addition to in-clinic therapy and appropriate medication and/or supplements, take-home devices like Assisi Loops are an excellent treatment option for pets with arthritis and back pain.

How You Can Use PEMF as Part of Your Pet's Treatment Plan

- PEMF can be used to support the healing of fractured bones. It is not recommended as a substitute for surgical repair.

- PST is a valuable treatment for arthritis and sometimes back pain. The effects of the treatment take months, so other forms of therapy are often needed, at least in the short term.

- Assisi Loops or devices like them work well for treating pain associated with soft-tissue injuries, arthritis, and back problems. They are also valuable to speed the healing of open wounds.

- You can look for veterinarians experienced with PEMF therapy through the American Holistic Veterinary Medical Association website: www.ahvma.org.

- PEMF therapy can take weeks to months for the full effects to become apparent. Be patient, as healing takes time.

Hyperbaric Oxygen Therapy

Hyperbaric oxygen therapy (HBOT) is a treatment in which a patient is placed in a sealed chamber that is filled with 100 percent oxygen at higher-than-atmospheric pressures. The high-pressure pure oxygen is breathed in and absorbed into the bloodstream. The high concentration of oxygen in the blood subsequently moves throughout the body, saturating tissues with oxygen.

Some people know about hyperbaric oxygen chambers only because of their use after scuba diving accidents, but this accounts for only a very small percentage of their use. In human medicine, most hyperbaric oxygen patients are those with chronic nonhealing wounds due to diabetes or difficult-to-control infections.

Oxygen is a vital part of the chemical reaction the body uses to make energy in the form of adenosine triphosphate (ATP). ATP is the chemical compound within cells that stores and supplies energy. Without adequate levels of oxygen, cells have a difficult time repairing and reproducing, which results in slowed healing or nonhealing conditions. In addition to facilitating ATP generation, the high levels of oxygen lead to the production of nitric oxide, a compound that stimulates growth of new blood vessels. These new vessels further provide blood supply to damaged tissues and facilitate healing.

Through HBOT, we eliminate the limiting factor to healing—tissue oxygen levels. The result of greatly elevated oxygen levels includes improved healing, decreased inflammation and edema, pain relief, and improved response to antibiotics.[9] Hyperbaric oxygen is an excellent example of a technological adaptation of holistic medicine.

Hyperbaric oxygen therapy works only when the patient is in a chamber breathing pressurized oxygen. The effects occur from breathing the oxygen, which is then distributed to the body tissues. There is no topical effect, so beware of therapies purporting to treat individual body parts with oxygen; they are ineffective.

Interestingly, hyperbaric oxygen therapy is actually pretty old tech. Believe it or not, the first hyperbaric chamber was invented in 1662. The first medical uses of hyperbaric medicine were in the mid-1800s, and by the mid-20th century research on the many uses of hyperbaric medicine was in full swing.[10]

Veterinary applications of HBOT are widespread. Any medical condition associated with severe swelling, edema (fluid buildup), trauma, or interruption of blood supply may benefit from HBOT. Some of the conditions that have been successfully helped in veterinary patients include:

- Postsurgical patients with severe swelling (especially orthopedics)

- Interruption of circulation

- Head trauma

- Spinal trauma including disc protrusion/rupture

- Snake bite/spider bite

- Resistant infection

Success Story: Jack versus the Spider

A few years ago, I received a call from a local internal medicine specialist. She was treating a 5-year-old Lab named Jack. Over a period of several days, Jack had developed severe swelling and edema (fluid accumulation) in his right hind leg. The swelling was so severe, it was cutting off circulation to the leg. The specialist feared they would be forced to amputate.

Jack's doctor was calling to see if I though HBOT would help. My answer was an enthusiastic yes!

When Jack came in later that day, his right hind leg was nearly twice the size of the left! It was painful, hot, and so swollen that fluid was seeping out of the skin. Poor Jack was miserable. We took measurements of his leg and immediately placed him in the hyperbaric chamber. Over the next three days, Jack was treated a total of five times. After each treatment, we measured his leg. Before the first treatment, Jack's thigh measured 50 centimeters around. Five days later, the same area was 36 centimeters and looking nearly normal. Jack was back to putting weight on the leg, and he was clearly well on his way to healing. In the span of five days he went from a dog whose primary treatment option was amputation to walking and being nearly healed! The only thing that changed was increased levels of oxygen in his blood and tissues. Hyperbaric oxygen saved Jack's leg and possibly his life.

During the course of treatment, Jack's owner was looking in the yard where Jack tends to sleep and found several black widow spiders under a log. A spider bite was most likely the cause of the severe swelling. In the end, Jack did great and his leg healed completely, without the need for surgery. Needless to say, Jack's owner has found him a new place for his afternoon naps.

How You Can Use HBOT
as Part of Your Pet's Treatment Plan

- HBOT works well for patients with conditions involving severe swelling, edema (fluid buildup), trauma, interruption of blood supply, infection, and nonhealing wounds.

- Successful use of hyperbaric medicine often requires frequent treatments. Anywhere from 5 to 30 treatments are often necessary. Healing takes time.

- While the availability of hyperbaric chambers for pets is limited, more and more are installed each year. You can find practitioners of this emerging technology by looking on the Hyperbaric Veterinary Medicine website: www.hvmed.com.

Laser Therapy

Many different types of lasers are used in medicine. Surgeons use lasers to cut or cauterize tissue in the operating room, while dentists use lasers to whiten teeth and treat tooth decay and gum disease. For the purposes of this discussion, laser therapy is used to treat pain and inflammation while promoting healing.

Some people dismiss laser therapy as ineffective quackery. After all, how can something like light change the way a living being functions? Consider photosynthesis. Plants convert light energy into chemical energy through the use of chlorophyll. In the animal world, humans synthesize vitamin D by absorbing sunlight through our skin. Clearly light energy can, and does, affect biological processes.

Distinct from surgical lasers, which use extreme heat to cut tissue, therapeutic lasers use light energy to affect the behavior and activity of living tissue. They go by many different names, including cold laser therapy or low-level laser therapy (LLLT), but a more accurate term would be photobiomodulation (PBM) lasers. PBM describes the process of light energy affecting the behavior and activity of living tissue.

PBM lasers work by stimulating biological processes within body tissues. Laser light increases circulation, which leads to increased oxygen and nutrients being delivered to the treated area. In addition, laser light increases metabolic activity within cells, leading to improved cellular function, generation of cellular energy, and tissue healing. For similar reasons, laser therapy is also beneficial in the reduction of swelling and edema, which, in turn, relieves pain and speeds healing.

Lasers come in varying power classes, from I through IV. Although they generally have similar effects on tissues, lower-powered lasers (such as class I and II) take much longer to achieve therapeutic results than higher-powered models. Conversely, a higher-powered class III or IV laser works faster, but must be used with caution to prevent overheating of tissues.

Inappropriate use of a PBM laser can lead to ineffective treatment or even tissue damage. Even "cold" lasers generate heat and, if used improperly, can cause burns. Safe and successful use of medical lasers is a function of training and experience on the part of your veterinarian.

How You Can Use Laser Therapy
as Part of Your Pet's Treatment Plan

- Laser therapy can be very beneficial for pets with orthopedic conditions, arthritis, back/neck pain, and a variety of wounds that are slow to heal or nonhealing.

- The effects of laser therapy are cumulative; in many cases, treatment several times per week is necessary in the early stages. The length of each treatment depends on the size of the area being treated and the power (class) of the laser being used.

- The physics of how and why laser therapy works is complex. However, there is no need to fully understand the intricacies of PBM laser therapy—that is your veterinarian's job.

- Cold laser therapy is widely accepted in veterinary medicine, and many veterinary offices have them even if they offer no other alternative medical options.

Stem Cell Therapy

While there are many exciting areas of medical research, regenerative medicine has to be one of the most promising. Scientists are now using a patient's own cells to stimulate healing. While the best is yet to come in the regenerative medical field, the use of stem cell therapy is here and available today for humans and pets.

Stem cells are cells within the body that have the ability to differentiate and become other, more specialized cells. (You might say that stem cells have not decided what they want to be when they grow up.) A stem cell could become a nerve cell, heart muscle cell, or any other cell within the body. The route it ultimately takes depends on the types of chemical signals it receives from the body. Harnessing the power of stem cells holds the promise of successful repair of severely damaged tissues, such as in spinal cord injuries. Stem cell researchers are also using these cells to literally regrow body parts and organs![11, 12]

There was controversy over the use of stem cells in the very early 2000s because at that time the best source of these undifferentiated cells was found in embryonic tissue. Thankfully, scientists have since discovered reservoirs of stem cells in the fatty tissue of adults. This new source has shifted much of the research focus and placed stem cell therapy on less controversial ground. However, because of FDA restrictions, stem cell therapy is still more readily available for veterinary medicine than for humans.

Stem cells are most commonly used to treat patients with arthritic joints. Cells can be injected directly into a damaged joint and/or given intravenously. The result is the stem cells differentiating into tissues such as cartilage, which helps repair the joint and thus relieves pain. Currently, the method involves a brief surgical procedure to collect fat from a patient, after which the stem cells are concentrated and prepared for injection. Extra stem cells can be banked for future use.

In addition to orthopedic applications, stem cells have been successfully used in cats with kidney failure. The cells are collected in the same way described above and then injected either intravenously or directly into the kidney via the renal artery. Results have been promising, and several cats I have personally treated have gone on to live for years after being diagnosed with kidney failure.

Research is ongoing for the development of allogeneic stem cells. These cells would be "universal donor" cells, thus eliminating the need for anesthesia and surgical collection of stem cells from patients. Once these allogeneic cells are available, stem cell therapy will undoubtedly become more widespread in its use.

How You Can Use Stem Cell Therapy as Part of Your Pet's Treatment Plan

- Stem cell therapy is currently being used to treat pets with arthritis. It is also commonly used to facilitate healing in pets that have had surgery on a joint such as a knee or elbow.

- Stem cells have been successfully used to help cats with kidney failure.

- Currently, stem cell therapy requires surgical collection of fat to harvest stem cells. FDA trials are in progress to approve the use of donor cells, which would eliminate the need for anesthesia and surgery.

- To learn more about stem cell therapy for pets and to find a veterinarian in your area experienced in using stem cells, visit www.VetStem.com.

Platelet-Rich Plasma

Like stem cell therapy, platelet-rich plasma (PRP) therapy is a form of regenerative medicine in which a patient's own cells are used to stimulate healing. Various factors contained within the blood promote healing, and many of these factors are found within the plasma.

- Plasma is the liquid portion of the blood; it is what remains after you remove all the cellular components (red blood cells, white blood cells, and platelets). Although it is mostly water, it also contains proteins, clotting factors, electrolytes, antibodies, and enzymes.

- Platelets are cells within blood that are responsible for clotting and tissue healing. When blood flows to the site of an injury, it is the platelets, along with proteins and clotting factors within the plasma, that begin the process of repairing what has been damaged.

- Platelet-rich plasma is derived from concentrating healing factors from blood. Blood is collected from a patient, and then the platelets and plasma are separated from the red and white blood cells.

PRP is used in much the same way as stem cells. Patients receiving PRP usually have either arthritis or an injury such as a ligament, tendon, or muscle tear. PRP is generally injected directly into the affected joint or site of injury to provide concentrated healing factors to the area. PRP is used commonly in both human and veterinary medicine—particularly for athletes.[13, 14]

Currently, PRP has a benefit over stem cells in that it does not require a surgical procedure to collect the material. Stem cells, on the other hand, may be more versatile given that the cells themselves are able to regenerate and create more cells and a better outcome. However, both modalities can be highly effective in pets. Stem cell therapy and PRP can be (and are) used together for even greater results.

How You Can Use Platelet-Rich Plasma as Part of Your Pet's Treatment Plan

- PRP is currently being used to treat pets with arthritis. It is also commonly used to facilitate healing in pets that have had surgery on a joint such as a knee or elbow.

- PRP is becoming popular among veterinary surgeons and veterinarians whose practices focus on orthopedic conditions. Contact your veterinarian for information on who you can talk to in your area regarding PRP for your pet.

Cancer Vaccines

The backbone of conventional cancer therapy is much the same as it has been for years, consisting of surgery, chemotherapy, and radiation. While the technology behind all three of these therapies continues to advance, the goals are largely the same: remove the cancer with surgery (if possible), then eradicate microscopic disease by killing cancer cells through chemotherapy drugs or through cellular damage with radiation.

While these cornerstone therapies continue to occupy most of the space in veterinary cancer care, new technologies are emerging. One of the most promising has been the development of a vaccine for cancer.

Under normal circumstances, vaccinations are used to prevent disease, stimulating the immune system to create protective antibodies that prevent the body from contracting a specific disease should they become exposed to it. A vaccine for cancer, however, is a bit different. Rather than promoting an immune response for disease prevention, cancer vaccines prime the patient's immune system to target specific markers on cancer cells.

Canine malignant melanoma is both locally aggressive and tends to metastasize (spread) to the lungs. These cancers are often not responsive to chemotherapy, and only 30 percent of dogs survive one year after surgical removal of the tumor.[15] Dogs with more advanced disease (Stage 2 or 3) have a survival time of less than six months after surgery.[16, 17]

In recent years, a melanoma vaccine has been developed for dogs. The canine malignant melanoma vaccine contains a version of a protein found on melanoma cells called tyrosinase. The vaccine stimulates an immune response to tyrosinase, which leads to the patient's own immune system attacking the cancer cells. The results of the melanoma vaccine have been promising. While the vaccine is not a cure, many of the dogs whose life expectancy would have been measured in months have gone on to live for years with good quality of life.[18, 19]

One of my own dogs, Elliott, developed an oral melanoma years ago. He had surgery to remove the tumor, but it metastasized and we lost him six months later. The vaccine became available only two years after we received Elliott's diagnosis. Had it been available at the time, I absolutely would have used it.

The canine melanoma vaccine is the first (hopefully not the last) cancer vaccine in the veterinary medical field. It is an excellent example of how researchers can hack the immune system and create hope where there previously was none.

How You Can Use Cancer Vaccines as Part of Your Pet's Treatment Plan

- The canine melanoma vaccine is widely available through veterinary oncologists. Your veterinarian can refer you to an oncologist should the need arise.

- The vaccine is most effective when melanoma is diagnosed and treated in its early stages. The vaccine protocol is begun following surgical removal of the tumor.

- Cancer therapy is most successful when a multifaceted approach is taken. Consult with an oncologist and a veterinarian knowledgeable about alternative cancer therapies. You can find alternative cancer care veterinarians through the American Holistic Veterinary Medical Association website, www.ahvma.org.

The Future of Medicine is "One Medicine"

The treatments discussed in this chapter represent a melding of technological advances and the holistic principle of encouraging the body to heal itself. It is likely the researchers developing these treatment options aren't thinking of them in this way, but that's okay. After all, a rose by any other name. . . .

There are many other examples of technology being used to stimulate healing in patients beyond the ones discussed here. The treatments chosen for this chapter were included because of their known efficacy and availability. You should be able to find many (if not all) of these options available to you if the need should arise.

As technology advances, scientists will continue to find more ways to encourage the body to prevent illness and heal itself when sick or injured. This is the progression toward what will ultimately be "one medicine."

PART III

COMMON DISEASES, THEIR CAUSES, AND INTEGRATIVE MEDICAL TREATMENT

Learning that a beloved pet has a medical condition can be frightening. It is in our nature to immediately search for ways to fix the problem. The first step when dealing with a medical issue is to understand what you are up against. Although symptoms can be treated independent of a deeper knowledge of how and why a medical condition occurs, the true key to successful therapy necessitates understanding the root cause of a disease.

Many pet owners come to see me requesting a second opinion. Although they may not know it, most are also searching for an understanding of the diagnosis. Sometimes this lack of clarity stems from the level of shock that occurred when a veterinarian delivered the bad news. People often just stopped hearing what was being said. Complicating this are the confines of the normal 15- to 20-minute veterinary appointment. There is no time for a veterinarian to dedicate to a detailed explanation of a diagnosis and treatment plan. Unfortunately this problem is pervasive throughout the health-care system, where doctors and veterinarians are afforded less and less time to spend with patients and clients.

Following a thorough examination, my first task is to sit down and explain the diagnosis, how it occurred, and what the progression is likely to be. In many cases, having a detailed understanding of the diagnosis sets pet owners at ease. Once light is shined upon the problem and the boogeyman is uncovered, things are less scary. Then we can have a productive conversation about treatment strategy. With a well-thought-out integrative treatment plan under way, everyone can breathe a little easier knowing that everything that *can* be done *is* being done.

What to Expect

The following chapters discuss common diseases in dogs and cats, how they affect the body system, and how and why each condition occurs. You can read this section straight through or use it as a reference guide by focusing only on the portions that relate to your pets. Either way, the material is here for your use, now and in the future.

The conditions in these chapters were chosen because they are encountered frequently and respond well to integrative care. Pets with these issues often have incomplete or unsuccessful responses to conventional therapy alone. These are the conditions for which integrative health care is most effective.

Each condition discussed will include an outline of conventional and alternative therapies. Treatment options will include accepted "standard of practice" care, cutting-edge therapies where they are available, and holistic options that are either commonly used or that I have personally had success with in my patients. For the most part, active ingredients in supplements rather than specific brands are discussed. In cases where a product is mentioned by name, it is because it is unique in its design and would not be readily available outside the brand name.

Given the scope of alternative medical care for any given condition, it is impossible to discuss every alternative. A holistic-minded veterinarian should be able to help you with methods of therapy not covered within these chapters.

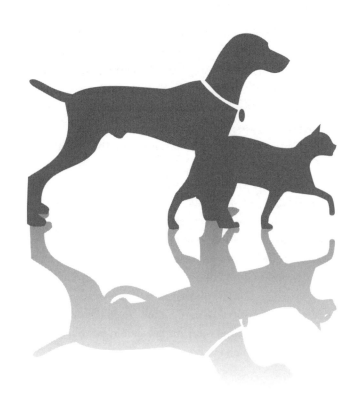

CHAPTER 11

ALLERGIES AND SKIN PROBLEMS

Health is much more dependent on our habits and nutrition than on medicine.

– JOHN LUBBOCK

The skin is an organ like no other. It protects the internal tissues, regulates body temperature, and absorbs or secretes materials into and out of the environment. Beyond that, skin is one of the primary sensory organs. What animals feel through their skin helps shape their perception of the world.

The skin is a sensitive organ; even mild inflammation can cause discomfort and affect quality of life. Dogs and cats with itchy, red, greasy, scabby, or flaky skin are regulars in every veterinary office. Dermatologic issues are not normally life-threatening, but they can be maddening for both the pet and the owner. Constant scratching and chewing is guaranteed to drive everyone in the house nuts! As you will see, there are many potential origins of skin problems, and diagnosing the underlying cause is key to the most successful treatment.

When Things Go Wrong: Allergies and the Allergic Threshold

Given that the skin is the protective covering for the body, it is no surprise it is often ground zero for immune response reactions to outside stimuli. The immune system keeps the body safe from infections, toxins, and other things that may do the body harm by recognizing what is "normal" and what is "abnormal" within the body and on the body surface. When immune cells detect something abnormal or foreign, they create an inflammatory response to surround and eliminate the harmful particles. These immune responses kept humans and animals alive for millions of years prior to the benefit of antibiotics and modern medicine.

Occasionally, however, the immune system will misidentify a harmless substance as a potential threat. When the immune system marks a harmless substance, like pollen, as a hazard to the body, it creates an inflammatory response every time it encounters that substance. If the response is mild, there may be no outward symptoms. But immune responses are additive, meaning that they combine on top of one another until they reach the *allergic threshold*, at which point allergy symptoms appear.

It is common for an animal with allergies to be sensitive to more than one thing, and each allergen creates an individual immune response in the body. If, for example, a pet has a pollen allergy *and* a little bit of food sensitivity, it's possible that the immune response to the food issue alone wouldn't be enough to manifest allergy symptoms. In this case, resolving the food issue could get your pet under the wire of the allergic threshold, greatly improving their symptoms. This is why it is crucial to eliminate as many potential allergens as possible. Food, for example, is an easier variable to manipulate than pollen.[1]

Know the Difference: Allergies versus Sensitivities

It's important to note that when it comes to pets and food, true allergic reactions are uncommon. While people sometimes experience potentially life-threatening reactions to peanuts, shellfish, etc., this rarely happens in animals. More frequently, animals experience a food sensitivity manifested as lower-level inflammation secondary to a reaction to a food ingredient, an ingested toxin, or artificial additives.

It is important to differentiate the terms *allergy* and *sensitivity*. Allergies are responses by the immune system that cause an immediate inflammatory reaction ranging from mild to severe. For example, a dog or a person with a severe bee sting allergy may experience an anaphylactic response that includes respiratory distress. On the other end of the spectrum, a mild allergy to fleas in dogs can lead to local or systemic inflammation and itchiness.

Sensitivities, on the other hand, tend to be subtler. These reactions often still lead to skin or gastrointestinal-related disease, but not in the immediate life-threatening sense a true allergy might.

The Immune Response and the GI Tract: Leaky Gut Syndrome

While diet plays a part in the overt stimulation of some allergies, it also has an indirect effect through the gastrointestinal tract (GI), because 70 percent of all immune cells in the body reside within the intestines.[2] So what better place to focus energy than where almost three-fourths of the immune system lives?

Under normal conditions, food particles are digested and broken down into components small enough to pass through and between the cells of the intestinal wall and into the bloodstream. When chronic inflammation in the GI tract causes increased permeability of the gut wall, this is called leaky gut syndrome. This condition allows the passage of larger molecules into the blood, which can cause an inflammatory immune response.

Leaky gut syndrome is primarily caused by a poor diet or dietary sensitivities, and the effects of the inflammation can occur anywhere in the body, including the skin. Although somewhat controversial in Western medicine, leaky gut syndrome is a well-recognized condition to practitioners of complementary and alternative medicine.[3, 4]

Determining Your Pet's Allergy or Sensitivity

Common symptoms of a pet's allergy or sensitivity are itching, pain, flaking, scabs, hair loss, and infection. In determining the underlying cause, your first clue is when your pet's symptoms began. Was there a new food or treat introduced around that time? Is your pet going somewhere new, or did you move to a new house? Are the symptoms seasonal?

If your pet's symptoms are seasonal, it's probably due to environmental allergens, which are often related to various pollens or the increased flea populations during warmer months. Symptoms that are nonseasonal may indicate food as a culprit, although environmental allergens and/or fleas cannot be ruled out purely on this basis.

The three most common causes of skin inflammation in pets are fleas, atopy, and food. In the following sections, we'll explore the symptoms and sources of inflammation and the means by which they are diagnosed.

Fleas and Flea Allergy Dermatitis

By far the most common skin allergy in dogs and cats is flea allergy dermatitis. As a flea bites your dog or cat, its saliva frequently causes an allergic reaction. Pets with flea allergy dermatitis often will be itchy and have red, scabby skin. Ground zero is often at the base of the tail, as this is where fleas tend to congregate. However, fleas are mobile and can be anywhere on your pet. In addition, the systemic reaction experienced by flea-allergic dogs and cats may make them itchy in places where there are no fleas.

Pets with flea allergy dermatitis may scratch and chew so much that they develop a secondary skin infection. The skin of these pets can be red and hot and often feels moist. Scabs and pustules may be present. Dogs in particular will sometimes scratch or chew and create a hot spot. The term *hot spot* refers to a focal area of traumatized and infected skin caused by licking or chewing.

Don't let the visible absence of fleas on your pet fool you into thinking that your pet can't have flea allergy dermatitis! Even strictly indoor cats can get fleas that are brought in on someone's shoes or clothes. If I had a dime for every time a pet owner came into the office and swore up and down that their pet did not have fleas but ultimately it did . . . Actually, I do have a dime for every one of those times. The point is, it happens a lot! This is because fleas are not always visible upon examination, and sensitive animals are able to groom them off very effectively. Therefore, even the most flea-allergic pets may have few, if any, actual fleas on them at any given time.

Atopic Dermatitis

Next to fleas, atopic dermatitis (atopy) is the most common cause of allergies in pets. Pets with atopy will commonly have itching on their face, feet, and armpits, or even their entire body. You might notice your pet often licking and biting their itchy feet and pawing at their itchy or infected ears. The excessive scratching can sometimes progress to a skin infection.

Atopy is caused by an allergy to environmental sources such as grasses, pollen, dust mites, and molds. An immune response can be triggered either by direct contact or as a systemic allergic response when the allergen is inhaled. (Just as humans get hay fever from inhaling pollen, dogs and cats can become itchy from inhaled allergens.) Atopy is often, but not always, seasonal in nature. In some pets, it may begin seasonally but then progress to year-round as the pet's sensitivities worsen over time.

Of the three most common causes of skin inflammation in pets, atopy is the most challenging to diagnose and treat. Determining exactly what your pet is reacting to is helpful, but this must be done via allergy testing with a veterinarian, which involves a blood test or intradermal testing.

In the blood testing method, a sample is submitted to a laboratory that tests for reactivity of the blood to various environmental allergens. Intradermal testing is accomplished by injecting a very small quantity of an allergen into the skin and monitoring for an inflammatory response. Either way, the greater the response, the more sensitive the patient is thought to be to a specific allergen.

All things being equal, the intradermal method is the gold standard for allergy testing. However, it is only available through specialized veterinary dermatologists, whereas blood allergy testing can be done in your regular veterinarian's office, and usually for less money. Both tests give valuable results, although the intradermal results may be a bit more precise. Regardless of the method, the practical use of allergy testing results is to begin a desensitization protocol (see the treatment section later in this chapter).

Food Sensitivity Dermatitis

Pets with food sensitivities frequently have inflammation and itching of the face, ears, and feet, although other parts of the body can be affected as well. Sometimes these pets will also have GI problems such as chronic soft stools or gas. The symptoms are nonseasonal for obvious reasons.

Despite accounting for only 10 to 30 percent of skin problems in pets, food sensitivity is frequently one of the initial topics discussed when a pet comes in for allergies. This is because, just as with fleas, food is a relatively easy variable to control. Furthermore, ideal nutrition is the foundation for good health and an optimally functioning immune system. So even if your pet does not have food sensitivities, upgrading the diet stands a good chance of improving their allergies. (Remember the allergic threshold!)

The most effective way to determine if allergies or chronic GI issues are caused by something your pet is eating is to conduct a diet trial, also known as a limited-ingredient diet (LID) trial or an elimination diet. As you remove ingredients in the diet and monitor for improvements, we can determine if your pet's condition is caused by something they are eating. I've outlined instructions for this diet in Appendix E.

A laboratory test, NutriScan, has recently become available that provides some guidance in choosing foods for sensitive animals. Developed by Dr. Jean Dodds and Hemopet labs, this test utilizes natural antibodies in saliva to test for reactivity to a variety of foods. Of all the saliva-based tests advertised for food and environmental allergies, NutriScan is the only one with scientific research to back its results.

The NutriScan test is useful in cases where a diet trial would be difficult to accomplish or where we want some direction regarding which foods to avoid for the trial. Given how difficult food trials can be, any information that might simplify the process is a plus.

Other Causes of Skin Problems

While fleas, atopy, and food sensitivity are the most frequent culprits, they are not the only causes of skin problems in pets. Other conditions that can manifest with skin abnormalities include:

- **External parasites:** Demodectic mange (demodex) and sarcoptic mange (scabies) require a skin scraping to diagnose and prescription medication to treat.

- **Ringworm:** Despite the name, ringworm is a fungal infection. Some species of ringworm are easily diagnosed, as they "glow" under a type of black light called a Wood's lamp. More often, a fungal culture or fungal DNA screening of the hair is required.

- **Hypothyroidism:** A low-functioning thyroid can manifest itself as chronic itchy, greasy skin. The skin issues frequently improve and/or resolve once thyroid hormone is adequately supplemented through your veterinarian. (See Chapter 21 regarding diagnosis and treatment of hypothyroidism.)

- **Nutritional deficiency:** A diet missing key micronutrients or adequate fatty acids can lead to skin problems. If the GI tract isn't healthy enough to absorb these nutrients (e.g., in the case of leaky gut), then the problem may not be diet as much as it is an issue of suboptimal GI tract health. (See Chapter 14 regarding diagnosis and treatment of gastrointestinal disease.)

Anyone with his or her own allergies knows treatment is a lifelong process. Except in cases of flea allergy or food sensitivity, where an allergen can be definitively removed from the environment, most pets with skin allergies will always have some level of persistent symptoms. Following are treatment options for specific conditions as well as more generalized therapies that are applicable to all forms of skin allergies.

Conventional Medical Treatment

Flea Control and Treating Flea Allergy Dermatitis

The decision of what kind of flea control to use depends on your pet's allergies and your own level of tolerance. For allergic animals, elimination of as many fleas as possible in the shortest time frame is paramount to successful treatment. So if you or your pet has flea allergies or you don't want fleas in the house at all, conventional flea treatment is necessary.

Nearly all pharmaceutical flea and tick products are oral or topical, although there are a few medicated collars as well. The wide range of oral and topical medications out there can make for a confusing landscape. In an effort to clear the waters a bit, here are a few important points to keep in mind.

- **Oral flea control:** All oral medications for fleas and ticks are available by prescription only. Since they are ingested, they are regulated by the FDA and are considered a prescription drug. Most of the newer-generation products (as of 2016) are very effective against fleas, and some kill ticks as well.

  As with any drug, the goal with oral flea control is to use the least amount possible. Geographic location, season, and your pet's lifestyle will dictate how often to use any flea control product.

  Oral flea control products are generally safe for the sizes and species of animals they are labeled for. Despite what you may read on the Internet, there are not scores of animals suffering severe side effects from these products. That said, no drug is without its potential side effects. Caution is advised for animals with known seizures, autoimmune disease, or any other serious illness. Consult with your veterinarian to learn about the safest and most effective oral flea control products currently on the market.

- **Topical flea control:** Some products treat only fleas and/or ticks and are generally sold over the counter. Other topical products also treat internal conditions such as heartworm or GI parasites. These medications are FDA regulated and accessible through prescription only.

  The efficacy and potential toxicity of topical flea control products vary greatly. Speaking generally, products sold exclusively through veterinarians tend to be the newer and more effective solutions. Ironically, the over-the-counter flea control products are sometimes the most dangerous. Some contain very strong chemicals, such as toxic organophosphate pesticides. The risk of toxicity from over-the-counter topical flea products is often higher than from the oral or topical products available through your veterinarian. Do research first and when in doubt, ask your veterinarian for advice. (Be particularly cautious with cats; *never* use a product on your cat unless it is specifically labeled for that purpose.)

Atopy

Once the underlying allergens for your pet's atopy are determined through blood or intra-dermal allergy testing, an allergy desensitization protocol can begin. Your veterinarian will use the results of the allergy testing to create custom oral drops or injections. These will be given to your pet to slowly desensitize their immune system to the allergens in question.

The process of desensitization generally takes months to accomplish, but most pets do improve. How much they improve is variable based on the individual, the accuracy of the allergy testing, and co-factors such as if they have other allergies or medical issues.

Food Sensitivity Treatment

After determining your pet's food sensitivity through a diet trial or a NutriScan food sensitivity panel, simply make sure that your pet does not eat that particular food. Carefully inspect ingredient lists or choose recipes that do not have the offending ingredients.

As discussed in Chapter 4, undeclared proteins sometimes "sneak" into foods, which leads to potential problems for sensitive pets. For this reason, a home-prepared, limited-ingredient diet is ideal.

Generalized Western Therapy for Skin Problems

There are times when the underlying causes of allergies in a specific pet cannot be determined or conventional therapy as described above is not completely effective. In these pets, therapy for particular symptoms is needed to minimize itching and keep them comfortable.

Topical Medication

Conventional topical therapy for skin issues generally consists of some combination of antibiotics, antifungals, and steroids. These products come as sprays, creams, ointments, and powders. It's always best to get a veterinarian's recommendation because the most effective treatments are tailored to a specific diagnosis, such as a bacterial or fungal infection.

While these products are effective, it can be a challenge to keep your pet from licking the medication off. Generally, it's not unsafe for your dog or cat to ingest; however, medication won't work if it's licked off! You'll need to keep the ointment on the skin for 10 to 15 minutes so that it has time to have a positive effect.

If your pet tends to lick off topical medications, a restraint collar may be necessary. There are multiple variations of the so-called cone of shame that can be purchased in a store or online.

The best time to use a topical medication on a dog without the use of a restraint collar would be right before you take him out for a walk. Apply the medication at the door, after you put the leash on. Your dog will be too occupied to lick the medication off. (Unless your cat can be walked on a leash, this method will not work for cat owners.)

Antihistamines

Allergic reactions cause specific cells within the immune system to release packets of inflammatory chemicals, including histamines and prostaglandins, into the tissues. Antihistamines help control allergy symptoms by limiting the number of inflammatory mediators released by immune cells.

The following are the most commonly used antihistamines in dogs and cats. The first three are available over the counter, while hydroxyzine is by prescription only. Know that efficacy of antihistamines can be spotty; sometimes they will help your pet, other times not. If you have any questions or doubts, please get clarification from your veterinarian.

Antihistamine	Dog	Cat
Cetirizine[5] (Zyrtec)	1 mg of medication per kilogram of dog's weight, given every 24 hours	5 mg of medication, given every 24 hours (dose is the same regardless of the cat's size)
Chlorpheniramine[6] (Chlor-Trimeton)	0.2–0.5 mg of medication per kilogram of dog's weight, given every 8–12 hours	2 mg of medication, given every 12–24 hours (dose is the same regardless of the cat's size)
Diphenhydramine[7] (Benadryl)	2.2 mg of medication per kilogram of dog's weight, given every 8 hours	Not typically used for cats
Hydroxyzine[8]	2.2 mg of medication per kilogram of dog's weight, given every 8 hours	Not typically used for cats

Antibiotics and Antifungals

Sometimes a dog or cat with allergies will develop a secondary skin or ear infection. The most common are staph (staphylococcus) and yeast (Malassezia) infections, although others do occur. Signs of infection include itching, pustules, oozing or discharge, and strong-smelling skin or ears.

The appropriate use of an antibiotic or antifungal medication can be highly beneficial for pets with infections. See your veterinarian for a diagnosis and the appropriate medication to use.

Steroids and Other Immunomodulating Drugs

Steroids are simultaneously the best and worst drugs in the world. There is nothing that can relieve swelling, inflammation, and itching faster than a steroid like prednisone. On the flip side, they suppress the immune system, put stress on vital organs, and can lead to heart failure or diabetes in susceptible animals.

The truth is that steroids can be highly beneficial in cases of severe allergy, although short-term usage of no more than a few weeks is preferred. Long-term steroid use can be detrimental to a pet's overall health. If long-term or frequent courses of steroids become necessary to control allergies, something is usually missing in the diagnostic and treatment plan.

In addition to steroids, other pharmaceuticals can be used in cases of severe allergies. The two most prevalent of these are cyclosporine (Atopica) and oclacitinib (Apoquel). These drugs can also be used instead of steroids in pets with severe allergic disease. They have fewer short-term side effects than steroids but still suppress the immune system. While these drugs have a place in the treatment of severely allergic pets, they should be a last resort.

While drugs like steroids and other immunosuppressants have potentially damaging consequences when used long-term, a newer form of targeted immunotherapy is available. One such medication, Cytopoint, is offered by veterinarians as a series of injections. It is an antibody that specifically targets IL-31, an important inflammatory mediator that plays a significant role in sending the "itch signal" to the brain. By neutralizing IL-31, Cytopoint is able to relieve itching in many atopic dogs (including my own itchy dog, Sammy). Because of the very specific targeted nature of the medication, the potential for side effects is minimal.

Complementary and Alternative Therapy

Flea Control

As much as I embrace holistic medicine, natural flea control can be disappointing. Natural flea products work up to a point; they will not eradicate *all* fleas from your pet or the environment. If you and your pets are fine with a few fleas here and there, go ahead and try natural flea control. The following are some of the most effective natural products available.

- **Essential oils:** Numerous types of essential oils can be used topically as a repellent for fleas, other insects, and ticks. Some examples are rosemary, eucalyptus, peppermint, clove, and citronella.

    Unless you are very experienced with essential oils, stick to products made specifically for pets. Products made for humans are often too concentrated and can be offensive or even toxic to animals. (For more information, refer to the section discussing essential oil therapy in Chapter 8.)

- **Pyrethrins:** Derived from the chrysanthemum, pyrethrins are toxic to fleas. Products containing pyrethrins can be found as sprays or topical "spot-on" products. In appropriate doses, pyrethrins are safe to use for both dogs and cats.

    Caution: Synthetic analogues of pyrethrin, such as permethrin and other pyrethroids, are highly toxic to cats. ***Never use a flea product on your cat unless it is labeled for use on cats.*** When in doubt, ask your veterinarian about any safety concerns.

- **Diatomaceous earth:** This granular powder is made up of crushed fossils of ancient marine life. It is so abrasive that it disrupts the coating of flea eggs, causing them to dehydrate and die. To use diatomaceous earth as flea control, sprinkle it on your pet and on furniture, bedding, and carpets. Although it is nontoxic, it can be dusty and is a potential respiratory irritant. Avoid inhalation of the dust by pets and humans.

  Food-grade diatomaceous earth can be taken internally and may help in the treatment or prevention of gastrointestinal parasites. (When taken internally, however, it has no effect on flea control.)

- **Flea combing and bathing:** Low-tech but effective are routine bathing and the use of a flea comb. The key with flea baths is contact time: Once lathered, keep the shampoo on your pet for 5 to 10 minutes prior to rinsing. Unless directed otherwise by a veterinarian, bathe your pet no more than once a week to avoid skin irritation through overbathing.

Atopy

- **Bee pollen:** Orally ingested bee pollen is sometimes recommended to treat allergies through the mechanism of oral tolerance. (See Chapter 7 for more details.) Use local bee pollen to be sure that you are desensitizing your pet to pollen from plants in your area.

  Caution: Do not use bee pollen or honey if your pet has a known severe allergy to bee stings.

Generalized Complementary and Alternative Therapy for Skin Problems

Skin allergies are so commonplace in animals and people, there is no shortage of products available. Listed below are some of the ingredients and products commonly and successfully used to help control allergic symptoms in dogs and cats. The list is by no means comprehensive and there are other helpful products out there. For safety's sake, double-check with a veterinarian before using anything that is not specifically labeled for pets.

Topicals

The goal of topical remedies, natural or pharmaceutical, is to relieve itching and discomfort and promote healing. Remember that topical remedies must remain on the skin for at least 10 or 15 minutes to be effective. (See the section earlier in this chapter about application tips.)

The following can be used either alone or in combination to soothe inflamed, itchy, or painful skin.

- **Aloe:** Promotes healing of wounds, burns, and dermatitis.[9]

- **Calendula:** Beneficial for wounds, burns, and dermatitis.[10]

- **Yarrow:** Facilitates healing of wounds.[11]

- **Black tea and nettle tea:** Black tea and nettle tea are astringents. At room temperature, either can be used as a rinse or compress to remove exudate (discharge) from hot spots and quell itchy spots and/or flea bites. The tannins in black tea are also anti-inflammatory and help with itching.[12]

- **Zymox:** Zymox is a brand of enzymatic products available as sprays, creams, ear drops, and shampoos. The enzymes provide antibacterial and antifungal action without the use of pharmaceutical drugs. These are good over-the-counter products to treat pets with allergies or mild ear and skin infections.

Nutritional Therapy

Nutritional therapy relates to improving allergic symptoms through nutrition. Offering a balanced, fresh, whole-food diet provides optimal nutrition with a minimum of unwanted additives and contaminants. Sometimes this is enough to resolve allergic symptoms.

Beyond the positive effects associated with optimal nutrition, there are a few food items to consider adding to your pet's diet, as they greatly improve skin health and immune system function in general.

- **Probiotics:** As discussed in detail in Chapter 6, probiotics support GI tract health and overall immune system health. Along with optimal nutrition, probiotics are part of the cornerstone of good health and subsequently good immune system function.

- **Fish oil:** Discussed in more detail in Chapter 6, fish oil provides essential fatty acids needed for healthy skin, supports normal immune system function, and is a natural anti-inflammatory when used in appropriate doses.

  Caution: Avoid fish oil supplementation in pets with excessively greasy skin, as it could make matters worse. It's best to avoid fish oil in pets with known sensitivities to fish protein. While the oil does not contain fish protein (only the fats), pets with severe sensitivities to fish should avoid it.

- **Whole-food supplementation:** The declining nutritional value of foods is well documented. Even a home-prepared, whole-food diet can be improved with additional nutrients. Companies such as Standard Process make supplements derived from all whole-food ingredients, and I particularly recommend adding their Canine Dermal Support to your pet's diet.

  Caution: Do not give Canine Dermal Support to pets who are sensitive to beef.

Herbal Therapy

Various herbs and combinations of herbs can be used to mitigate allergic response. Like everything else, their efficacy tends to be specific to the individual, and some herbs work better than others for specific conditions. Below are some of the most commonly used and effective herbs for skin allergies.

- **Nettles:** Nettles can be ingested as dried whole herb, tea, or a tincture to help itchy, allergic dogs.[13]

- **Systemic cleansing herbs:** Combinations of herbs are often used to help the body remove toxins from the blood and tissues, which, in turn, can reduce inflammation and signs of allergy.

- **Dandelion:** This powerful herbal diuretic can be beneficial in flushing toxins and allergens from the body.[14]

- **Red clover:** This herb facilitates lymphatic drainage. In other words, it helps move fluids through the tissues and cleans out compounds that may be causing allergy symptoms.[15]

- **Yellow dock:** Yellow dock stimulates bile production, which facilitates better liver function. An optimally functioning liver is vital to normal immune response.[16]

- **Licorice root:** Licorice is a natural anti-inflammatory, which can be used for both dermatitis and arthritis.[17]

Integrative Treatment Plan

Although not life-threatening, allergies can have a major impact on quality of life. Finding a path to controlling allergic skin disease can be an exercise in patience. While allergies are seldom cured, they are routinely controlled with well-thought-out integrative care that includes a combination of allergen avoidance, improving the immune response, and symptomatic care.

When treating your pet with allergic skin disease, keep the following in mind.

- Control for fleas using highly effective conventional flea control to begin with, then monitor for effect.

- Convert your pet to a fresh, whole-food diet.

- Treat symptoms with natural herbs and supplements.

- Treat any secondary bacterial or yeast infection.

- Treat symptoms with conventional therapy, as needed.

- Consider testing for atopy for food sensitivity, and begin therapy accordingly.

- Ask your veterinarian about targeted immunotherapy such as Cytopoint.

- Use long-term immunosuppressive drugs as the last resort.

CHAPTER 12

DEGENERATIVE JOINT DISEASE/ARTHRITIS

None are so old as those who have outlived enthusiasm.

– Henry David Thoreau

Moving parts are always the quickest to break down in any machine. Biological replacement parts, however, are a lot more difficult to come by than mechanical ones. Learning how to maintain and preserve the body's moving parts is a big factor in preserving quality of life for our pets.

Degenerative joint disease (DJD), commonly known as arthritis, often affects older large-breed dogs, although it occurs in dogs of any size as well as cats. The term *arthritis* literally means inflammation of joints. As with any medical issue, the key to successful treatment lies in understanding exactly what the problem is.

Joints: Form and Function

Everywhere in the body where two bones come together, there is a joint. (Think of the elbow, knee, etc.) The ends of the bones are lined with a smooth, slick surface called cartilage, which allows the joint surfaces to move freely over one another. Synovial fluid occupies the space between the bones within the joint capsule and provides additional lubrication. Similar to motor oil in a car, this fluid provides a viscous, fluid barrier between two hard surfaces to minimize friction and wear.

When Things Go Wrong

DJD develops when inflammation and/or injury occurs within a joint. When joints are inflamed, the synovial fluid loses viscosity, leading to friction and pain.[1] When the cartilage is damaged and its slick surface is missing in spots, the resulting bone-on-bone contact creates friction, inflammation, and pain. Over time, inflammation leads to the formation of bone spurs, decreased range of motion, muscle loss, and progressively worsening discomfort.

Compensating for a painful joint can be very subtle and difficult to pick up on, even for professionals. Dogs and cats are very good at this, and they may appear to walk normally even when they have completely changed the weight distribution on their feet. For example, a dog with sore hips or knees will shift their weight forward onto their front legs as a pain avoidance measure.

Although it is occasionally caused by infection or autoimmune disease, DJD in animals is nearly always a function of traumatic injury, wear and tear, or congenital and developmental abnormalities.

Dysplasia

Congenital and developmental abnormalities such as hip or elbow dysplasia are very common precursors to DJD in dogs. The term *dysplasia* defines a body part or organ that did not form properly. The joints of dysplastic pets wear rapidly, which leads to inflammation and premature degeneration of cartilage, followed by DJD.

Dysplasia of the hips and/or elbows is caused by a combination of genetics and nutrition. While the genetic die is cast at fertilization, nutrition is a variable that is under our control. Feeding large-breed puppies an optimal diet in appropriate amounts is crucial to ensuring maximum joint development and stability.[2, 3, 4] If you have a large-breed puppy, please refer to the detailed discussion of optimal feeding of these dogs by nutritionist Dr. Susan Lauten in Appendix C.

Weight and Age—Life Happens

Beyond early-onset issues associated with dysplasia, DJD most frequently occurs as a function of age and mileage. As pets get older, normal wear and tear on joints leads to arthritic changes. This is more so the case in larger, heavier animals or when a pet has had an injury of some kind. Once a joint is injured, it is often never quite the same and becomes prone to developing arthritis months or years down the road.

Being overweight is a common problem with arthritic dogs. The excess weight may be both a cause and effect of joint pain. The extra pounds make it tougher for them to get around and can lead to more rapid progression of DJD because of the increased stress on the affected joint(s). Achieving optimal body weight is critical for these animals.

Cranial Cruciate Ligament Injury

A frequent injury in dogs that can lead to DJD if left untreated is damage to the cranial cruciate ligament (CCL). The CCL, which is analogous to the ACL (anterior cruciate ligament) in humans, is a ligament that helps with knee stabilization. If your larger dog suddenly limps on a hind leg after exercise, they may have experienced damage or a tear to this ligament. Ongoing or intermittent hind limb lameness in a large dog is highly suspect for a CCL injury and should be evaluated by your veterinarian.

Diagnosis of DJD and CCL Injury

DJD is commonly diagnosed through a combination of symptoms and X-rays. Arthritic dogs may have a decreased activity level, be slow to get up in the morning, and generally act stiff and sore. As their activity level decreases, they often lose muscle mass. X-rays frequently show signs of joint degeneration including bone spurs, irregular joint spaces, and changes in bone density around the joint.

Pets with an injury to the CCL will have specific symptoms beyond the generalized pain and soreness seen with DJD. Dogs with a CCL injury or tear frequently have joint instability, which can be evaluated by your veterinarian through palpating the knee joint and conducting a cranial drawer test or tibial thrust. Several months after being injured, pets with a damaged CCL will develop scarring on the inner surface of the knee called medial buttressing, the presence of which can also be used to assess whether the CCL has been damaged.

Even though pets with a suspected CCL tear routinely get X-rayed, the ligament itself cannot be seen. Instead, X-rays show fluid (effusion) within the joint, which is almost always a sign of a CCL injury. In pets with a long-standing CCL injury, the knee may also show signs of DJD.

Treatment of DJD

Underlying issues aside, DJD is a painful condition that often gets progressively worse over time. As arthritis becomes increasingly severe, pets downregulate their activity level and/or shift their weight away from the affected leg.

When a leg is used less due to DJD, the result is muscle atrophy, loss of range of motion, and pain. To make matters worse, compensation causes the joints in the other limbs and the spine to become sore due to overuse and poor biomechanics. In other words, the natural progression of the disease leads to its becoming exponentially worse.

Unchecked, DJD can become so debilitating that euthanasia is discussed as a "treatment" plan. There are few things more tragic in the veterinary world than an otherwise healthy pet that has to be euthanized because of debilitating arthritis.

If I have successfully scared you about what arthritis can do, that's good. I promise it doesn't have to go that way. DJD can be managed to maintain the quality and quantity of life for nearly any pet. The keys to successful treatment are prevention of joint damage when possible, improving the environment within a damaged joint, and aggressive, lifelong integrative care for affected pets.

Conventional Medical Treatment

The very long list of treatment options for DJD speaks to how widespread the condition is throughout the pet population. In some cases, arthritis is linked to breed-specific injury or genetic-related orthopedic issues. In many cases, however, it's merely the vagaries of age. If a pet lives long enough, they are going to get some degree of DJD.

Conventional medicine has developed a wide variety of options to aid in the management of DJD. Most are pharmaceuticals, although surgery is an option in specific circumstances. The following list is most of what Western medicine has to offer for pets with DJD.

Surgery

Most surgical procedures related to DJD are intended to prevent degeneration of a joint that is either congenitally malformed or injured. The goal is to improve joint function and thus decrease wear and tear. Surgical procedures for hip dysplasia, elbow dysplasia, and CCL damage are commonplace. There are also minimally invasive procedures such as arthroscopy that are sometimes an option.

When deciding whether surgery is a good option for your pet, it is best to focus on long-term expectations. Specifically, is the procedure likely to make your pet more comfortable, less arthritic, and more mobile in the long term? If the answer is yes, then the benefits may outweigh the short-term discomfort of the surgery. Whenever possible, consult with a board-certified veterinary surgeon.

Nonsteroidal Anti-Inflammatory Drugs

By far the most commonly used pharmaceuticals for DJD are nonsteroidal anti-inflammatory drugs (NSAIDs). Most pet owners are familiar with carprofen (Rimadyl) and meloxicam (Metacam).

NSAIDs provide relief for many dogs, but they are not without their drawbacks. They can cause GI upset and, in some cases, stress and damage to the liver and kidneys. Dogs on long-term NSAIDs should have their blood checked at least annually to monitor for problems. As of 2016, there is no FDA-approved NSAID for long-term use in cats.

While NSAIDs interrupt some of the chemical pathways that lead to inflammation and pain, they do not alter the environment within the arthritic joint and have no positive effect on the long-term progression of DJD. Because of this, NSAIDs are best combined with other therapies.

Caution: Multiple NSAIDs cannot be given at the same time due to a risk of severe GI ulceration and possibly liver or kidney damage.

Steroids

Steroids are some of the most powerful anti-inflammatory medications available. Because of this, they used to be a commonplace treatment for pets with DJD. You may be familiar with the common steroids prednisone and prednisolone.

However, despite steroids' ability to reduce inflammation, their long-term side effects far outweigh their benefits. Steroid use for more than a few weeks can cause muscle loss, joint laxity, suppression of the adrenal glands, and enlargement of the liver.

Occasionally, extenuating circumstances necessitate a short-term course of steroids for DJD. In these pets, the goal is to keep the course of therapy as short as possible to minimize negative effects.

Caution: Steroids cannot be given concurrently with NSAIDs.

Pain Medications

In addition to NSAIDs and steroids, there are other pain-relieving medications for arthritic pets. Remember that while these drugs help with pain, they will not change the course of arthritis within the joint and should be used in combination with other therapies.

Caution: Over-the-counter pain medications meant for humans (Advil, Tylenol, Exced-rin, Aleve, etc.) can be very dangerous in pets. Aspirin can be used in certain circumstances, but even that may cause stomach issues. Administer over-the-counter pain medication for humans *only* after consulting with your veterinarian.

- **Tramadol:** Tramadol is most commonly used in dogs whose pain is not adequately controlled with NSAIDs alone. The drug acts on opiate receptors in the brain (although it is not an opiate) and has the potential to cause drowsiness or make dogs a little loopy.

There is some controversy among veterinarians regarding tramadol's efficacy. The perceived pain relief may merely be due to the drug's sedative effects. Ultimately the benefits of tramadol should be evaluated based on how the individual responds.[5]

- **Gabapentin:** Gabapentin inhibits specific neurotransmitters to interfere with the transmission of pain signals to the brain. While the literature suggests gabapentin should be used for nerve pain, veterinarians have found it useful in the treatment of DJD pain as well. Other than sometimes making dogs and cats a little sleepy, there are few, if any, concerning side effects. Begin gabapentin therapy once daily in the evening, so your pet can sleep through the drowsiness.

- **Amantadine:** A relative newcomer in veterinary medicine, amantadine shows real promise in the treatment of pain. One way it works is by affecting nerve receptors within the central nervous system. Amantadine is most useful in the treatment of chronic pain such as DJD and is nearly always used in conjunction with other pain drugs such as NSAIDs or gabapentin.[6]

- **Buprenorphine:** Opiates are infrequently used in veterinary medicine for chronic pain because of their unreliable absorption when given orally and side effects such as sedation or dysphoria. The one exception to the rule is buprenorphine, which can be particularly beneficial for cats.[7]

Treating chronic pain in cats with Western medicine is challenging. There are no approved NSAIDs for long-term use. Tramadol and gabapentin may produce unacceptable side effects. Buprenorphine, however, does provide good pain control in kitties and is odorless and tasteless, making it easy to administer. Even better, it is absorbed directly through the mucous membranes of the mouth, so cats don't have to swallow it. Buprenorphine can be used similarly in dogs, but the quantities needed often make it cost prohibitive.

From a Western medical perspective, buprenorphine (with or without gabapentin) may be the best orally administered drug for cats living with chronic DJD pain.

Chondroprotective Agents

The primary objective of DJD therapy should be improving the environment within the joint. In other words, rather than treat the symptom, treat the primary problem. Chondroprotective agents are one way to literally protect cartilage from damage, slowing joint degeneration and resulting in less pain and inflammation.

One of the most readily available and effective means we can use to improve the condition within an arthritic joint is administering polysulfated glycosaminoglycan (PSGAG). It decreases the activity of the enzymes that break down cartilage and thus reduces joint inflammation and damage. I use so much of this in my practice, we have a hard time keeping it on the shelf.

The most commonly used PSGAG is a product called Adequan. It is given by injection, but don't let that scare you; it's so easy, you can even give the injections at home. You don't even have to inject anywhere near the affected joint. It can be given under the skin or into any muscle; the animal's own physiology will put it where they need it. Adequan essentially has no negative side effects. I can't speak highly enough about the benefits of PSGAG for arthritic dogs and cats.

Joint Injections

Injecting medication into painful, arthritic joints is commonplace in human and equine medicine. It is rarely done for dogs and cats, although it can be highly effective in controlling inflammation and pain.

The two most common medicines injected into joints are steroids and hyaluronic acid. The latter is a major component of synovial fluid. Inflamed, arthritic joints tend to have poor-quality synovial fluid, so by injecting hyaluronic acid into the joint space, viscosity is restored and the joint can move with less friction and discomfort.[8]

While I am not a fan of the use of systemic steroids in arthritic pets, there can be value in joint injections. A direct injection concentrates the medicine in the affected area, so the patient can reap the potent anti-inflammatory benefits of steroids without the myriad systemic side effects.

Joint injections need to be performed by a veterinarian who is experienced with the procedure to ensure efficacy and limit the chance of adverse reactions, such as creating a joint infection.

Complementary and Alternative Therapy

Dogs and cats with orthopedic issues are by far the most frequent cases that come to my office for holistic care. There are such an incredible number of alternative therapies to help pets with DJD that sometimes the most challenging aspect is deciding where to start. First, you have to consider what is most practical for you and your pet, particularly when it comes to logistics and finances. Beyond that is where the art of medicine comes into play, and the experience of your veterinarian will help guide your way.

Food

DJD is inseparable from chronic inflammation, so any decrease in foods with potentially inflammatory compounds is a big positive. Feeding a fresh, whole-food diet is an excellent way to limit nutritional sources of inflammation.

In addition to what is in the food, consider the number of calories ingested. For some arthritic pets, weight is a big issue. The inability to exercise leads to weight gain and increased stress on already inflamed joints. The DJD diets for dogs and cats found in Appendix C are designed to help support lean body mass and contain additional levels of omega fatty acids for their anti-inflammatory properties.

Nutritional Supplementation and Herbal Therapy

Beyond a highly nutritious, minimally inflammatory diet, there are vast benefits to be gained from nutritional and herbal therapy. The list of beneficial herbs and supplements is seemingly endless. The following supplements have a proven track record, and I have personally had success with them.

Your pet does not need to take everything on the list—and besides, it's not realistic to give armloads of supplements every day. Often the best route of action is to use high-quality supplements that incorporate multiple ingredients. It is an excellent way to broaden the spectrum of treatment while keeping things manageable.

—**Chondroprotective agents:** In addition to the injectable products described above such as PSGAGs (Adequan) and hyaluronic acid, oral supplementation can support cartilage as well.

- **Glucosamine and chondroitin:** These compounds are the most widely used oral chondroprotective agents. Glucosamine is derived from shellfish cartilage, and chondroitin is made from mammalian or avian cartilage. The bodies of many arthritic dogs and cats will repair damaged cartilage if provided with these nutritional building blocks.

   Although the use of these supplements is widespread in both human and veterinary medicine, the science is noncommittal. Some reports show efficacy and others do not.[9, 10, 11, 12] In my clinical experience, I have found high-quality glucosamine and chondroitin supplements to be effective in many pets with DJD.

- **Methylsulfonylmethane (MSM):** MSM is a compound found in the body, and the supplement is sometimes used in a similar fashion to glucosamine and chondroitin. There may be some benefit to using MSM after joint injury or trauma, but for long-term DJD therapy, it is likely not necessary.

- **Hyaluronic acid:** Oral hyaluronic acid is not as direct as the injections described earlier. However, ingested hyaluronic acid can be effective in supplementing joint fluid and thus protecting cartilage and joint health.

—**Whole-food supplementation:** When treating DJD, consider whole foods that supply the nutritional components needed to repair joint tissue and minimize inflammation. Canine Musculoskeletal Support, produced by Standard Process, is an excellent example of a combination supplement utilizing whole-food items to support dogs and cats with DJD and joint-related pain.

—**Omega fatty acids:** Omega fatty acids such as those found in various types of marine oils have a wide variety of medical benefits (see Chapter 6). With respect to pets with DJD, appropriate doses of these essential fatty acids have anti-inflammatory properties.

—**Antioxidants:** When body tissues are damaged by inflammation, it is often due to oxidative damage. The body generates its own antioxidants to counterbalance these effects, and we can tip the balance further in our favor through the addition of antioxidants in the form of food or supplements.

The best antioxidants are the ones Mother Nature makes. Most brightly colored fruits and vegetables are well stocked with them, and feeding these to pets can be a big help. In addition to food-based antioxidants, supplementing with one or more (not necessarily all) of the following can be helpful:

- Glutathione[13]
- Coenzyme Q10 (CoQ10)[14]
- Alpha-lipoic acid (ALA)[15]
- Resveratrol[16]
- Vitamins A, C, E, and D

—**Natural anti-inflammatories:** The benefits of natural anti-inflammatories are much the same as NSAIDs, without many of the side effects. While nature's versions may not act as fast as those brought to us by big pharmaceutical companies, managing DJD is about the long view. Use NSAIDs on an as-needed basis; for daily use, stick with the natural variety. Some commonly used and effective natural anti-inflammatory herbs are:

- Curcumin[17]
- Boswellia[18]

- Ginger[19]
- Bromelain[20]
- Yucca[21]

—**Cannabis:** The mechanisms of action and range of uses of medical cannabis are covered in detail in Chapter 9. Its use for patients experiencing moderate to severe chronic pain is well documented in the literature on human patients, and it works just as well in animals.

The key to success with medical cannabis is in using the right product. THC-to-CBD ratio and concentration are paramount to efficacy and avoiding toxicity. Before making any attempt to administer cannabis to your pet, please refer to Chapter 9 and, if possible, speak to a veterinarian with experience using medical cannabis in pets.

Homeopathy

Homeopathic remedies including arnica are commonly used to treat soreness and pain due to arthritis. For comprehensive homeopathic therapy, a full constitutional analysis by a classically trained homeopath is required.

Traditional Chinese Veterinary Medicine

Chinese medicine has been used to treat DJD for literally thousands of years (see Chapter 8). A combination of acupuncture and Chinese herbs can make a huge difference in the life of an arthritic pet.

When it comes to Chinese medicine, frequency of treatment, specific acupuncture points used, and best herbal combinations are highly specific to the individual pet. It can take upward of four to six weekly treatments to see significant improvement in pets with long-standing DJD. Please be patient.

Chiropractic

Long-standing DJD leads to decreased range of motion, which alters the way an animal moves and often puts excessive stress on other joints, resulting in further complications. Chiropractic mobilizes the joints to restore joint mobility and normal motion.

Physical Rehabilitation

Consider physical rehabilitation for your pet. Just like a physical therapist for humans, a rehab-trained veterinarian or therapist treating animals assesses their patient and makes a treatment plan using the various modalities at their disposal. Your therapist may utilize physical activity such as swimming, underwater treadmills, and various obstacle courses, as well as technologies like laser or therapeutic ultrasound. (For more information, see Chapter 8.)

Technological Advancements in DJD Therapy

Many of the technological advancements in holistic medicine discussed in Chapter 10 are applicable to the treatment of pets with DJD. The following are some of the technologies routinely employed:

- Stem cell therapy and platelet-rich plasma
- Pulsed signal therapy and other PEMF technologies
- Photobiomodulation laser therapy (also known as cold laser therapy)

Integrative Treatment Plan

With so many treatment options, choosing what is best for your pet can seem daunting. While every pet is an individual, there are some constants you can use to guide you through the treatment of DJD.

First, look for therapies that will improve the environment within the damaged joint(s) rather than just treating symptoms. In other words, address the root of the problem whenever possible. Consider the following methods:

- Supplements containing glucosamine and chondroitin
- PSGAG injections (I recommend Adequan)
- Hyaluronic acid (administered orally or through joint injections)
- Pulsed signal therapy
- Stem cell therapy and/or platelet-rich plasma

Gravitate toward therapies with a good chance of efficacy and a minimum of potential adverse side effects, such as the following:

- Nutrition and nutritional supplementation

- Antioxidants and natural anti-inflammatories

- Homeopathic arnica (or products containing arnica, such as T-Relief from MediNatura)

- Acupuncture

- Chiropractic

- Physical rehabilitation

Don't be afraid to use pharmaceuticals when needed, but use them only on an as-needed basis. Treat for the here and now, but make a long-term plan as well.

The best therapy for DJD is the combined approach. By utilizing more than one modality, we approach the problem from multiple angles and improve the chance of success. Most pets with DJD can live long and happy lives years after being diagnosed.

CHAPTER 13

TRUE GRIT

Urinary Tract Infections, Crystals, and Stones

*It isn't the mountain ahead that wears you out;
it's the grain of sand in your shoe.*

— Robert W. Service

Conditions of the lower urinary tract, including bladder infections, crystals, and stones in the urinary tract, can present either short-term or lifelong problems for some pets. While these issues can occur within the kidneys, they are relatively infrequent by comparison to the occurrence within the urinary bladder.

When Things Go Wrong

Under normal circumstances, urine is sterile. When bacteria find their way into the urinary tract, the resulting urinary tract infection (UTI) can be a source of discomfort, stone formation, and/or kidney damage.

Urinary Tract Infections

While occasionally a UTI comes through the blood, the majority of UTIs occur due to an ascending infection. This term describes when bacteria on the external surfaces of a pet's urogenital area work their way up the urethra into the urinary bladder. Just as in humans, ascending infections are almost exclusively seen in females. This is due to the urethra in females being shorter than in males, which makes for less of a journey for bacteria to travel into the bladder. Conversely, the longer and narrower urethra in males makes them more susceptible to urethral obstructions from stones.

Crystals and Stones

The formation of crystals and stones within the urinary tract of dogs and cats is relatively common and causes problems ranging from simple irritation to urinary obstructions requiring emergency surgery. Crystal and stone formation are often, but not always, related to kidney function. Genetics, hydration, nutrition, urine pH, and infection are all factors in how and why these issues occur. Urine concentration, mineral content, and presence of bacteria are all factors regarding the formation of crystals and stones in the kidneys and bladder.

The presence of crystals in the urine (crystalluria) is problematic for several reasons. Consistent crystalluria can be an indication of chronic dehydration, which is not healthy for the body as a whole. Crystals can also be irritating and cause inflammation in the urinary tract. (Think of sand tumbling around on the very delicate surfaces of the bladder.) The irritation may lead to pain and/or bleeding. In cats, it can lead to feline lower urinary tract disease (FLUTD).

It is common, however, for a dog or cat to have a small number of crystals seen on a urinalysis. Their presence does not necessarily indicate a problem, especially if there are no symptoms. The greater concern is for pets showing large numbers of crystals consistently in their urine or exhibiting signs of urinary distress.

The relationship between crystals and stones is simple: Stones grow from crystals formed by the precipitation of supersaturated crystals in urine. Unlike humans, who most commonly form stones in their kidneys, dogs and cats more often form them within the urinary bladder. Pets with bladder stones most commonly will show signs associated with inflammation in the urinary bladder such as blood in urine, increased urge to urinate, and licking the urogenital area. It is worth noting that these are the exact same signs you would see in a pet with a urinary tract infection. Urinary tract crystals and/or stones are always on the list of differential diagnoses when these signs are present.

Stones in dogs and cats range in size from "grains of sand" up to "rocks" that are several inches in diameter. Very small stones may pass upon urination, but larger ones become trapped in the bladder and lead to inflammation, discomfort, blood in the urine, etc.

Similar to the way crystals can lead to a urinary obstruction in male cats, stones in the bladder of a male dog can pass into the urethra and cause a urinary obstruction. (In cats, urinary obstruction due to stones is rare.) These pets have difficulty urinating and will have a diminished urine stream or none at all. *An inability to urinate for any reason is a life-threatening medical emergency.*

FLUTD/ Urinary Obstruction in Cats

FLUTD occurs when highly concentrated urine and/or crystals within the urinary bladder and urethra cause inflammation, leading to discomfort and a constant urge to pee. Infection is very rarely present in these cases, although the symptoms are the same: straining to urinate while producing small, often blood-tinged drops of urine.

Dehydration and/or dietary issues are major factors in the development of FLUTD. Environmental stresses often contribute to the dehydration, as stressed-out cats don't eat or drink as much as they should. Such stresses may be caused by anything that upsets the cat's normal routine. The kidneys, in response to dehydration, conserve water and create highly concentrated urine that is supersaturated with minerals, leading to the formation of crystals. Once the inflammatory process starts, it often lasts for days.

FLUTD is an uncomfortable but self-limiting condition that usually resolves on its own within a matter of days, with one important exception: Male cats with FLUTD will sometimes develop a urinary obstruction.

The tip of a male cat's urethra is very narrow; when inflamed, it gets even narrower. If crystals and/or mucus from the bladder form a plug in the urethra, the cat can't urinate. This is a *medical emergency.* Regardless of time of day, if your male cat is straining to urinate, take him to a veterinarian. Cats can die within hours of developing a urinary obstruction if not treated.[1, 2]

Types of Urine Crystals and Stones

With the exception of those caused by infections, urinary tract stones are a function of genetic predisposition. There are six types of crystals and stones that can form in the urinary tract of dogs. Four of them are rare and are generally due to breed-associated genetic anomalies: urate, cystine, calcium phosphate, and silicate.

The most common types of crystals and stones found in both dogs and cats are struvite and calcium oxalate. Although both struvite and calcium oxalate crystals can grow to form stones, their composition, environment in which they form, and methods of treatment are very different.[3]

Struvite

These are the most common crystals and stones in dogs and cats; they are composed of magnesium, ammonium, and phosphate. Struvite stones have a tendency to form in alkaline (high-pH) urine.

- **In dogs:** Urinary tract infections cause up to 90 percent of struvite stones in dogs due to the presence of a bacterial enzyme (urease) that causes an increase in urine pH. Prevention and treatment of struvite crystals and stones in dogs hinges on the treatment of the urinary tract infection, correction of urine pH, and nutrition.

- **In cats:** Struvite crystals and stones in cats are generally not related to infection and instead are more a function of genetics, diet, and inadequate hydration.[4, 5]

Calcium Oxalate

As the name implies, these crystals and stones are composed largely of calcium. The causes of their formation, however, differ between dogs and cats.

- **In dogs:** The formation of calcium oxalate crystals in dogs is due to neither diet nor infection, but rather a genetic anomaly. Over 70 percent of dogs affected by calcium oxalate crystals are male, and breeds at greatest risk include Lhasa Apsos, miniature schnauzers, Yorkshire terriers, miniature poodles, shih tzus, and bichon frises.

    Another cause of elevated calcium levels in the urine is hypercalcemia (elevated blood calcium). If blood calcium levels are elevated, the kidneys will work to restore that balance by pulling calcium out of the blood and into the urine. Hypercalcemia can be a sign of potentially serious underlying medical issues ranging from kidney disease to various types of cancers. When hypercalcemia is present, further testing is always indicated to determine the cause.[6]

- **In cats:** While still relatively uncommon, calcium oxalate problems in cats occur more frequently than they used to. Because of the high incidence of struvite crystal–induced FLUTD and urinary obstructions in cats, commercial feline diets were reformulated to acidify the urine. The effort was a success when it came to reducing struvite-related FLUTD and urinary obstructions, but the lower urine pH may promote the formation of calcium oxalate crystals.

    Genetics plays a role in cats as well. Certain breeds of cats, including Burmese and Himalayans, are more susceptible to the formation of calcium oxalate crystals.[7, 8, 9, 10, 11]

Diagnosis of UTIs, Urinary Crystals, and Stones

Urinary tract infections, FLUTD, and stones can all present with exactly the same symptoms. While treatment frequently involves a combination of Western and alternative care, diagnosing these conditions can only be accomplished through Western medicine.

Any pets that shows signs of urinary distress or has urine that looks or smells unusual should evaluated by a veterinarian. Based on their physical examination findings, the following diagnostic tests may be indicated.

- **Urinalysis:** This is an evaluation of your pet's urine to determine its pH, concentration, presence of crystals, and/or bacteria. It's important to note that many veterinary hospitals send urine samples to an outside laboratory for analysis. While this is normally fine, crystals in urine are temperature dependent and tend to form in cooler temperatures. In other words, once the urine is outside the body and begins to cool, crystals may form that were not present within the animal. Pets with a history of crystals in their urine should have their urine samples evaluated immediately after collection rather than after hours of refrigeration.

- **Urine culture:** Bacteria are not always visible in a urine sample and sometimes they need to be cultured. In addition, a urine culture can be used to determine which antibiotics will be most effective.

- **Blood sampling:** If there are questions about kidney function in pets showing signs of urinary distress, monitoring kidney function is recommended.

- **Imaging:** When stones are suspected, an X-ray and/or ultrasound is necessary. Ultrasound tends to be better than X-rays for detecting very small stones in the bladder or kidneys. However, X-rays may be needed if there is a suspicion of stones in the urethra.

Treatment of UTIs, Urinary Crystals, and Stones

Management of urinary crystals and stones is a truly integrative process. While diagnosis is accomplished through Western care, successful long-term treatment often requires a combination of Western medicine, nutrition, and complementary therapy.

Conventional Medical Treatment

UTIs

For most pets, UTIs are a one-off condition and are easily remedied with an appropriate course of antibiotics. When an infection does not resolve or it recurs, further diagnostics are indicated. A urinalysis, urine culture, and imaging can illuminate underlying causes that present an obstacle to clearing the infection.

Chronic or recurring UTIs are commonly due to underlying systemic illness such as kidney failure or diabetes. Sometimes, however, a pet's anatomy makes infections more likely to occur. Depending on the nature of the abnormality, surgical correction is sometimes possible. Regardless of the cause, chronic or recurring UTIs can lead to kidney damage and/or the formation of stones. These pets require definitive (and sometimes ongoing) treatment.

FLUTD

Feline lower urinary tract disease generally resolves without treatment within a few days. Given that it's rather uncomfortable, however, your veterinarian may recommend some short-term treatment options such as subcutaneous fluids to help dilute the urine and flush away irritating crystals or short-term use of an NSAID or a painkiller such as buprenorphine.

Urinary Obstruction

Urinary obstructions due to FLUTD or stones are a medical emergency. To relieve the obstruction, a urinary catheter must be placed and left in for a minimum of 24 to 48 hours. These pets should be hospitalized and often require IV fluid therapy and pain control while they are recovering. Depending on the severity of the obstruction, kidney damage may need to be addressed as well. The long-term prognosis is generally good, provided treatment was initiated in time.

In cats with recurrent urinary obstructions, there is a surgical procedure called a perineal urethrostomy that will prevent them from happening in the future. However, appropriate preventive integrative care for cats with FLUTD usually keeps things from progressing this far.

Pets with urinary obstructions due to stones frequently require surgery to relieve the obstruction. The type of surgical procedure is dependent on whether the stones can be pushed from the urethra back into the bladder.

Struvite Crystals and Stones

It is possible to dissolve struvite stones, although it can be time-consuming and last a period of months. In male dogs, there is a risk of developing a urinary obstruction should one of the stones fall into the urethra and get stuck. Also, because not all stones are 100 percent homogenous, the part not composed of struvite may not dissolve.

The key to dissolving either struvite crystals or stones is to first resolve any UTI, then dilute the urine, keep pH down, and begin dietary restriction of the minerals that make up struvite. Surgery is also an option in the case of struvite stones.

- **UTI:** The information above regarding UTI therapy applies here. In cases where a UTI is present, your pet's urine should be checked at regular intervals. Struvite stones can harbor bacteria within them, so regular urine cultures are necessary to determine if ongoing antibiotic therapy is needed.

- **Dilute the urine:** Offering your pet a diet with more moisture and increasing their water consumption will help dissolve crystals and even prevent them from forming. Your veterinarian can easily do routine monitoring of your pet's urine concentration. The goal is to keep urine concentration below 1.020 for dogs and 1.025 for cats.

- **Restrict minerals and lower pH:** Feed your pet a diet that is restricted in the minerals magnesium and phosphorus. While veterinary prescription diets can do this, it can also be accomplished with higher-quality, whole-food diets. Once the diet change has been implemented, routine monitoring of the urine is necessary to measure pH and urine concentration, and to look for the presence of crystals. For pets with infection-related struvite stones, long-term dietary management is not necessary.

- **Surgery:** There are cases in which dissolution of struvite stones is not practical or effective. Dissolving a large stone can take six months or more and require frequent urine checks and X-rays or ultrasounds to measure progress. Believe it or not, in many cases it is easier, quicker, and less expensive to surgically remove the stones. Talk with your veterinarian about the relative risks and expenses of each option.

Calcium Oxalate Crystals

Much like in pets with excessive struvites, the key to controlling calcium oxalate formation lies in diluting urine concentration, raising urinary pH, and dietary restriction of the minerals composing the crystals. Although many veterinarians will recommend one of several prescription diets for these pets, a fresh, whole-food diet is preferable. Once a diet change has been implemented, routine veterinary monitoring of the urine is necessary to measure pH and urine concentration (known as "specific gravity"), and to look for the presence of crystals. Ideally, urine should have a pH greater than 6.5, have a specific gravity of 1.020 (in dogs) or 1.025 (in cats), and be negative for crystals.

Calcium Oxalate Stones

Unlike struvite stones, calcium oxalate stones cannot be dissolved through dietary management. Usually veterinarians must remove calcium oxalate stones surgically.

Dietary management can help prevent the formation of future stones and crystals. The goal is to dilute the urine through increased water consumption and diet change to achieve a urine specific gravity below 1.020 and a urine pH above 6.5. Monitor urine parameters several times per year to reduce the chance of calcium oxalate crystal and/or stone recurrence. Despite appropriate diet changes, up to 50 percent of dogs will develop new stones within three years due to the strong genetic predisposition in affected animals.[12, 13, 14, 15, 16]

Complementary and Alternative Therapy

Urinary Tract Infections

An active UTI should always be treated with antibiotics. I've always declined when pet owners have asked me to treat their pet's UTI exclusively through natural methods. Not only is the risk of a life-threatening kidney infection too high, but also there is very little risk in a short-term course of antibiotics. (The worst-case scenario is likely to be GI upset.)

When the goal is integrative health care, you have to know which tools to use. Herbs and supplements can be used *in conjunction with* antibiotics and can also help prevent future UTIs from occurring. Following is a list of supplements I have found helpful for treating and preventing UTIs in pets.

- **Probiotics and prebiotics:** These help mitigate possible GI upset related to antibiotic usage.

- **Uva ursi:** This herb has antimicrobial and diuretic properties and can be used to help treat or prevent UTIs. Long-term use, however, can *cause* urinary tract irritation.[17]

- **Marshmallow:** Useful in UTIs for its antimicrobial effect.[18]

- **Yarrow:** Useful in UTIs for its antimicrobial effect.[19]

- **Plantain:** Useful in UTIs for its ability to protect mucous membranes such as the urinary bladder wall.[20]

- **Slippery elm:** Useful in UTIs for its anti-inflammatory effect.[21]

- **Couch grass:** Useful in UTIs for its antimicrobial, anti-inflammatory, and diuretic effect.[22]

- **Echinacea:** Useful in UTIs for its antimicrobial effect.[23]

- **Oregon grape:** Useful in UTIs for its antimicrobial effect.[24]

- **Cranberry extract:** The compounds in cranberry extract have been shown to interfere with adherence of several species of bacteria to the bladder wall.[25, 26]

Urinary Obstruction

Urinary obstruction is a life-threatening emergency. If your male cat is straining to urinate, do not attempt to treat him at home; a delay of hours can make the difference between life and death.

FLUTD

As previously stated, FLUTD usually resolves on its own within a few days. The single most effective symptomatic and preventive therapy for cats with FLUTD is to get more water into them to dilute the urine and diminish crystal formation. (See Chapter 2 for detailed advice.) Also consider the struvite diets for cats in Appendix C to reduce the crystal formation that can lead to FLUTD.

Remember that an ounce of prevention is worth a pound of cure. FLUTD is frequently caused by inadequate water consumption, which may be due to the effects of stress, lack of access to clean water, or feeding low-moisture food. Minimizing stress in the house and feeding a fresh, whole-food diet that is naturally high in moisture will lessen the chances of problems.

To treat FLUTD symptoms, some of the same supplements noted above for UTIs are helpful due to their protective and anti-inflammatory effect on the urinary bladder.

- **Plantain:** Useful in FLUTD for its ability to protect mucous membranes such as the urinary bladder wall.

- **Slippery elm:** Useful with FLUTD for its anti-inflammatory effect.

- **Couch grass:** Useful with FLUTD for its antimicrobial, anti-inflammatory, and diuretic effect.

High-strung cats whose stress level may make them prone to FLUTD may also benefit from herbal therapy to reduce their stress and anxiety, such as with the following herbs:

- **Skullcap**[27]
- **Valerian**[28]
- **Passionflower**[29]
- **Cannabis** (see Chapter 9)

Crystals and Stones

From a holistic perspective, the best treatments for urinary crystals and stones are food and water. Please see Chapter 2 for detailed advice on increasing your pet's water intake. In addition, diets restricted in specific minerals help prevent the formation of struvite or calcium oxalate crystals. Please see Appendix C for specific diet advice.

Dogs with struvite stones as a result of a urinary tract infection do not require a therapeutic diet. Other than dissolution or surgical removal of the stones, control of the UTI is all that is needed to prevent their recurrence.

There are herbs in the Chinese medical formularies designed to help speed the dissolution of struvite stones. Their use should be recommended and supervised by someone trained in traditional Chinese veterinary medicine.

Integrative Treatment Plan

As with many medical conditions, prevention of crystals and stones is achieved through good nutrition and regular medical care. If problems do occur, appropriate utilization of Western and holistic care provides the most direct path to resolution. With the exception of infections, there is a genetic component we are up against. While we can't fight the genetic components of crystal formation, we can change the environment within the urine to tip the odds in our favor.

The most successful therapy for struvite stones and crystals is prevention—feeding the right diet and getting enough water into the dog or cat. Both fresh, whole-food diets and prescription diets can be used to help dissolve struvite stones. In the bigger picture sense, the fresh diets are better for your pet.

Dogs and cats with excessive crystals and cats with FLUTD often can be treated primarily with diet and alternative therapy. When it comes to infections and stones, however, the balance tends to swing the other way. Struvite stones due to infection must be treated with antibiotics. Adjunctive herbal therapy can be helpful, but it is not a substitute for the real thing.

CHAPTER 14

CHRONIC GASTROINTESTINAL CONDITIONS

All disease begins in the gut.

– HIPPOCRATES

Your pet's gastrointestinal tract breaks down large, highly complex materials into components that their body uses as building materials and fuel. It takes undigested materials, wastes, and toxins from the body and excretes it all as feces. This amazingly elegant process is the cornerstone of good health. Understanding how the process works is the first step in effectively preventing and treating diseases of the GI tract. This chapter lays the groundwork for optimizing health thorough a healthy digestive system.

The GI Tract: Form and Function

Digestion begins in the mouth, where enzymes in the saliva begin to break down food before it is even swallowed. As food passes into the stomach, strong gastric acids further break it down and transform it into liquid. From here, food enters the small intestine and is acted upon by the gallbladder and pancreas. These small organs inject powerful digestive enzymes into the intestine, further breaking down food to the point where it can be absorbed through the intestinal wall. Absorbed nutrients enter the bloodstream, which distributes them throughout the body. Unabsorbed materials continue into the large intestine as waste and, ultimately, all that is left is feces.

The most interesting aspects of the GI tract are the parts that are often not talked about. To begin with, approximately 70 percent of all the body's immune cells are housed in the GI tract.[1] Also, the GI tract cannot function without a helping hand from microorganisms. They're referred to by many names, including intestinal bacteria, gut flora, and gut microbiota. A large population of bacteria is necessary for digestion and nutrient assimilation. They aid in the breakdown of nutrients prior to absorption, are necessary for the synthesis of vitamins B and K, and protect the body against harmful bacteria. An estimated 100 trillion bacteria are found within the human intestinal tract, with similar figures in dogs and cats.[2] That's more than 10 times the number of cells in the body!

What your pet eats affects the numbers and species of bacteria within the gut. GI tract health is dependent on healthy flora, and healthy flora requires an optimal diet. Everything is interconnected. An imbalance of GI flora (dysbiosis) can lead to short- or long-term inflammation and GI upset. When the intestines are inflamed, 70 percent of the immune system is right there on the front lines. It doesn't take a Ph.D. in gastroenterology to see the direct link between nutrition, immune function, and overall health.[3]

When Things Go Wrong

Malfunctions of the GI tract have many potential causes, but frequently the common thread is inflammation. The symptoms of inflammation depend on the location in which it occurs. The following are common inflammatory processes that can occur within the GI tract.

- **Stomatitis** (inflammation of the mouth) causes oral pain and poor appetite.

- **Gastritis** (stomach inflammation) often leads to vomiting and appetite changes.

- **Enteritis** (small intestinal inflammation) may cause vomiting, diarrhea, and altered nutrient absorption. It is sometimes associated with concurrent pancreatic inflammation (pancreatitis).

- **Colitis** (inflammation of the large intestine) often causes diarrhea with blood and/or mucus.

Frequently, inflammation is a reaction to food, bacterial imbalance, or parasites. Determining the underlying cause of chronic GI tract inflammation can sometimes be a challenge, but it's necessary for successful treatment. It's important to address the underlying cause rather than merely treating symptoms.

Leaky Gut Syndrome

Under normal conditions, food particles are digested and broken down into components small enough to pass through and between the cells of the intestinal wall and into the bloodstream. When chronic inflammation in the GI tract causes increased permeability of the gut wall, this is called leaky gut syndrome. This condition allows the passage of larger molecules into the blood, which cause an inflammatory immune response.

Leaky gut syndrome is caused primarily by a poor diet or dietary sensitivities, but the effects of the inflammation can occur anywhere in the body, including the skin. Although somewhat controversial in Western medicine, leaky gut syndrome is a well-recognized condition to practitioners of complementary and alternative medicine.[4, 5]

Inflammatory Bowel Disease

Dogs and cats with chronic intestinal inflammation are frequently diagnosed with inflammatory bowel disease (IBD). As the name implies, part or all of the intestines are inflamed in these pets. The condition often causes chronic vomiting and/or diarrhea and weight loss. IBD is usually diagnosed with tissue samples collected using ultrasound, although sometimes endoscopy or surgery is needed.

IBD is very similar to the condition in humans known as inflammatory bowel syndrome (IBS). In the purest sense of the word, IBD or IBS is not actually a disease but instead a description of symptoms. The underlying cause of the bowel inflammation in most patients is unknown.

Some pets with IBD are responsive to diet changes, while others are not. For the latter, long-term antibiotics and steroids are often recommended. In my experience, many of these pets can be helped greatly through complementary and alternative care with minimal long-term pharmaceuticals.

Diagnosis of Gastrointestinal Disorders

Like most other medical issues, the diagnosis of chronic GI tract conditions begins with a thorough physical examination and medical history. The specifics of how your pet manifests signs of illness are often a major clue to the underlying problem. Some factors to consider are:

—**General physical condition:** Because the GI tract is related to general health and immune function, pets with chronic digestive disease often are "unthrifty." Their hair coat may be dry or greasy, and cats often do not groom themselves well. A generalized unkempt appearance is a sign of illness in pets.

—**Appetite:** Is your pet's appetite increased, decreased, or normal?

- *An increased appetite* may indicate inadequate digestion or absorption of food or possibly a hormonal imbalance such as Cushing's disease in dogs (Chapter 22), hyperthyroidism in cats (Chapter 21), or diabetes in either species (Chapter 16).

- *A decreased appetite* suggests nausea and/or pain associated with eating and digesting. Lack of appetite can also be caused by any number of systemic medical issues.

—**Vomiting:** When and how often is your pet vomiting? This can be a sign of nausea, foreign material stuck in the GI tract, or more systemic medical problems.

—**Stool quality:** Does your pet have diarrhea or constipation?

- *Diarrhea with blood or mucus* is indicative of large intestinal diarrhea, whereas diarrhea without these components may originate from the small intestine. Treatments between the two may differ.

- *Chronic constipation* occurs most frequently in Manx and geriatric cats. Pets who have eaten foreign material (such as cloth) or a large amount of bone may also become constipated.

—**Weight loss:** Weight loss is due to decreased absorption of nutrients, not enough nutrients taken in, or both. Weight loss without obvious GI signs may be due to a more systemic condition.

Diagnostic Testing

Testing for pets with chronic GI conditions ranges from very simple to highly complex. Which tests your veterinarian recommends hinges on your pet's medical history and symptoms.

The following tests are grouped by what is being tested. Each group is listed roughly in the order in which they would be recommended, based on the severity and chronicity of the symptoms. Not surprisingly, the further down the list you go, the more costly things tend to get.

- Ova, parasites, and giardia tests look for common parasitic diseases.

- Fecal cultures or polymerase chain reaction (PCR) tests look for pathogenic (bad) bacteria in the GI tract.

- Routine blood testing is used to evaluate causes of symptoms not directly related to GI disease.

- A canine or feline pancreatic lipase (cPL or fPL) test is used specifically to diagnose pancreatitis in dogs and cats, respectively. (See Chapter 15 on pancreatitis.)

- Trypsin-like immunoreactivity (TLI), vitamin B12 (cobalamin), and folate testing evaluates pancreatic function and looks for signs of bacterial overgrowth in the small intestine.

- X-rays evaluate abdominal organ abnormalities and GI foreign bodies. (However, ultrasound is usually a better choice than X-rays in pets with GI conditions.)

- Ultrasound-guided aspirates or biopsies are ways of collecting samples of abnormal tissues for analysis without the need for surgical intervention.

- An endoscopy or colonoscopy provides direct visualization of the upper and lower portions of the GI tract. Biopsies can be collected during the scoping. (Note that anesthesia is required for scoping pets.)

- Exploratory surgery is the most invasive option but also allows the greatest visualization and the highest-quality biopsies to be collected. Of course, anesthesia is required.

Conventional Medical Treatment

Dietary Therapy

Along with food-related skin allergies, gastrointestinal conditions are perhaps the only instance where conventional medicine uses nutrition as a primary means of therapy. In response to this need, pet food companies have developed several prescription diets for animals with chronic diarrhea and/or vomiting. Frequently, these are animals diagnosed with IBD who may have a sensitivity to one or more dietary proteins, although we do occasionally see carbohydrate sensitivities as well.[6]

Given that there is no definitive treatment for IBD, the goal is to find a diet the animal can do well on. From the prescription diet perspective, there are three ways to do this:

- **Bland diet:** Switch to a bland, easily digestible diet that is nutritionally balanced for long-term feeding. (See Appendix E for instructions.)

- **Limited-ingredient diets (LIDs)**: Also known as novel protein diets, LIDs use protein and carbohydrate sources not commonly found in commercial pet foods. The presumption is that a pet is unlikely to have an inflammatory reaction to food ingredients they have never had before. This is why you'll find unusual combinations like duck and potato or venison and green pea. I once had a client feeding canned beaver to her dog!

- **Hydrolyzed diets:** These diets use a common protein such as chicken, but processed in such a way that the protein molecule is chopped up into smaller pieces that are unrecognizable by the immune system.[7]

When utilizing any of these diets, it is critical to not feed your dog or cat anything else for the first three to eight weeks. If they are truly food sensitive, any treats or other "illegal" snacks may trigger inflammation and perpetuate symptoms. Instructions for successful administration of a diet trial can be found in Appendix E.

Antibiotics

The use of antibiotics for pets with diarrhea is more common than you may think. While these medications are sometimes overused, there are instances where they may be necessary therapy.

- **Short-term:** When a dog or cat has pathogenic bacteria in their small or large intestine, a course of antibiotics may be necessary as part of a larger treatment plan. Veterinarians frequently use the antibiotic metronidazole to treat diarrhea in pets. It is used to treat the parasite giardia, or sometimes for nonspecific diarrhea. The drug is generally safe at appropriate doses, and it works due to its ability to cut down on pathogenic bacteria as well as its mild anti-inflammatory effect on the large intestine.[8]

- **Longer-term:** Metronidazole, or another antibiotic called tylosin, is sometimes used in pets as an alternative to steroids to control long-term diarrhea, such as in cases of IBD. While they can be effective, long-term antibiotic use is never ideal. Often the use of complementary medical options limits or eliminates the necessity of long-term antibiotics.

Steroids and Immunomodulating Drugs

Pets with severe forms of IBD are frequently prescribed steroids such as prednisone or prednisolone for their powerful anti-inflammatory effect. In severe cases of IBD, internal medicine specialists will sometimes use drugs like cyclosporine or chlorambucil. These powerful drugs suppress the immune system and are similar to chemotherapy drugs for cancer patients. These drugs should be avoided in favor of integrative care whenever possible.

Complementary and Alternative Therapy

There are many dogs and cats with chronic GI issues, and the common thread between nearly all of them is inflammation, though the causes of the inflammation may differ. While it is helpful to know the root cause, a definitive diagnosis is not necessary for treatment with alternative medicine. Remember, IBD is not a definitive diagnosis; it is a description of symptoms. From a complementary and alternative perspective, the key to success is changing the environment within the GI tract so as to limit the inflammation.

While this chapter focuses primarily on chronic conditions, the dietary and symptomatic therapies for pets with diarrhea within this group are generally applicable to the occasional acute episode of vomiting or diarrhea. Acute GI upset in pets (particularly dogs) is very common and is most often due to them having eaten something they shouldn't have. Usually these episodes resolve within a few days with supportive care.

Nutritional Therapy

This is one of the few times when conventional and alternative medicines agree on what the first step in treatment should be. In pets with dietary sensitivities, GI tract inflammation is caused directly by food. Removing ingredients that your pet is sensitive to will reduce inflammation and greatly improve (or resolve) the symptoms.

If you suspect your pet has a dietary sensitivity, conduct a diet trial, also known as a limited-ingredient diet trial or an elimination diet. You'll feed your pet a restricted ingredient diet for three to eight weeks to monitor them for improvement. Diets for the trial can be commercially prepared prescription diets or a fresh, home-prepared diet. (The fresh diet is the preferable option, of course. Appendix E outlines how to successfully conduct a diet trial.)

A laboratory test called NutriScan has recently become available that provides some guidance in picking foods for sensitive animals. Developed by Dr. Jean Dodds and Hemopet labs, this test utilizes natural antibodies in saliva to look for reactivity to a variety of foods. Of all the saliva-based tests advertised for food and environmental allergies, NutriScan is the only one with scientific research to back its results.

The NutriScan test is useful in cases where a diet trial would be difficult to accomplish or where we want some direction regarding which foods to avoid for the trial. Given how difficult food trials can be, any information that might simplify the process is a plus.

Note that not all pets with chronic GI conditions have food sensitivities. Regardless, many of them improve on fresh, whole-food diets, whether home-prepared or commercial raw, freeze dried, or dehydrated. When starting any diet change, a gradual transition of 7 to 14 days is recommended to allow the GI tract to adjust to the new food.

Nutritional Supplementation

- **Probiotics:** As discussed in detail in Chapter 6, probiotics support the GI tract and overall immune system health. Optimizing both leads to better digestion, nutrient absorption, and decreased GI inflammation. Along with optimal nutrition, probiotics promote good intestinal flora and are a cornerstone of good health and immune system function.

- **Whole-food supplementation:** The declining nutritional value of foods is well documented. Even a home-prepared, whole-food diet can be improved with additional nutrients. Companies such as Standard Process make supplements derived from all whole-food ingredients, and I particularly recommend adding their Canine Enteric Support to your pet's diet.
    Caution: Do not give Canine Enteric Support to pets who are sensitive to beef, pork, or lamb.

- **Bovine colostrum:** Derived from cow's milk, colostrum is well documented to improve inflammation within the GI tract. In humans, it has been shown to improve the symptoms of inflammatory bowel disease and chronic colitis.[9, 10] It has even been shown to protect the GI tract against damage induced by NSAIDs.[11]
    Caution: Do not give colostrum to pets that are sensitive to dairy proteins.

- **Fish oil:** Discussed in Chapter 6, fish oil provides essential fatty acids, supports normal GI and immune system function, and is a natural anti-inflammatory when used in appropriate doses.
    Caution: While fish oil does not contain fish protein (only the fats), pets with severe sensitivities to fish should avoid it. Other essential fatty acids such as mussel oil, krill oil, or algal DHA may be less problematic in these pets.

- **Clay powder:** Bentonite clay and montmorillonite clay are great supplements for acute or chronic diarrhea. The clay binds to bacterial toxins and helps to normalize stool quality. Clay helps resolve conditions caused by bacterial imbalance (dysbiosis) with minimal side effects.[12, 13, 14]

Herbal Therapy

The following section describes herbs beneficial for pets with chronic GI inflammation or IBD. Don't try to use *everything* on the list at once. More is not necessarily better; when it comes to chronic GI conditions, take it slow. Consider using a product that combines multiple herbs in appropriate proportions.

- **Cannabis:** Medical cannabis is first on the list because of the overwhelmingly positive results many patients experience. Some pets do well with a hemp-based CBD product, although more severe conditions may require a product with a 1:1 THC-to-CBD ratio. See Chapter 9 for more information regarding the safe use of medical cannabis.

- **Aloe extract:** Aloe stimulates healing of GI ulceration in much the same way that it helps with burns on the skin.[15]

- **Digestive enzymes:** Enzymes can be helpful for pets with excessive gas and diarrhea. For general GI support, fungal-derived enzymes rather than the more expensive porcine enzymes are usually adequate.

  Be very sparing with the dosing of enzymes; too much will cause GI upset. Usually giving one-quarter to one-half of the recommended dose on the label is sufficient.

- **Ginger:** Ginger is well known to support digestion and relieve nausea.[16, 17]

- **L-glutamine:** This amino acid helps protect the mucosal lining of the gastrointestinal tract.[18]

- **Licorice (deglycyrrhizinated):** Licorice is known to have anti-inflammatory properties and protects mucous membranes such as those of the GI tract. Look for "DGL" licorice that has the potentially toxic compound glycyrrhizin removed from it.[19]

- **Marshmallow:** Protects the mucous membranes of the GI tract.[20]

- **N-acetyl glucosamine:** Similar to the glucosamine used in the treatment of arthritis, n-acetyl glucosamine makes up part of the mucosal layer of the GI tract. Supplementing with it supports a healthy mucosa.[21]

- **Oregon grape:** This herb is antibacterial and supports digestion by stimulating the secretion of bile and digestive enzymes into the GI tract.[22]

- **Plantain:** Protects the mucosal layer of the GI tract and has anti-inflammatory properties.[23]

- **Slippery elm:** Protects the mucosal layer of the GI tract and has anti-inflammatory properties.[24]

Traditional Chinese Veterinary Medicine

Acupuncture, Chinese herbs, and Chinese medicine–based food therapy have been used effectively for thousands of years to treat people with chronic gastrointestinal problems. As with all Chinese medical therapy, treatment protocols depend on the patient. Consultation with a practitioner experienced in TCVM is recommended prior to starting any therapy.

Fecal Transplantation

The concept of fecal transplantation is simple, albeit gross: By transplanting feces from a healthy patient, we seed the sick patient's GI tract with more beneficial flora and help resolve underlying inflammation and the symptoms of IBD. Even within the human medical field, fecal transplantation is gaining ground as a treatment for patients with long-term bacterial imbalances.[25]

Integrative Treatment Plan

Pets with chronic GI conditions have a chronically inflamed intestinal tract. It's like a raw, open sore: painful and sensitive. Because the GI tract is unable to function correctly in its current state, many GI-supportive supplements will actually worsen symptoms if they are used too early in the process. Success depends on a gradual rehabilitation of the GI tract to a noninflamed state.

Depending on the severity of the symptoms, Western antibiotics and steroids are sometimes necessary in the short term to provide relief. Decreasing the worst of the inflammation provides some wiggle room when starting supplementation as well. In pets with severe inflammation, start slowly with very gentle supplements one at a time. Begin with a probiotic or clay powder and slowly add in other supplements while keeping a close watch for worsening symptoms.

My go-to protocol for IBD or other chronic GI upset is as follows:

- Treat symptoms with Western medication, if necessary.

- Begin judicious use of supplements such as colostrum, Canine/Feline Enteric Support by Standard Process, probiotics, etc. Start with just one or two supplements, as too many at once can cause GI distress.

- Slowly transition your pet to a fresh, whole-food diet.

- Consider cannabis oil.

- Slowly introduce further supplements on an as-needed basis. Introduce no more than one supplement (or combination supplement product) every three to four weeks.

Chronic GI disease in pets or people is a crappy problem to have (pun very much intended). Using herbal medicine for pets with chronic GI conditions can have dramatically positive results. Pets who have done poorly on nearly every conventional medical option often improve with the right combination of diet and supplements. In most cases, the key is to take it slow.

CHAPTER 15

PANCREATIC DISEASE

Pancreatitis and Pancreatic Insufficiency

The pancreas is by far the most complex organ in the body.
— PATRICK SOON-SHIONG, SURGEON AND MEDICAL RESEARCHER

If you appreciate a highly effective multitasker, have I got an organ for you! Allow me to introduce you to a rather unassuming organ within the upper right quadrant of the abdomen known as the pancreas. If you didn't know what to look for, you would miss this thin strip of cream-colored tissue. It may not look like much, but this organ is a powerhouse.

The Pancreas: Form and Function

The endocrine pancreas, which consists of small clusters of cells within the larger organ, secretes hormones into the bloodstream. These hormones—insulin and glucagon—play a pivotal role in the movement of blood sugar between the blood and nearly every cell in the body. Malfunctions of the endocrine portion of the pancreas nearly always result in diabetes, which is covered in detail in the next chapter.

The majority of pancreatic tissue, however, plays a pivotal role in digestion; it is known as the exocrine pancreas. The exocrine pancreas secretes digestive enzymes into the duodenum, the first portion of the small intestine, which break down food and allow its nutrients to be absorbed through the intestinal wall into the bloodstream.

When Things Go Wrong

There are two ways the exocrine pancreas can go awry. The organ can either be under-functioning, causing exocrine pancreatic insufficiency, or it can become inflamed, leading to pancreatitis.

Pancreatitis

The most common condition affecting the exocrine pancreas is pancreatitis. Pancreatitis, or pancreatic inflammation, is encountered in both dogs and cats and ranges in severity from moderate GI upset to a life-threatening disease.

The causes of pancreatitis are often vague, although it may be triggered through consumption of foods containing large amounts of fat. These foods cause excessive secretion of pancreatic enzymes, leading to pancreatic inflammation. Another contributing factor may be the consumption of spoiled or bacterially contaminated food, such as when pets get into the garbage. Bacteria from the food move from the intestine through the pancreatic duct and into the pancreas, causing infection and inflammation.

Pets with concurrent disease of the liver or intestines, diabetes, or hypothyroidism (low thyroid function) may be more prone to pancreatitis. Middle-aged to older overweight dogs seem to be the most affected; miniature schnauzers, dachshunds, and Yorkshire terriers are most at risk.

Symptoms of a dog or cat with pancreatitis include severe abdominal discomfort, vomiting, diarrhea, and/or lack of appetite. These signs occur when digestive enzymes that are normally secreted by the pancreas begin to seep into the pancreatic tissue as a result of inflammation and/or infection. When this occurs, the pancreas itself becomes subject to its own digestive fluids.

Most cases of pancreatitis are acute and relatively short-lived, although chronic pancreatitis in some pets does occur. In chronic cases, smoldering inflammation within the pancreas can flare up at any time. These flares are sometimes associated with a diet change or your pet getting into food they were not supposed to eat. For pets that are overweight, returning them to a more ideal body weight may limit or resolve chronic pancreatitis.

Exocrine Pancreatic Insufficiency

Exocrine pancreatic insufficiency (EPI) is primarily a condition of dogs. While feline EPI occurs, it is rare. In these pets, the pancreas is underproducing or not producing the enzymes required to break down foods for digestion. EPI is frequently genetic but can occur as a result of chronic pancreatitis leading to inflammatory destruction of the exocrine pancreas. Either way, the result is that food is not properly broken down and thus passes through the GI tract without being absorbed.

The classic symptoms of EPI are low body weight, ravenous appetite, and voluminous, light-colored stools. EPI is most commonly seen in German shepherds, but is seen in other breeds of dogs as well as in cats.

Diagnosis of Pancreatitis and EPI

Pets with pancreatitis frequently have symptoms of vomiting, diarrhea, and/or abdominal pain. They may or may not have a known history of a diet change or dietary indiscretion (that's a nice way of saying they ate something gross). When your pet's history and physical symptoms suggest pancreatitis, the following diagnostic tests may be used to confirm the diagnosis.[1, 2, 3]

- **Blood tests:** Your veterinarian will check systemic body function with a complete blood count (CBC) and blood chemistries. Also, a specific test for pancreatitis called canine pancreatic lipase (cPL) or feline pancreatic lipase (fPL) is a valuable tool.

- **Abdominal ultrasound:** Ultrasound is an excellent (and widely available) method of visualizing the pancreas in a noninvasive way. Most pets do not even require sedation. Many veterinary radiologists believe that ultrasound is a better diagnostic indicator of pancreatitis than cPL or fPL.

Because EPI is not a condition that occurs all that frequently, veterinarians will rightly want to eliminate more common conditions first by doing a standard screening to rule out gastrointestinal parasitic diseases (ova, parasites, and giardia) prior to testing for EPI.

- **Trypsin-like immunoreactivity (TLI):** TLI testing is the definitive diagnosis for EPI. TLI testing is frequently combined with a check of cobalamin and folate (both B vitamins) levels to concurrently evaluate for bacterial overgrowth in the small intestine. The presence of all that undigested food is a feast for microorganisms.

Conventional Medical Treatment

Pancreatitis

There are no drugs that specifically treat pancreatitis. Therapy involves a combination of controlling the infection and inflammation and providing symptomatic care.[4, 5, 6]

Depending on the severity of the case, some pets will require hospitalization, IV fluids, and medication to help with nausea and pain until they feel well enough to eat and keep food down. Sometimes fluids are administered subcutaneously (under the skin) to keep pets hydrated if they are not hospitalized.

- **Antibiotics:** Infection is commonly a component of pancreatitis. Despite the fact that antibiotics can sometimes cause GI upset, short-term use is recommended for acute pancreatitis.

- **Nonsteroidal anti-inflammatory drugs (NSAIDs):** Much like antibiotics, NSAIDs can cause GI upset. However, their value in reducing pancreatic inflammation often outweighs this concern.

- **Pain control:** Opiates like buprenorphine or sometimes a slow-release patch of fentanyl can be used for pets with severe pain.

EPI

- **Pancreatic enzyme replacement:** The primary therapy for EPI is the addition of enzymes to your pet's food to replace what their own pancreas is not producing. There are two types of digestive enzyme supplements available: porcine and fungal.

  Pets with EPI need the supplements made from desiccated porcine (pig) pancreas. You can mix the powdered enzyme supplement with their food. Positive effects are very quickly evident; stools become more normal within days of starting.

  Fungal-derived enzymes can be effective for pets with mild digestive issues, gas, and sometimes IBD. However, they are not sufficient to treat EPI.

- **Antibiotics:** Pets with TLI will sometimes have an overgrowth of intestinal bacteria due to all the undigested food in their GI tract. Antibiotic therapy with drugs like metronidazole or tylosin is sometimes recommended.

- **Vitamin B12 (cobalamin) and folate supplementation:** Pets with bacterial overgrowth within the small intestine often concurrently have B vitamin deficiencies. This overgrowth of bacteria can lead to a deficiency of vitamin B12 (in cats and dogs) and folate (in cats), so supplementation is necessary. Initially, your veterinarian may give B12 or folate supplementation via injection, and then switch to oral administration later.[7, 8, 9]

Diet for Pancreatitis and EPI

- **Acute pancreatitis:** Many pets with pancreatitis will not eat or will vomit if they do. Once they get to a point where they *can* eat, a bland diet is often recommended. A prescription bland diet or a mixture of boiled chicken and rice is the most frequently recommended (see Appendix E for further information). Either is fine in the short term, although home-prepared is always superior.

- **Chronic pancreatitis:** Pets with chronic pancreatitis often are very sensitive to high-fat diets. Conventional medicine generally recommends a prescription bland diet.

- **EPI:** Depending on the severity of the EPI, a change in diet may or may not be recommended within the scope of conventional medicine. If it is, most likely the recommendation will be for an easily digestible prescription diet.

Complementary and Alternative Medical Therapy

Acute pancreatitis requires acute medical care. This is the time for Western medical intervention. Without Western treatment, pets can become dangerously dehydrated, making their situation progressively worse. The following recommendations focus on managing chronic pancreatitis in pets who are able to eat and keep food down. (Hyperbaric oxygen and cannabis, however, do offer relief for pets with acute pancreatitis.)

Pancreatitis

- **Diet:** Ideal diets for pets with chronic pancreatitis are very low in fat, as these are easily digestible and do not require as much pancreatic activity. Diets to help manage canine and feline pancreatitis can be found in Appendix C.

- **Hyperbaric oxygen therapy:** The anti-inflammatory and antimicrobial effects of HBOT make it highly effective in the treatment of acute pancreatitis or flareups of chronic pancreatitis.[10] HBOT is described in detail in Chapter 10.

- **Cannabis:** Medical cannabis is first on the list of herbs for chronic GI conditions and pancreatitis because of the overwhelmingly positive results many patients experience. Cannabis can be used for both acute and chronic pancreatitis. Some pets do well with a hemp-based CBD product, although more severe conditions may require a product with a 1:1 THC-to-CBD ratio. See Chapter 9 for more information regarding the safe use of medical cannabis.

EPI

- **Pancreatic enzyme replacement:** Even from the holistic perspective, supplementation with porcine-derived digestive enzymes is the best plan. It is all-natural, directly addresses the condition (rather than treating symptoms), and has no side effects when used in recommended doses.

- **Diet:** Regardless of the level of success of enzyme supplementation, anything we can do to improve the nutritional profile of pets with EPI is going to be a plus. Remember, most of them are underweight and malnourished at the time of diagnosis. Feeding EPI pets a fresh, whole-food diet provides a highly digestible and nutritious meal that will ultimately provide the kind of nutrients their body needs with a relative minimum of digestive effort.

  Caution: EPI pets are digestively challenged, and the goal is to feed the easiest foods to digest. Raw foods, however, require more energy to digest than cooked, and therefore may not be the first choice for pets with EPI. If you are really determined to feed raw, start with cooked and slowly transition to a raw diet to see if your pet with EPI can handle it.

- **Vitamin supplementation:** Given that EPI pets may not be digesting their nutrients optimally, they often need vitamin/mineral supplementation. They may require long-term supplementation of folate and B12 (see conventional therapy section for EPI).

Nutritional Supplementation for Pancreatitis and EPI

- **Probiotics:** As discussed in detail in Chapter 6, probiotics support the GI tract and overall immune system health. Optimizing both leads to better digestion, nutrient absorption, and decreased GI inflammation. Along with optimal nutrition, probiotics promote good intestinal flora and are a cornerstone of good health and immune system function.

- **Clay powder:** Bentonite clay and montmorillonite clay are great supplements for acute or chronic diarrhea. The clay binds to bacterial toxins and helps to normalize stool quality. Clay helps resolve conditions caused by bacterial imbalance (dysbiosis) with minimal side effects.[11, 12, 13]

- **Whole-food supplementation:** The declining nutritional value of foods is well documented. Even a home-prepared, whole-food diet can be improved with additional nutrients. Companies such as Standard Process make supplements derived from all whole-food ingredients, and I particularly recommend adding their Canine Enteric Support, Pancreatrophin PMG, and/or Zypan to your pet's diet to support digestion and pancreatic function. To determine which products are best, talk to a practitioner who is familiar with using Standard Process supplements.

    Caution: Do not give these supplements to pets that are sensitive to beef, pork, or lamb.

- **Bovine colostrum:** Derived from cow's milk, colostrum is well documented to improve inflammation within the GI tract. In humans, it has been shown to improve the symptoms of inflammatory bowel disease and chronic colitis.[14, 15] It has even been shown to protect the GI tract against damage induced by NSAIDs.[16]

    Caution: Do not give colostrum to pets that are sensitive to dairy proteins.

- **Fish oil:** As discussed in Chapter 6, fish oil provides essential fatty acids, supports normal GI and immune system function, and is a natural anti-inflammatory when used in appropriate doses. Despite its benefits, fish oil should be used with caution in pets with pancreatitis or EPI, as fat digestion stimulates pancreatic function. Begin with very small doses, then increase the amount slowly.

    Caution: While fish oil does not contain fish protein (only the fats), pets with severe sensitivities to fish should avoid it.

- **Herbal therapy:** In theory, many of the herbs recommended for IBD in Chapter 14 may be applicable for pets with pancreatitis or EPI, although they may not be necessary. Be cautious, as the addition of anything has the potential to cause GI upset.

    When it comes to pets with pancreatitis, sometimes less is more. The goal is to make the digestive process as easy as possible. View the supplement recommendations on this list as a reference guide. If you or your pet's health-care provider believes they are indicated, proceed slowly and with caution.

    The intestines of EPI pets, unlike those of pets with IBD, are usually fine. The signs of GI upset frequently resolve once the primary treatment measures described above are under way.

Integrative Treatment Plan

For such a small organ, a malfunctioning exocrine pancreas sure can make a big mess. Successful therapy of either EPI or pancreatitis depends on accurate diagnosis and the right combination of therapies. Consider the integrative treatment plans listed as suggestions. Every individual is going to be different and therapy will need to be adjusted accordingly.

Acute Pancreatitis

Managing pancreatitis can be a one- or a two-stage process. Many pets that develop acute pancreatitis will never progress to a chronic condition. For these pets, short-term care is all they need.

- Depending on your pet's level of pain and ability to keep food down, they may need in-patient hospitalization and supportive care. IV fluids, antibiotics, and anti-inflammatory and pain medications will likely be necessary.

- The next step is outpatient supportive care, including subcutaneous fluids (under the skin), antibiotics, and anti-inflammatory/pain medication as frequently as necessary.

- Hyperbaric oxygen therapy is an excellent way to speed recovery from acute pancreatitis.

- Feed your pet a bland diet, at least in the short term. This can either be homemade (see Appendix E) or a prescription bland diet, to be fed for several days or weeks. Ideally, homemade is better.

- Consider medical cannabis for nausea, pain, and inflammation.

Chronic Pancreatitis

Pets with chronic or recurring bouts of pancreatitis need long-term care to keep inflammation to a minimum. It is best, however, to start with a less-is-more approach with chronic pancreatitis.

- Long-term appropriate dietary therapy is a cornerstone of treating chronic pancreatitis. Fresh, whole-food recipes for canine and feline pancreatitis can be found in Appendix C.

- Probiotics and clay powder provide very gentle supplementation and excellent GI support.

- Cannabis can be used regularly or symptomatically for GI upset or discomfort.

- Be cautious in considering additional supplementation—you run the risk of upsetting the apple cart. View the supplement recommendations in this chapter as a reference guide. If you or your pet's health-care provider believes they are indicated, proceed slowly and with caution.

EPI

EPI is one of those conditions for which there is general agreement between conventional and alternative care.

The only disagreement may be in cases where long-term antibiotic use is recommended. Instead of long-term antibiotics, a better approach is to change the environment in the GI tract to create a friendly space for beneficial bacteria and inhibit the proliferation of pathogenic (bad) bacteria.

The following is a good integrative approach to EPI.

- Immediately start your pet on porcine-based digestive enzyme supplementation.
- Switch to a fresh, whole-food diet that is designed to be easily digestible. Refer to "low-fat" and "pancreatitis" sections of Appendix C.
- Begin vitamin supplementation, especially B vitamins (folate and B12).
- If the lab work indicates bacterial overgrowth, start short-term antibiotic use.
- Add probiotics to your pet's diet.
- If you feel it is necessary and your pet tolerates it well, add fish oil to their diet.
- If GI signs persist, consider whole-food supplementation and/or colostrum.
- If GI signs persist, consider herbal therapy for GI support.

CHAPTER 16

DIABETES

The physician should not treat the disease but the patient who is suffering from it.

– Maimonides

The pancreas, an unassuming organ with high-level responsibilities, is located within the upper right quadrant of the abdomen and performs two pivotal body functions. The majority of pancreatic tissue, known as the exocrine pancreas, plays a significant role in digestion by secreting powerful enzymes into the small intestine. (Disruptions of the exocrine pancreas are discussed in detail in Chapter 15.)

The other, equally vital function of the pancreas is the endocrine pancreas. It consists of small clusters of cells called the islets of Langerhans. Although they sound like a desolate group of islands in the North Sea, these cells are of enormous importance to everyday living. They secrete hormones—insulin and glucagon—that regulate blood sugar and are the key to every cell in the body getting fed.[1, 2, 3]

When an animal eats, food is broken down into nutrients and glucose (energy) and absorbed into the bloodstream. In order for the nutrients and energy to enter the cells, they need transportation. In other words, just because they are in the neighborhood does not mean the cells can use them. It's kind of like putting a filled gas can next to a car with an empty tank. Unless someone is around to pour it in the tank, the car is not going anywhere. The hormone insulin acts as that transporter, controlling the rate of movement of glucose from the bloodstream into the cells. (There are several hormones involved with glucose transport, but insulin is the one directly related to the onset of diabetes.)

When Things Go Wrong

When there is a lack of insulin, or the body is not responding appropriately to insulin, glucose builds up in the blood and leads to diabetes mellitus—often called diabetes for short. (There is also a disease of dogs called diabetes insipidus, but it is relatively rare, has nothing to do with insulin, and is completely unrelated to diabetes mellitus.)

When a dog or cat is diabetic, the classic symptoms are drinking excessive amounts of water, urinating large volumes, and often having a ravenous appetite. In veterinary medicine, the term for increased urination is *polyuria* (PU), increased water intake is *polydipsia* (PD), and increased appetite is *polyphagia* (PP). When veterinarians describe these symptoms, they are often referred to collectively as PU/PD/PP.

PU/PD/PP in diabetic pets is the body's response to the inability to move glucose from the blood into the cells. Under normal circumstances, the kidneys keep glucose in the blood and out of the urine. In diabetics, however, the blood glucose is so high that it overwhelms the kidneys' abilities, so glucose spills over into the urine. Once that happens, excessive water is drawn into the urine. More water in the urine leads to increased urine volume (PU). In response to PU, the body must balance the fluid loss or risk dehydration. If it can't keep the water from leaving through the kidneys, the only alternative is to increase water consumption through thirst (PD).

PP occurs because the body is starving despite being awash in cellular food in the form of blood glucose. The lack of insulin (or lack of response to it) prevents glucose from entering cells, so the cells send signals to the brain indicating they are hungry. The brain moves to remedy the situation by increasing appetite and food intake. Despite PP, significant weight loss can occur due to lack of accessible blood sugar.

When an untreated diabetic pet stops drinking and eating excessively, it is a bad sign. This usually indicates that your pet has become so sick, they do not want to eat or drink regardless of the influence of excessive blood glucose. These pets rapidly become severely dehydrated and may develop a condition called diabetic ketoacidosis (DKA). DKA is a life-threatening complication of untreated diabetes that requires immediate medical care.

Know the Difference: Type I vs. Type II Diabetes

There are two general forms of diabetes: type 1 and type 2. Type 1 diabetics do not produce insulin. (In humans, this is also referred to as juvenile diabetes or insulin-dependent diabetes.) Type 2 diabetics produce insulin, but not enough to get the job done. Type 2 may be a function of genetics, obesity, or diet; in many individuals, it's likely a combination of all three.

While diabetes occurs in both dogs and cats, species has everything to do with the incidence of type 1 versus type 2.

- **Type 1 diabetes** is almost exclusively seen in dogs. These dogs' bodies cannot produce insulin. Once diagnosed, type 1 diabetes is irreversible; these dogs require lifelong insulin therapy. Even with relatively good diabetic control, some dogs will develop diabetic cataracts, leading to impairment or loss of vision unless the cataracts are surgically removed.

  Most frequently, pet owners first realize there is a problem due to the onset of some combination of PU/PD/PP and/or weight loss. Prior to the onset of symptoms, these dogs often appear to be normal and healthy.

- **Type 2 diabetes** is exclusively a disease of cats. These cats don't produce enough insulin to maintain their blood sugar. Uncontrolled diabetes in cats can sometimes lead to diabetic neuropathy, which causes weakness and pain in the hind limbs.

  Obesity often plays a role here. Increased body mass necessitates that the pancreas produce more insulin in order to maintain blood sugar balance. Research in humans shows that increased body fat leads to the production of chemicals within the body that promote inflammation and insulin resistance.[4] It's probably a combination of insulin resistance resulting from obesity and genetic predisposition that leads to type 2 diabetes.[5, 6] Because type 2 diabetes is, at least partially, caused by nongenetic factors such as poor diet and obesity, the condition can sometimes be reversed.

Diabetic Ketoacidosis

DKA is a life-threatening emergency that can occur with diabetic dogs and cats.

When cells are starved for glucose (due to a lack of insulin), the body responds by metabolizing fat stores for energy. Fats are broken down into chemicals called ketones, which are used for fuel. As large numbers of ketones are burned, the result is a profound metabolic derangement in which pH and electrolyte levels change, leading to severe dehydration and shock. If untreated, DKA is fatal.

DKA occurs in pets whose diabetes is uncontrolled, so it is most common in newly diagnosed and poorly controlled diabetics. Usually DKA is encountered in pets with a concurrent inflammatory or infectious condition such as a urinary tract infection or pancreatitis.

Hypoglycemia

Low blood sugar is also known as hypoglycemia. Signs of hypoglycemia include weakness, loss of balance, loss of consciousness, and seizures. Left untreated, your pet can go into hypoglycemic shock—and die.

There are many causes, but the most common is an overdose due to an insulin injection. If hypoglycemia is suspected in a diabetic pet, or if too much insulin was accidentally administered, put a little corn syrup on their gums (it will be absorbed into their blood stream) and get them to a veterinarian immediately!

Cataracts

Similar to humans, diabetic dogs (not cats) will sometimes develop cataracts. Chronically elevated blood sugar levels lead to opacification (whitening) of the lenses of the eyes. Diabetic cataracts can lead to visual impairment or blindness. The only treatment for cataracts is surgical removal by a veterinary ophthalmologist.

Diagnosis of Diabetes

Diagnosing diabetes is a piece of cake (pun intended). Treatment, however, requires your full commitment for the life of your pet.

The methods of diagnosing diabetes are the same regardless of whether it is type 1 or type 2. Any pet that is PU and PD, with or without PP, should be suspect. Overweight cats are especially prone to diabetes.

Ultimately, diabetes is diagnosed through testing blood and urine.

Blood Testing

- **Blood glucose:** A full blood panel is necessary in suspected diabetic patients because any number of complicating factors, such as pancreatitis, liver disease, or kidney disease, may be present. The key factor in diabetics is blood glucose. Normal blood glucose levels are around 100, but the blood glucose of uncontrolled diabetic animals can be as high as 300–500.

   One complicating factor in diagnosing diabetes from blood sugar levels is the phenomenon of stress hyperglycemia—which can easily be triggered by a visit to the veterinarian. In dogs and especially cats, stress leads to a normal physiologic response of an increase in blood glucose. It is very common to see blood glucose levels in the 200s for healthy animals. I have seen levels into the 400s in highly stressed, nondiabetic cats.

- **Fructosamine:** A fructosamine level is often performed to confirm a diagnosis of diabetes. Fructosamine gives a rough indication of how high blood sugar has been for the previous two weeks, thus clearing any doubts about elevated blood glucose having been caused by stress. (Fructosamine is similar to A1c testing in people.)

Urinalysis

If your pet has elevated blood glucose and fructosamine levels, then a definitive diagnosis of diabetes can be made. There is, however, a lot of valuable information to be gained from a urine sample.

The presence of glucose in urine in conjunction with elevated blood glucose and fructosamine levels helps confirm the diagnosis of diabetes. Any amount of glucose in the urine is considered abnormal, although transient urine glucose can occur in highly stressed cats due to stress hyperglycemia.

Furthermore, having all that sugar in the urine makes a wonderful medium for bacteria to grow, so a urinalysis may find a urinary tract infection, which is very common in uncontrolled diabetics. Diagnosing a UTI through urinalysis and/or urine culture is important for two reasons. First, an uncontrolled UTI can cause pain, kidney damage, and the development of bladder stones (see Chapter 13). Second, any kind of infection can lead to insulin resistance, making diabetic control much more difficult.

Conventional Medical Treatment

Once the diagnosis of diabetes has been made, the first thing you must do is commit to treatment. Just as in people with diabetes, therapy is lifelong and, at the very least, involves insulin, nutritional changes, and routine monitoring through lab work. Diabetes is not a disease that can be treated casually.

Insulin Therapy

Supplementing insulin is the most effective way to control diabetes. Unfortunately, all diabetic dogs will require long-term insulin. On the other hand, while all diabetic cats should be started on insulin at diagnosis, some can be converted to a non–insulin-dependent state. Weight loss and nutrition are integral to achieving and maintaining this non–insulin-dependent state in cats. While strategies differ a little between dogs and cats, there is one constant to keep in mind:

**Too much insulin is far worse than not enough.
An overdose of insulin can lead to hypoglycemic shock and death.**

To prevent hypoglycemia, always give insulin immediately following a meal. If insulin is administered before and then your pet doesn't eat, your pet could go into hypoglycemic shock.

If you suspect your pet has hypoglycemia, put a little corn syrup on their gums and immediately go to the veterinarian's office or emergency room.

When beginning insulin therapy, your veterinarian will start your pet on a very low dose to reduce the risk of hypoglycemia. You will then slowly work up to giving the optimal dose. Insulin injections are given every 12 hours, and your veterinarian will provide you with specific instructions regarding dosing.

Insulin therapy must be administered by injection, but don't let that frighten you. The injections are nearly painless and are very easy to administer. In some ways, it's easier than having to give oral medication twice daily (especially in cats).

There are many different types of insulin available for humans, but most are not used for pets. Your veterinarian will determine which type of insulin is best for your diabetic pet. *Never use any insulin that was not recommended by your veterinarian.*

The two types of insulin most frequently used for pets are:

- **Porcine zinc insulin (Vetsulin):** This veterinary-specific insulin is most commonly used for dogs.[7]

- **Glargine insulin (Lantus):** This insulin is produced for humans but can be used in both dogs and cats.[8]

Be cautious when it comes to the concentration of your insulin. All human insulin products are 100 units per milliliter (U-100). Some veterinary-specific insulins, including Vetsulin, are 40 units per milliliter (U-40). There are specific syringes designed for use with each concentration of insulin. If you use a U-100 syringe with U-40 insulin, you will underdose the insulin. Much worse, using U-40 syringes with U-100 insulin may lead to a fatal insulin overdose.

While conversion charts are available, I strongly advise using the syringe designed for the insulin prescribed. Syringes are cheap, and it's too easy to make a serious mistake if you use the wrong kind.

Oral Medications

Most veterinarians (including myself) would agree that all newly diagnosed diabetics require insulin therapy. There is, however, an oral drug called glipizide that is used in human type 2 diabetics. Glipizide and drugs like it stimulate insulin production in humans; in some cases, this eliminates the need for insulin injections.

Glipizide has very limited use in veterinary medicine. Under the best of circumstances, it only works for type 2 diabetes. Research on type 2 diabetics indicates that only 20 to 30 percent of cats respond to the medication by increasing insulin production. It is impossible to predict which cats will respond or how well they will respond.[9]

If you have a cat with type 2 diabetes and for whatever reason you are unable to give insulin injections but are able to give an oral medication twice a day, then ask your veterinarian about glipizide. However, the bottom line is I wouldn't recommend it. Insulin is, by far, the better option.

Nutrition

As different foods are digested and assimilated, they affect blood sugar in different ways. Blood glucose spikes when a diabetic pet eats a meal with high levels of simple carbohydrates or sugars. The solution (as you may have guessed) is to modulate the diet to prevent these elevations in blood sugar.

In particular, optimal diets are ones providing appropriate levels of energy while limiting blood sugar elevation to a slow and predictable rate. This allows for lower insulin doses, more consistent diabetic control, and decreased requirements for monitoring.

Diabetic Nutrition for Cats with Type 2 Diabetes

Nutritionally speaking, canine and feline diabetics have completely different needs. The evolutionary difference between the two species is the cornerstone of nutritional management of diabetes and is the reason why feeding strategies for diabetic dogs and cats are so different.

Cats are primarily carnivores who are equipped to consume a high-protein, moderate-fat, low-carbohydrate diet. High levels of dietary carbs lead to blood sugar spikes and make diabetic regulation unnecessarily difficult. A diet consisting largely of protein and fat provides a better plateau of blood sugar and a lower insulin requirement.

Feeding a proper diet to diabetic cats has a dual effect on insulin requirements. First, low levels of dietary carbohydrates decrease the blood sugar spike after eating, thereby decreasing the insulin requirement. Second, a low-carbohydrate diet leads to weight loss. Lower body fat reduces the amount of insulin that the pancreas needs to secrete to maintain blood sugar levels. The goal is to create an environment within the body in which the amount of insulin being produced becomes adequate to regulate blood sugar without insulin injections.

Overall, the nutritional goal in diabetic cats is a diet high in protein with moderate to low fat and very low carbohydrates. The low fat helps prevent pancreatitis, which diabetic animals are prone to developing, is a contributing factor to insulin resistance, and may lead to diabetic ketoacidosis. The effects of a changing diet can lead to the reduction and possibly elimination of insulin injections in these patients.[10] Diabetic cats can lose their insulin dependence literally overnight. However, there is no easy way to see this change coming, and the results of giving an unnecessary dose of insulin can lead to life-threatening hypoglycemia. This is one of the many reasons why both pet owners and veterinarians must be *very* diligent during the regulation process.

As for most medical conditions requiring nutritional management, Western medicine has a solution in the form of a prescription diet. In the case of feline diabetes, these diets tend to be higher in protein. Interestingly, these diets come in both canned and dry forms. Given that the manufacturing of kibble necessitates its being high in carbohydrates (see Chapter 4), these diets seem off track. The only use of a kibble in diabetic cats would be in a kitty that is "addicted" to dry food and refuses to eat canned or fresh food.

Diabetic Nutrition for Dogs with Type 1 Diabetes

Dogs are evolutionarily able to assimilate dietary carbohydrates much more effectively than cats (see Chapter 2). Research has shown that feeding diabetic dogs a "feline-style" low-carbohydrate diet has little benefit with regard to diabetic control.

The most successful nutritional strategy for diabetic dogs is a diet containing moderate protein, low fat, and high levels of complex carbohydrates and fiber. Avoid simple carbohydrates like sugars and refined starches (white rice, pasta, etc.) because they are too easily digested, leading to unacceptable spikes in blood sugar. Keep fat levels low to limit the possibility of pancreatitis, which can lead to insulin resistance and diabetic ketoacidosis.

The addition of dietary fiber to a diabetic dog's regimen is beneficial. Dietary fiber, which is also a complex carbohydrate, slows the digestion of digestible complex carbohydrates within the intestines and promotes healthy weight loss. By slowing carbohydrate digestion, glucose absorption is delayed, and there is a more gradual infusion of glucose into the blood. Fewer fluctuations in blood glucose after a meal helps reduce the insulin requirement and ultimately makes diabetic regulation easier.[11]

Veterinarians frequently recommend weight-loss diets for diabetic dogs. These diets tend to be low in fat and high in fiber, which fits the parameters of diabetic nutrition for canines. Either prescription or over-the-counter weight-loss diets are sometimes recommended.

Therapeutic Monitoring of Diabetes

For many pet owners, keeping up with diabetic monitoring for their pet is the most challenging aspect of their pet's health care. In the early stages of treatment, blood and urine often need to be checked every two weeks or so. Adjustments in insulin doses are based on changes in symptoms and lab results. Once your pet is well regulated, monitoring can be done less frequently.

Diabetic humans normally check their blood sugar levels multiple times per day to help them keep a tight rein on their diabetic control. Due to the unfeasibility of checking blood glucose so often in pets, the goal of diabetic therapy in dogs and cats is to keep them slightly hyperglycemic. (Remember, too much insulin is much more dangerous than not enough.)

Pet Owner Observations

One of the most critical means by which diabetic control is measured is through your own observations of how your pet is doing at home. In particular, pets undergoing treatment for diabetes should show significant improvements with regard to PU/PD/PP. They may still drink a little more than they did prior to becoming diabetic, but the overall water consumption and urine production should go way down. In addition, carefully monitor for signs of hypoglycemia. Any sign of weakness or loss of balance, especially after an insulin shot, requires immediate evaluation by a veterinarian.

Blood

Monitoring blood work utilizes the same tests that are used in diagnosis. A reading of a single blood glucose level in a diabetic receiving insulin can be difficult to interpret because the level can fluctuate wildly based on how long ago the insulin was given, when your pet last ate, and the interactions of stress hyperglycemia. The addition of a fructosamine level is valuable in that it tells us about the general level of blood glucose control over the previous two weeks.

A blood glucose curve is a series of blood glucose measurements taken over six to eight hours. The goal is to evaluate the curve, or how the blood sugar responds over time after insulin is given. It provides a window into how well your pet is responding to the current type and dose of insulin. Also known as BG curves, these tools are not without their problems. Stress hyperglycemia can be a big complicating factor, and curves don't always seem to correlate with real-world diabetic control.

For some owners and pets, checking blood glucose at home is possible. Usually this is done through pricking the margin of your pet's ear with a needle and testing the blood glucose. The potential benefits are that it minimizes stress hyperglycemia, so you have more accurate results, and it provides more data points because you can do more frequent checks.

Being able to check blood glucose on a diabetic pet at home is not a requirement. If it is done, however, use a glucometer specifically designed for pets to ensure accurate readings.

Urine

Evaluating urine for glucose, infection, and ketones is important in the early stages of diabetic treatment and if your pet seems sick for any reason. Your veterinarian will recommend a schedule for periodic urine evaluation.

Some pet owners use urine dipsticks at home to check for glucose and ketones in their diabetic pets. The amount of glucose noted on the dipstick can be a valuable tool in determining blood glucose on a day-to-day basis. Remember, the higher the blood glucose, the more glucose in the urine.

Ideally, diabetic pets should have "trace" or "1+" glucose in the urine. This implies good diabetic control while ensuring that blood glucose is not too low. A dipstick that is negative for glucose cannot differentiate between normal blood glucose and life-threatening low levels.

Complementary and Alternative Medical Therapy

Nutrition

In the case of diabetes, Western medicine has done an excellent job working out what each species needs to help with diabetic control. (Please see the nutrition information in the conventional treatment section.) Of course, fresh, whole-food diets provide the same nutritional profiles needed for diabetic dogs and cats without the drawbacks of the highly processed prescription diets.

Nutritional Supplementation

There are myriad Internet "cures" and "treatments" for diabetic pets claiming to get pets off insulin. Don't believe them. Dogs with diabetes require lifelong insulin therapy, period. While it is possible to get some cats off insulin, it is a function of nutrition and appropriate insulin therapy begun immediately at diagnosis.

Diabetic pets are metabolically challenged due to their disease, so consider a high-quality multivitamin and mineral supplement if you are feeding your pet a commercially prepared diet. Well-balanced home-prepared diets such as the ones in this book do not require additional supplementation.

Traditional Chinese Veterinary Medicine

Traditional Chinese veterinary medicine, including acupuncture and herbal therapy, can be a good adjunctive treatment for diabetic pets as it may improve their overall well-being. In addition, some Chinese herbs can assist in blood sugar regulation; their use should be recommended and supervised by someone trained in TCVM. That said, TCVM cannot act as a substitute for insulin and nutritional therapy.

Integrative Treatment Plan

When it comes to treating a diabetic dog or cat, there are relatively few steps in the treatment plan. Following a comprehensive treatment plan, however, is critical to a positive outcome. The most successful treatment plans include:

- Nutritional therapy using a fresh, whole-food diet appropriate for a type 1 diabetic dog or type 2 diabetic cat

- Insulin therapy

- Diligent monitoring to optimize diabetic control (Monitor cats closely as they may become non–insulin-dependent.)

- Adjunctive therapy, such as Chinese medicine, if your pet seems to benefit

Managing a diabetic requires a commitment of both time and financial resources for the life of your pet. With diligence, many pets can be regulated successfully and have an excellent quality of life. That said, all you can do is the best you can for these pets. Complications do occur and the best advice is to approach these challenges as they come.

CHAPTER 17

HEART DISEASE

Please help me mend my broken heart and let me live again.

– Barry and Robin Gibb

Within the center of the chest resides an organ that is the metaphorical seat of the soul. This distinction was surely made because the heart must work every second of every day of life. Loss of function for even a few seconds is often fatal. There is literally not a moment's rest.

The Heart: Form and Function

Simply put, the heart is a muscle whose purpose is to move blood. Blood carries nutrients to, and waste products away from, every cell in the body.

In humans, the heart beats about 100,000 times per day; it's slightly more for dogs and cats.[1] In mammals, the cardiac (heart) muscle contains four chambers. The top chambers are called the left and right atriums; the bottom chambers are the left and right ventricles. Each beat of the heart represents a contraction of the cardiac muscle.

When the heart contracts, blood is pushed throughout the body. The blood picks up oxygen in the lungs and delivers it, along with other nutrients, to the cells. With the same contraction, carbon dioxide is delivered to the lungs for exhalation and the liver and kidneys extract various waste products from the blood. This process takes place every second of every day without interruption.

A series of one-way valves within the heart maintains blood flow in a single direction. Blood enters the heart through the right atrium and travels to the right ventricle, the lungs, the left atrium, and finally the left ventricle before exiting the heart and back into circulation. Maintaining unidirectional flow of blood is important; it ensures efficient circulation and minimizes workload on the heart.

When Things Go Wrong

When most people think of heart disease, they think of a heart attack. A heart attack, or myocardial infarction, is a condition in which the blood supply to a portion of the heart is interrupted, causing damage. Fortunately, heart attacks don't occur in dogs and cats. However, pets are susceptible to other forms of heart disease.

Heart disease in dogs and cats is related to changes within the cardiac muscle or valves, or disturbances of electrical conduction. Diseases of the heart muscle are known as cardiomyopathy. Cardiomyopathy occurs in both dogs and cats, although the specifics of how the heart muscle is affected differ greatly between species. Abnormalities within the heart valves frequently lead to heart murmurs and sometimes congestive heart failure. Electrical disturbances can disturb the regularity of the heartbeat and may lead to life-threatening arrhythmias.

Regardless of the cause, heart disease is a serious matter, and the sooner it is diagnosed and treatment is begun, the better the long-term outcome.

Hypertrophic Cardiomyopathy in Cats

Hypertrophic cardiomyopathy (HCM) is the most common heart disease of cats. Cats with HCM develop thickening of the heart muscle, most frequently the left ventricle. While there is a genetic component to HCM that makes some pets prone, any cat can be affected.

Thickening of the cardiac muscle from HCM decreases the size of the heart's chambers and limits the ability of the heart to fill with blood when it relaxes. This decreased filling capacity leads to less blood being pushed through the body when the heart contracts and causes a backup of fluid that may ultimately lead to congestive heart failure. (We'll discuss congestive heart failure later in this chapter.)

Changes in the shape of the heart due to HCM may also lead to turbulence of blood. Blood turbulence, or lack of directional flow, can lead to blood clot formation within the heart. The effects can be catastrophic if a clot leaves the heart and enters the circulatory system—a clot to the lungs or the brain can be instantly fatal. More commonly, however, clots are ejected from the left ventricle, travel down the aorta, and lodge at the point where the aorta divides to supply blood to the hind legs. This condition is known as "saddle thrombus" because the clot sits at the branching of the blood vessels.

Saddle thrombi cause instantaneous disruption of the blood supply to the hind legs. Cats with a saddle thrombus will often appear completely normal and then, within just a few seconds or minutes, they'll lose the ability to move their hind legs. The condition is painful, and treatment options are limited. Prognosis in these cats is guarded due to the effects of the clot, the risk of additional clots, and the severity of the underlying cardiac disease.

Restrictive Cardiomyopathy in Cats

Restrictive cardiomyopathy (RCM) is a relatively uncommon condition occurring in cats. Cats with this condition have changes in the heart that affect the elasticity of the cardiac muscle. This lack of elasticity leads to an inability of the heart to fill with adequate amounts of blood, which in turn can lead to congestive heart failure. There is no specific therapy for RCM; diagnostic and treatment options are the same as for cats with HCM.

Dilated Cardiomyopathy in Dogs

Dilated cardiomyopathy (DCM) occurs most frequently in large-breed dogs, most commonly Doberman pinschers, although other breeds are affected as well. In contrast to HCM, this is a condition in which the heart muscle stretches and thins. When this occurs, muscle contractions (heartbeats) are weak and do not efficiently push blood through the body.

Enlargement of the heart due to stretching may affect one or more of the heart valves, leading to turbulence of blood (lack of directional flow), further enlargement, and progression toward congestive heart failure. The stretching of the cardiac muscle in DCM may also cause abnormal heart rhythms, which can lead to fainting episodes.[2, 3] Similar to HCM, the end result of DCM is the heart's inability to move blood, causing fluid backup and congestive heart failure.

Note: Although primarily a disease of dogs, DCM *can* be seen in cats with a taurine deficiency. This is exceptionally rare because taurine is included in all commercially prepared cat diets. It is even added to commercial dog food as a preventive, in case people feed dog food to their cat. Realistically, the only way to cause a taurine deficiency in a cat these days would be to feed them a taurine-deficient home-prepared diet for the long term.

Valvular Disease in Dogs

Heart problems can occur due to a poorly functioning valve, and the mitral valve (MV) is the most common cause of the trouble. The MV sits between the left ventricle and the left atrium. Under normal circumstances, blood from the lungs enters through the left atrium and flows down through the MV into the left ventricle, where it is ultimately pushed out of the heart and into circulation.

Degenerative changes in the MV are known as myxomatous mitral valve degeneration. This is a genetic condition in which the valve slowly deforms over time. The valve leaflets become thickened and misshapen so that it no longer functions efficiently as a one-way valve. When the heart contracts, some of the blood from the left ventricle moves backward and up into the left atrium in a process called regurgitation.

Over time, this turbulent blood flow causes excessive wear on the heart muscle because it has to work harder to maintain adequate circulation. The regurgitation of blood into the left atrium increases pressure within the atrium and causes this part of the heart to stretch and enlarge. The inefficiency of the MV and wear on the heart muscle can ultimately lead to fluid backup and congestive heart failure.

Mitral valve degeneration is most commonly seen in smaller dogs. Some of the more commonly affected breeds are King Charles spaniels, miniature poodles, and cocker spaniels.

Heart Murmurs in Dogs and Cats

The regurgitation of blood through a faulty valve is audible with a stethoscope. The sound is kind of a whooshing and is referred to as a heart murmur. The most common cause of a murmur in small dogs is mitral degeneration. In cats or larger dogs, it is usually due to a poorly functioning valve as a result of HCM or DCM. Some murmurs in pets will remain unchanged over time, while others will progress to congestive heart failure. Any newly diagnosed murmur should be evaluated, particularly those that are progressing.[4, 5]

Young animals can sometimes have an "innocent" murmur. These are mild murmurs that are not indicative of a larger problem. They are caused by normal physiologic changes that occur in the heart shortly after birth, and many will resolve over a period of weeks. Make sure to conduct regular monitoring with your veterinarian, as murmurs that do not resolve or seem to get worse should be evaluated further.

Arrhythmia in Dogs and Cats

Like every other muscle in the body, the heart's activity is controlled by electricity. In order for blood to be moved efficiently throughout the body, contractions (heartbeats) must be regular and coordinated. Contraction of the cardiac muscle begins at the top of the heart and works its way down to the bottom. An inefficient or an irregular heartbeat can be life-threatening.

When electrical conduction through the heart is interrupted or disorganized, the result is an abnormal rhythm, or an arrhythmia. The most common arrhythmia is known as AV block, and it occurs when there is a delay or complete interruption of electrical signals from the top of the heart to the bottom. The condition ranges from mild (first-degree) to severe (third-degree) AV block. In severe cases, medication or even a pacemaker may be required to maintain heart rhythm.

Note that there is a normal physiologic phenomenon called a respiratory sinus arrhythmia. Dogs or cats at rest will frequently have an irregular heart rhythm that goes up and down in time with their respiration. You can feel this by putting your hand on their chest while they are relaxed. The arrhythmia should go away once their heart rate increases, such as when they get up and move around. A respiratory sinus arrhythmia is normal and nothing to worry about.

Congestive Heart Failure in Dogs and Cats

Congestive heart failure (CHF) occurs when the heart muscle can no longer compensate for the stress placed on it by cardiomyopathy or valvular disease. Regardless of the primary cause, the malfunctioning heart muscle is unable to move blood efficiently, so blood backs up in veins with ever-increasing pressure, leading to fluid leakage into parts of the body.

If you have ever done any gardening, you may be familiar with something called a soaker hose. It looks like a garden hose, but it drips water though the walls of the hose to slowly water your garden. In a similar fashion, blood vessels will weep fluid from their walls when pressure within them is high enough.

Depending on the specific nature of your pet's heart disease, this fluid can build up within the lungs (pulmonary edema), outside of the lungs (pleural effusion), or within the abdomen (ascites). Regardless, CHF is an indication of a severely damaged heart muscle and must be treated in order to control the fluid buildup and maintain quality of life.

Diagnosis of Heart Disease

Outward Symptoms

Ideally, cardiac disease in dogs and cats should be diagnosed before there are any symptoms to notice. Once pets are symptomatic, treatment is significantly more complicated.

- **HCM:** Cats with HCM will frequently show no outward signs of problems until they develop CHF or saddle thrombus. Cats with CHF will have lower activity levels due to increased fluid in or around their lungs, which makes it difficult for them to breathe. Cats with a saddle thrombus will be acutely "down" in the back end and frequently experience a lot of pain their hind limbs. Pulses in the hind limbs will be weak, as the clot is obstructing blood flow to the hind legs. The nail beds of the hind feet will also be white or bluish (rather than pink) due to the interrupted blood supply.

- **DCM:** Dogs with DCM most frequently show signs of lethargy as their heart muscle progressively loses its ability to efficiently pump blood through the body. In advanced cases, pets may cough due to fluid buildup in the lungs from CHF or have fainting episodes as a result of arrhythmias.

- **Mitral valve degeneration:** Most dogs with a valve problem have mitral valve degeneration. As turbulence within the heart becomes more severe, the left atrium enlarges and puts pressure on the dog's airways. This leads to coughing, most frequently occurring when the dog is lying down. Dogs experience an overall decrease in energy level due to poor circulation. Eventually, some dogs will progress to CHF, which leads to a worsening cough and breathing difficulties.

- **Arrythmia:** Pets with mild arrhythmias frequently have no outward symptoms. In severe cases, there may be episodic weakness or fainting due to interruption of blood flow to the brain.

Physical Examination

Most heart conditions in dogs and cats are diagnosed during a physical examination. Your veterinarian will use a stethoscope to listen to your pet's heart rhythm and heart sounds.

- **Heart rhythm:** Heart rhythm should be regular. Depending on the stress level of your pet, the rate should be between 80 and 150 beats per minute. Highly stressed cats can have a heart rate of up to 200 beats per minute. Any irregularity in rhythm is cause for further investigation.

    When dogs and cats are very relaxed, they may have an irregular rhythm that increases and decreases in time with their breathing. This is a completely normal phenomenon called a "respiratory sinus arrhythmia," and the arrhythmia should resolve when the animal gets up and moves around.

- **Heart sounds:** Changes in heart sounds often indicate something abnormal within the heart. The abnormality may be primary, such as with mitral valve degeneration, or secondary due to changes in the shape of the heart, such as is seen in HCM or DCM. Once your pet is diagnosed with a murmur, your veterinarian should discuss the possible causes and outcomes with you and whether the murmur necessitates further evaluation.

    The severities of cardiac murmurs are graded on a scale from I to VI. Grade I murmurs are very mild. Grade VI murmurs are so severe, they can be heard in a quiet room without a stethoscope. The more severe the murmur, the greater the chance of your pet developing complications such as CHF.

- **Lung sounds:** Lung sounds may also suggest heart problems in dogs and cats. Listening to the lungs with a stethoscope may reveal "crackles" and "wheezes" that indicate fluid buildup due to CHF. In these cases, your pet's gum color may be pale or even slightly bluish in response to poor circulation.

X-rays

Chest X-rays are a valuable tool for diagnosing suspected heart disease. The images provide an evaluation of heart size and determine if there is fluid buildup in the lungs due to CHF.

Dogs with DCM or mitral valve disease often have visible enlargement of part or all of the heart on X-rays. However, the thickening of the heart muscle in HCM cats tends to happen from the outside in, which leaves the cardiac silhouette unchanged.

Fluid within the chest is also visible radiographically. Fluid is white on X-rays, while the lungs are much darker. Fluid buildup within the lungs (pulmonary edema) due to CHF can be seen as whitening of the lungs on X-rays. Buildup outside the lungs (pleural effusion) appears as white around the lungs and partial lung collapse.

Echocardiogram

A cardiac ultrasound, or echocardiogram, is the best method of definitively diagnosing the type and severity of heart disease. Through this technology, a veterinarian (usually a veterinary cardiologist or radiologist) is able to visualize the beating heart and take measurements that are pivotal in determining treatment options and prognosis.

Electrocardiogram

An electrocardiogram (ECG or EKG) is a graphical representation of the electrical activity of the heart. Everyone has seen these; they are very prominent in TV and movie hospital dramas. Electrodes are attached to the patient's skin, and the connected monitor displays the heart's electrical activity as a little dot that traces peaks and valleys across the screen. An ECG is a valuable tool in evaluating both heart rhythm and electrical activity within the heart. Causes of arrhythmias are diagnosed using ECGs.

Blood Tests

Depending on the severity of the heart disease, abnormalities on a routine blood panel may or may not be present. Even in cases where values are normal, a blood panel is often a valuable tool that establishes a baseline for your pet, because some heart medications can put stress on the kidneys.

A specific test called proBNP (pro B-type natriuretic peptide) can be used to help determine the severity of your pet's heart disease. This test measures an enzyme that elevates when cardiac muscle fibers are stretched or otherwise stressed. The value in proBNP is that it can be used to help evaluate the prognosis of animals with heart problems.

Conventional Medical Treatment

When humans have heart surgery, it is most commonly in the form of a bypass, which restores blood supply to the heart muscle after a heart attack. Pets don't have heart attacks; with the exception of pets in need of a pacemaker, heart surgery is almost never performed. Although there has been some experimentation with mitral valve replacements in dogs, this procedure is far from being perfected.

Heart disease in pets is usually managed medically. Given the spectrum of cardiac diseases and possible medications, a board-certified veterinary cardiologist or veterinary internal medicine specialist with cardiology experience should evaluate your pet whenever possible. While general practitioners can (and do) manage pets with heart disease, subtle nuances in treatment and monitoring through a specialist can make a difference.

The following section describes a few of the most common cardiac drugs used. (The full formulary of cardiac medications is much too long to outline within this chapter.) Your veterinarian will guide you toward the most effective drugs and dosages and an appropriate monitoring schedule.

Hypertrophic Cardiomyopathy

- **Beta-blockers:** Current research indicates that the progression of HCM is not improved by medical therapy.[6, 7] In severe cases, however, cats are frequently started on atenolol (a beta-blocker), which theoretically may improve the function of the mitral valve and thus improve cardiac efficiency.[8]

Saddle Thrombus

Other than time, there is no known effective medical therapy to dissolve a blood clot that has already formed.[9] In some cats, clots will begin to break up within 48 to 72 hours of the onset of symptoms. A cat with a thrombus usually receives pain control while waiting for the clot to dissolve.

- **Clopidrogrel:** This drug is commonly administered to cats who have either previously formed a thrombus or whose heart disease puts them at high risk to form one. The drug is thought to prevent clot formation, but will not dissolve an existing clot.[10, 11]

Dilated Cardiomyopathy

- **ACE inhibitors:** A class of drugs known as ACE inhibitors dilate blood vessels, thus decreasing the pressure that the heart pumps against. They have been shown to prolong the onset of congestive heart failure in dogs with DCM. ACE inhibitors such as enalapril and benazepril are used in the treatment of DCM.[12, 13, 14]

- **Beta-blockers:** The benefits of beta-blocking drugs such as sotalol in pre-CHF dogs is controversial. They *may* help arrhythmias but could also lead to low blood pressure or even CHF. The decision to use these drugs should be made by a veterinary cardiologist.[15, 16]

- **Pimobendan:** This veterinary-specific drug improves the strength of heart contractions and dilates blood vessels. Pimobendan has been shown to prolong survival times in dogs with DCM.[17, 18]

Mitral Valve Degeneration

Mild to moderate mitral valve degeneration requires no treatment from the conventional medical perspective. Treatment strategies for severe disease are the same as for congestive heart failure.

Arrhythmias

There are so many potential causes of arrhythmias in dogs and cats, it is impractical to discuss every potential medication. Drug classes including sodium channel blockers, beta-blockers, and potassium channel blockers are all used for different types of rhythm disturbances. Your veterinarian will decide on the most appropriate medication.

- **Pacemakers:** An interruption of the conduction of electricity between the top of the heart and the bottom is called AV block. When that interruption is severe, the best solution is to place a pacemaker in the chest surgically. This small computer sends regular electrical impulses to regulate the heart rate.

Congestive Heart Failure

The goals of CHF therapy are to decrease pressure within blood vessels to stop the seeping from the walls and facilitate the reabsorption of fluid. Whether the fluid buildup is within the lungs (pulmonary edema), outside the lungs (pleural effusion), or within the abdomen (ascites), treatments for CHF are intended to relieve the fluid congestion and lighten the load on the heart. Most CHF therapies are nonspecific to the underlying cardiac problem.

- **Diuretics:** These drugs, which include furosemide and spironolactone, stimulate urine production and thus decrease total body water. The result is decreased pressure within the blood vessels, leading to reabsorption of fluids built up in the tissues.[19, 20]

- **ACE inhibitors:** These drugs, which include enalapril and benazepril, dilate blood vessels, thus decreasing blood pressure and subsequently stopping the oozing of fluid through vessel walls. If pressure is reduced sufficiently, fluid is reabsorbed into the vessels and, with the help of a diuretic, removed through urination.[21]

- **Positive inotropes:** These drugs, which include digoxin, increase the strength of the contraction of the cardiac muscle. More efficient contractions move blood and limit fluid congestion. Positive inotropes are also used in patients with failure of the cardiac muscle, such as dogs with DCM.[22]

- **Pimobendan:** Going by the brand name Vetmedin, this drug is unique in that it is both a positive inotrope and a vasodilator. Pimobendan is used for both dogs and cats with many types of heart disease.[23]

- **Calcium channel blockers:** These drugs, which include amlodipine, work in a similar way to ACE inhibitors. They specifically dilate arteries, thereby lowering blood pressure and relieving fluid congestion.[24]

Nutrition

Nutritional therapy for heart disease is not a cornerstone of Western medical therapy; often dietary recommendations are not part of a conventional treatment plan. There is a prescription diet for dogs that is low in sodium (to maintain blood pressure) and supplemented with amino acids (L-carnitine and taurine) and antioxidants (to support the heart muscle). No prescription diet currently exists for cats.

When a pet with heart disease loses weight and muscle mass, it is known as cardiac cachexia. This condition is associated with decreased quality of life and decreased survival times.[25] Therefore, be sure to provide a highly palatable diet with a high energy density so that your pet maintains appropriate body weight and muscle mass.

Therapeutic Monitoring

Monitoring the progress of pets being treated for heart disease utilizes the same testing methods that are outlined in the diagnosis section.

- **X-rays:** Monitor overall heart size and the presence (or absence) of fluid within or around the lungs.

- **Echocardiogram:** Objectively measures heart function and progression of heart disease.

- **Electrocardiogram:** An ECG provides valuable information regarding the status of an arrhythmia.

- **Blood testing, including proBNP:** Monitoring general health is important for heart patients on medication. Blood work helps evaluate kidney function, which can be stressed by drugs like ACE inhibitors and diuretics. The proBNP test can provide data regarding ongoing or worsening stress on the heart muscle.

Complementary and Alternative Medical Therapy

There are many potential complementary and alternative therapies for pets with cardiac disease. None of them should be used as replacements for recommended veterinary pharmaceuticals in pets with clinical heart problems. However, many can be used in conjunction with conventional heart medication.

The ideal therapeutic plan is to treat pets before they are symptomatic. For pets with a known familial history of heart disease or those who may be genetically predisposed by breed, early supplementation might delay the onset of disease.

For most pets, however, early treatment means starting supportive therapy at the first sign of trouble—usually the onset of a new murmur. Most early heart murmurs do not warrant pharmaceutical intervention, so this is when complementary therapy may offer its greatest benefit, possibly delaying the beginning of congestive heart failure.

Nutrition

Providing a fresh, whole-food diet to pets with cardiac disease offers a number of advantages. Heart disease puts a lot of stress on the body, which has to expend excess energy to keep the heart functioning at an acceptable level. Just about any fresh, whole-food diet can provide higher-quality, better nutrition than highly processed foods.

Cardiac-specific diets have the added benefit of being lower in sodium, which minimizes fluid retention. In addition, the stress of cardiac disease can lead to depletion of vitamins, minerals, omega fatty acids, and amino acids. The canine and feline cardiac-specific diets listed in Appendix C are designed to provide optimal nutritional support for these pets. Further supplementation as described below may be of benefit depending on the nature and severity of the heart condition your pet has.

Nutritional Supplementation and Herbal Therapy

The following section describes numerous nutritional and herbal supplementation options for pets with heart conditions. Combination products contain many of the following ingredients; however, not every supplement listed below is appropriate for every pet. The stage and nature of the heart problem as well as individual responses to therapy are important factors to monitor.

Remember that heart disease is a serious matter. Maintaining regular veterinary supervision for any treatment (both Western and complementary) is paramount to a successful outcome.

- **Whole-food supplementation:** The primary goal for pets with heart disease is to provide nutritional components to maintain the heart muscle and support the body as a whole. Products like Canine Cardiac Support and Feline Cardiac Support from Standard Process are designed with this in mind. In my experience, Standard Process products are a good example of supplements with little or no downside.

  Caution: Standard Process's Feline Cardiac Support contains hawthorn, which may be problematic for some cats with HCM. If you choose to use this for your HCM cat, monitor for any increase in heart rate and discontinue if it occurs.

- **Vitamins and minerals:** Vitamins, including B and E, and minerals, including magnesium, potassium, and selenium, are all critical in maintaining normal heart function. Look for combination supplements made specifically for pets with heart conditions, as they frequently contain these vitamins and minerals.

- **Amino acids:** For both dogs and cats with heart disease, supplementing with L-carnitine and taurine helps provide the cardiac muscle with the building blocks it needs to stay healthy.[26, 27]

- **Fish oil:** Omega fatty acids seem to have endless benefits in the body, including the heart. Research indicates that fish oil helps maintain a healthy heart and improves function in damaged or diseased heart muscles.[28, 29, 30, 31]

Herbal Therapy

There are many herbs that potentially affect cardiac function in positive ways. Below is a list of herbs that can be used effectively in pets; some products will offer a combination of the following useful herbs. However, any herbal regimen for heart disease should be given under veterinary supervision.[32, 33]

- **Hawthorn:** Of all the herbs used for heart conditions, hawthorn is the most well known. Hawthorn flowers and berries have many of the same effects as pharmaceuticals, including dilating blood vessels, increasing contractility of the heart muscle, and normalizing heart rhythm.[34] These effects are subtler than pharmaceuticals and may benefit pets whose condition does not yet warrant drug intervention.

  There is some concern among veterinarians and herbalists regarding the use of hawthorn in cats with HCM, because hawthorn's ability to increase the force of heart contraction could worsen the condition. The best advice regarding hawthorn and cats is to proceed with caution and discontinue use if heart rate increases.

- **Dandelion leaf:** Pets with advanced cardiac disease or CHF often benefit from a diuretic, and dandelion is the strongest herbal diuretic available.[35] While pharmaceutical diuretics have a more pronounced effect, dandelion leaf may benefit pets with an early-stage disease, prior to their need for medications like furosemide.

  Caution: Any diuretic can put strain on the kidneys. Regularly monitoring kidney values is recommended in these pets.

- **Ginkgo:** Ginkgo is commonly used as a memory aid for humans, but it also dilates blood vessels and improves circulation, making it a good herb to support cardiac health.[36]

- **Yarrow:** Much like ginkgo, yarrow dilates blood vessels and improves circulation, making it a good herb to support cardiac health.[37]

Traditional Chinese Veterinary Medicine

Acupuncture and herbal therapy can be good adjunctive treatments for pets with heart disease to improve their overall well-being. Some herbs can assist in cardiac function and fluid balance. That said, Chinese medicine cannot act as a substitute for pharmaceuticals when they are clinically indicated.

Integrative Treatment Plan

When it comes to heart disease, early diagnosis and treatment are key. Be sure to have regular evaluations by your veterinarian to help pick up on the early signs of a heart murmur or abnormal heart rhythm. Once a patient is in CHF or has developed a saddle thrombus, treatment is more challenging.

Remember that pets with early heart disease look and act normal. The classic mistake made by pet owners is not taking early action. While it is impossible to predict the course any individual's heart disease will take, early treatment through veterinary cardiology evaluation along with complementary care is the best course to an optimal outcome.

For Pets with No Symptoms or Murmur

Consider beginning nutritional and complementary therapy prior to any sign of problems for pets with a familial history of heart disease or breeds with known genetic predispositions such as King Charles spaniels, boxers, Dobermans, and cocker spaniels.

- A fresh, whole-food diet that does not necessarily need to be heart specific
- Whole-food therapy such as Standard Process supplements
- Vitamin and mineral support
- Fish oil

For Pets with Early Heart Disease

These pets may have a mild murmur or arrhythmia. (Any new murmur or arrhythmia should be evaluated by your veterinarian or, if possible, a veterinary cardiologist.) Pets with early disease often do not require pharmaceutical intervention. Begin with the dietary and nutritional therapies listed for pets with no symptoms, then consider the following.

- Prior to the use of pharmaceuticals, consider supplements containing hawthorn, dandelion, ginkgo, and yarrow. If using combination supplements, make certain not to double up on herbs like hawthorn.
  Caution: Hawthorn in cats with HCM is somewhat controversial. If you choose to use it, monitor your cat carefully.
- Traditional Chinese veterinary medicine, especially herbs, may be of benefit.

For Pets with Moderate to Severe Heart Disease

These pets have progressed to requiring pharmaceuticals to maintain their cardiac function and are either already in CHF or are at risk for CHF.

- Begin with dietary and nutritional therapy as previously described—these pets should be on a cardiac-specific diet.

- Use all heart medications exactly as instructed by your veterinarian.

- Exercise caution when using herbs in conjunction with pharmaceuticals, particularly in cats. Combination therapy can be done, but *only* with veterinary supervision.

- Traditional Chinese veterinary medicine, including acupuncture and herbs, may be of benefit in supporting heart function and overall quality of life.

CHAPTER 18

LIVER AND GALLBLADDER DISEASES

Is life worth living? It all depends on the liver.

– WILLIAM JAMES

Tucked up under the diaphragm is a large, brown, lobular organ known as the liver. To the uninitiated, it may look like an amorphous lump, but this vital organ is a real workhorse.

The Liver: Form and Function

The primary role for the liver is to serve as a filter to clean the blood. But that's just the beginning. Liver functions include regulation of glycogen (cellular food) storage, decomposition and recycling of blood cells and blood proteins, hormone production, and detoxification. In addition to all of this, the liver produces bile (stored in the gallbladder), which is vital for digestion and absorption of fats. All told, the liver has at least 500 functions in the body.[1] No wonder it's called the *liver*. We certainly cannot *live* without it!

Unlike some vital organs such as the kidneys, the liver has an amazing ability for self-repair. Liver cells (hepatocytes) are routinely regenerated. As the body's primary organ for detoxification, the liver frequently suffers toxic insults that lead to inflammation, damage, and even death of liver cells. Despite this, the liver endures and is able to maintain its function under most circumstances.

When Things Go Wrong

There are times when the liver is overwhelmed by toxins, infection, or other medical conditions that impair its function. In these cases, a pet may feel sick and need intervention with Western and complementary medical care. The following are some of the most common liver and gallbladder diseases of dogs and cats.

Congenital Liver Disease: Portosystemic Shunt

Small breeds of dogs are sometimes born with a congenital defect called a portosystemic shunt (PSS). In these pets, blood is shunted around the liver rather than being filtered through it. Decreased blood supply prevents the organ from developing properly, and PSS dogs experience problems because of their underdeveloped liver as well as due to unfiltered toxins in their blood.

Acute Liver Disease: Infection and Toxicity

Acute conditions often seem to come out of nowhere, causing a healthy dog or cat to become very sick within hours to days of their onset. Pets with acute liver disease often show general signs of malaise such as low energy, poor appetite, vomiting, and a general loss of well-being. As the condition worsens, the patient may become jaundiced (icteric). This yellowish coloration, caused by a buildup of bilirubin in the blood (see below), shows up in the eyes, mouth, and skin. In severe cases of liver failure, neurologic symptoms such as loss of coordination or seizures may occur as toxic products building up in the blood affect the brain. Liver failure is ultimately fatal if treatment efforts are unsuccessful.

Most commonly, acute liver disease is due to either infection or toxicity. Regardless of the cause, it is called hepatitis, which refers to inflammation within the liver.

- **Infectious hepatitis:** In the case of infectious hepatitis, bacteria get into the liver either through the blood or the gallbladder. (Bacteria from the small intestine can work their way up the bile duct into the gallbladder and then subsequently into the liver.)

  A particular bacterium known as leptospirosis can affect both the liver and kidneys of dogs. Lepto, as it is called, is transmitted when a pet comes in contact with the urine of infected animals, such as through drinking from a contaminated puddle. A leptospirosis infection is quite serious and can be tricky to diagnose and treat.

- **Toxic hepatitis:** Toxic hepatitis can be caused by a wide range of ingested substances including spoiled food, various types of molds, and even certain mushrooms. Both veterinary and human drugs can also cause liver toxicity. Acetaminophen (Tylenol), for example, is highly toxic to cats. The severity of acute toxic hepatitis ranges from mild to life-threatening, depending on the nature of the toxin and the amount ingested.

  One particular toxin to look out for is the artificial sweetener xylitol, which can cause dangerously low blood sugar levels and liver toxicity in both dogs and cats. Xylitol can be found in many low-calorie foods such as sugar-free gum.

Acute Liver Disease: Hepatic Lipidosis

Hepatic lipidosis, or fatty liver disease, is a unique form of liver disease in cats that is caused when they stop eating for any reason. After days or weeks of not eating, the body goes into starvation mode and begins moving fat to the liver for use as fuel. As fat accumulates in the liver, the organ becomes overwhelmed and can no longer function, resulting in acute liver failure. Regardless of why the cat has stopped eating, hepatic lipidosis is a serious condition that must be treated aggressively.

Chronic Liver Disease: Chronic Active Hepatitis

The most common cause of chronic liver disease in dogs is chronic active hepatitis (CAH). (CAH in cats is uncommon.) CAH describes long-standing liver inflammation, which can result from many possible sources: toxicity, infection, and pharmaceuticals such as non-steroidal anti-inflammatory drugs (NSAIDs). Some dogs have a genetic predisposition toward accumulating copper in the liver, leading to copper storage disease and CAH.

Long after the initial cause for the CAH is gone, chronic inflammation persists. The inflammatory process in these pets is an ongoing, self-perpetuating condition requiring long-term care. Chronic liver inflammation can lead to cirrhosis (severe scarring of the liver) and ultimately liver failure. The goals of treatment for pets with CAH are to minimize scarring and maintain liver function.

Due to the slow, smoldering nature of chronic liver disease, these pets tend not to have dramatic symptoms. They are often not jaundiced and may not show overt clinical signs for months or even years. The effects can be low energy, a poorly functioning immune system, and ultimately premature aging, since the liver is not able to efficiently detoxify the body (never mind performing the 499 other functions it's supposed to do).

Hepatic Encephalopathy

Hepatic encephalopathy occurs in animals when greater than 70 percent of their liver function is compromised.[2] Toxins in the blood build up, causing neurologic symptoms that include an altered mental state, loss of motor coordination, seizures, and even death.[3]

Gallbladder Disease

One of the 500 (give or take) functions of the liver is to produce a yellowish, greenish fluid called bile, which accumulates in the gallbladder and is secreted into the small intestine, where it aids in the digestion of fats. If bile is prevented from exiting the gallbladder, the resultant backup leads to inflammation and malfunction of not only the gallbladder but the liver as well. The following are the most common malfunctions of the gallbladder.

- **Cholecystitis:** If bacteria from the intestines work their way into the gallbladder, it can cause an inflammatory process called cholecystitis. Infection of the gallbladder and/or liver can lead to serious complications such as rupture of the gallbladder or compromised liver function.

- **Bile duct obstruction:** The bile duct is a very small tube that traverses from the gallbladder through the pancreas, and ultimately empties bile into the intestine. The most common cause of bile duct obstruction is pancreatic inflammation. Swelling from pancreatitis (see Chapter 15) can compress the bile duct and prevent the flow of bile. The obstruction usually resolves with resolution of the pancreatitis.

- **Gallstones:** Bile is made up of mineral salts, which can crystallize and form small stones. Although rare, gallstones can obstruct the common bile duct, preventing bile from emptying into the intestines.

- **Bile sludging and gallbladder mucocele:** In some pets, bile within the gallbladder will thicken and become sludge. This process slows the flow of bile and may lead to inflammation of the gallbladder and/or liver. The goal of therapy is to reliquefy the bile and restore normal flow.

  Unique to dogs, a gallbladder mucocele is when the normally liquid bile becomes thicker and solidifies into a discrete mass. This obstructs the bile flow and, in severe cases, leads to rupture of the gallbladder, causing severe pain and caustic bile leaks into the abdomen.

Diagnosis of Liver and Gallbladder Disease

When liver cells are damaged or inflamed, they release enzymes into the blood, making liver malfunction readily diagnosable via a blood panel. The following is a look into the interpretations of various liver function tests.

Blood and Urine Analysis

- **Alkaline phosphatase (ALP):** ALP is a nonspecific liver enzyme. In other words, liver damage may cause an elevation in ALP, but a number of other conditions can raise ALP, including Cushing's disease (see Chapter 22), certain types of kidney disease, bone disorders, and gastrointestinal problems. ALP also tends to be elevated in young, growing animals because of their increased bone metabolism. While ALP is a valuable indicator of liver health, its significance must be evaluated alongside other parameters of liver function.

- **Aspartate transaminase (AST):** Like ALP, AST may also be elevated for reasons other than liver problems, such as red blood cell destruction or muscle damage. AST is used to indicate liver disease only in concert with other liver function parameters.

- **Alanine aminotransferase (ALT):** ALT is the most diagnostically important of the liver enzymes because of its specificity to the liver. Elevations in ALT always indicate inflammation, damage, or destruction of liver cells. The higher the ALT, the more severe the liver damage.

- **Gamma glutamyl transferase (GGT):** GGT is an indication of bile flow through the liver. Because bile flows through both the liver and gallbladder, elevations in GGT may indicate problems with either or both organs. Liver damage may lead to an interruption of bile flow and elevated GGT. In these cases, we would expect significant elevations of ALT and the other liver enzymes as well.

  In other circumstances, the liver may be relatively normal and gallbladder disease is preventing bile from emptying into the small intestine. The subsequent backup of bile into the liver will lead to elevated GGT levels with potentially less profound elevations of the other liver enzymes.

- **Bilirubin:** Bilirubin is a breakdown product of hemoglobin from red blood cells. As red cells are destroyed or recycled within the body, the yellow bilirubin is normally filtered by the liver and excreted through the bile. If the liver does not filter bilirubin efficiently, it builds up in the blood. As bilirubin levels increase, the yellow pigment becomes visible as icterus (jaundice) in the mouth, skin, and eyes.

Elevated bilirubin can also be caused by conditions not related to the liver. Specifically, conditions such as autoimmune hemolytic anemia, which causes destruction of red blood cells within the blood vessels, will cause jaundice.

- **Bile acids:** Levels of bile acids in the blood measured before and after eating are used to evaluate liver function. Normally there is a slight elevation of bile acids after eating; however, in animals with poor liver function, bile acid levels may be significantly elevated after food is ingested. Bile acid testing is frequently used to diagnose dogs with suspected portosystemic shunts.

- **Leptospirosis titers:** Specific blood testing can be done in dogs with suspected leptospirosis. The most common test is for antibodies to the lepto bacterium. Since antibody levels indicate exposure and not necessarily active infection, test results can be tricky to interpret. A diagnosis of leptospirosis is often made when testing and symptoms are both suggestive of the disease.

- **Urinalysis:** The presence of bilirubin in urine is potentially an indicator of liver problems in dogs and cats. While a small amount of bilirubin in the urine of dogs can be normal, any amount in cat urine indicates a problem.

Liver Visualization and Tissue Sampling

- **Abdominal ultrasound:** The best method of visualizing the liver of a dog or cat is through abdominal ultrasound. (X-rays offer a more limited view, while surgery is a much more invasive procedure.) With an ultrasound and an experienced veterinarian, the liver and gallbladder can be explored to determine size, shape, and presence of tumors, gallstones, mucoceles, and sometimes even a portosystemic shunt. Ultrasound can also determine the texture of the inside of the liver, which can provide clues as to the underlying problem, such as Cushing's disease or cancer.

    Please note that ultrasound is highly subjective—perhaps more than any other diagnostic test in medicine. I strongly recommend using a board-certified veterinary radiologist (or internal medicine specialist) to perform ultrasounds, as they have the greatest level of training and experience and are therefore most likely to obtain accurate diagnostic information.

- **Tissue sampling:** The collection of tissue samples can be invaluable for diagnosing liver disease. While samples can be obtained through surgery, more frequently they are collected with ultrasound. Using the ultrasound probe for visualization, a needle or biopsy tool is inserted into the liver, and small samples are collected. While there is never a guarantee of an answer, sending samples to the lab is frequently the best way to get a definitive diagnosis of liver disease.

- **Nuclear medicine:** With this technique, a radioactive dye is injected into your pet and a specialized device called a gamma camera is used to watch as the dye filters through (or around) the liver. The pattern and location of the blood movement can help determine if surgical correction is an option. This technique is usually employed when a young dog displays symptoms and blood work suspicious for a portosystemic shunt and an ultrasound is unable to locate it.

Conventional Medical Treatment

Portosystemic Shunt

The only definitive resolution to a PSS is surgical correction, which involves the use of a device called a constrictor band. The band is placed around the abnormal blood vessel and slowly constricts over time, cutting off the blood supply and restoring normal circulation to the liver. It has to be slow because the underdeveloped liver is not able to handle the new onrush of blood all at once.

For some pets, the location and specific nature of their shunts may make surgery impossible, or the risk of restoring full blood supply to their underdeveloped liver is too great. Outside of surgery, all other therapies for PSS focus on the prevention and/or control of hepatic encephalopathy.

Acute Liver Conditions

Depending on the nature of the liver insult, specific therapy to address the underlying cause is sometimes possible. In all cases, however, supportive care that allows the liver time to heal and regenerate is a major part of successful therapy.

The level of supportive care necessary for these pets is dependent on how severe the liver condition is. Severity is determined by a combination of outward symptoms and laboratory results. Very sick pets may require hospitalization, while others can be treated on an outpatient basis. The most common methods of supportive care are fluids, antinausea medications, antibiotics for opportunistic infections, drugs to support bile flow, and a bland, easily digestible diet. The goal is to keep your pet eating and feeling okay during the time their liver needs to recover.

- **Bacterial infection:** In many cases, the specific type of bacteria causing a pet's bacterial hepatitis is not determined, so broad-spectrum antibiotics are used. Two of the most commonly used antibiotics are enrofloxacin (Baytril) and metronidazole (Flagyl). If a dog has contracted leptospirosis, he will frequently require hospitalization, IV fluids, antibiotics, and supportive care during the course of the infection. Sadly, not all dogs survive the infection. There is a vaccine for leptospirosis, although it is not 100 percent effective. Leptospirosis infection in cats is possible but very rare.

- **Toxicity:** Treatment for liver toxicity is generally supportive in nature; specific treatment depends on the nature of the toxicity. Dogs that get into garbage or spoiled food frequently do fine with minimal supportive care. When it comes to more severe toxicity, such as exposure to the artificial sweetener xylitol, or cats exposed to acetaminophen, more aggressive therapy is necessary, including hospitalization, IV fluids, and other supportive measures until the toxicity abates.

- **Hepatic lipidosis:** Therapy for cats with hepatic lipidosis begins with diagnosing and treating any physical problems that led to loss of appetite. In many cats, the underlying cause is never determined, and treatment focuses on getting nutrition into these kitties. Once they start eating again, the condition commonly resolves.

  In mild cases, outpatient treatment including fluids injected under the skin to maintain hydration as well as antinausea and appetite stimulation medications is enough. In more severe cases, however, cats may require hospitalization, IV fluids, antibiotics, and supportive care. Placing a feeding tube is necessary in cats that won't eat. As the lipidosis begins to resolve, often cats will feel better and begin to eat on their own.

Chronic Active Hepatitis

Chronic liver disease frequently does not have a discernible underlying cause. Therapies such as the following focus on long-term liver support.

- **Immunosuppressive therapy:** Drugs like prednisone, azathioprine, or cyclosporine are sometimes used to minimize inflammation as long as there is no infection present.[4, 5, 6]

- **Antifibrotic therapy:** Colchicine has been used in dogs with CAH to limit scar tissue formation in the liver, although its efficacy is unproven.[7]

- **Bile flow:** Ursodeoxycholic acid (Actigall) promotes bile flow through the liver and may decrease inflammation in the process.[8]

- **Copper reduction:** For dogs with copper storage disease, specific therapies like penicillamine are required.[9]

Hepatic Encephalopathy

The goal of therapy for hepatic encephalopathy is to minimize toxicity through addressing the primary liver issue (if possible) and limiting the production of toxic products within the body.

- **Nutrition:** Feeding a highly digestible diet with reduced protein levels limits the production of toxic products such as ammonia. In addition, the more digestible the diet, the less food there is to feed bacteria, further limiting toxic waste products.

- **Antibiotics:** Antibiotics such as metronidazole decrease levels of bacteria in the GI tract, thus limiting their production of toxic waste products.[10]

- **Catharsis:** Regular enemas or a cathartic drug such as lactulose reduces the numbers of colonic bacteria and subsequently the toxic waste products they produce.[11]

Gallbladder

Diseases of the gallbladder are either related to infection or disruption of bile flow. The following are the most common ways to treat these issues.

- **Antibiotics:** Drugs such as enrofloxacin (Baytril) and metronidazole (Flagyl) are used to treat an infected gallbladder in the same way as bacterial hepatitis. Frequently, the conditions are concurrent.

- **Ursodeoxycholic acid:** Ursodeoxycholic acid (Actigall) is used to promote bile flow through the liver and gallbladder. Actigall is commonly used to treat biliary stasis and early mucoceles. It should not be used in cases where bile flow is completely obstructed or a mature mucocele is present. The increased bile flow in such pets can lead to rupture of the gallbladder.[12]

- **Surgery:** Surgery is indicated for pets with signs of biliary obstruction such as those with mature mucoceles or some gallstones.

Complementary and Alternative Therapy

As is the case with Western medical therapy for liver conditions, the goal of complementary and alternative medicine is support. Through nutrition and natural supplementation, we can promote liver healing and limit the side effects of severe liver dysfunction. Any pet with elevated liver enzymes or other signs of liver disease may benefit from complementary care.

Nutrition

It's not uncommon for pet foods to become contaminated with bacterial and/or fungal organisms, both of which can produce toxins that affect the liver. Bacterial endotoxins and afla-toxins are two common problems in commercially prepared diets. In otherwise healthy animals, levels of such toxins in most foods often do not pose a health threat. In pets with underlying liver disease, however, even a small amount can lead to problems.[13, 14, 15, 16, 17, 18]

The goal of a liver support diet is limiting the body's toxin load. Thus, what a liver support diet doesn't contain is as important as what it does. Successful dietary therapy includes a combination of restricting the intake of toxins by feeding a fresh, whole-food diet and providing easily digestible nutrients.

For pets with liver disease, optimal nutrition means a diet moderately restricted in protein and designed specifically to be highly digestible. The lower protein and high digestibility decrease toxins by limiting the production of ammonia and other harmful by-products of the digestive process.[19, 20] Diets formulated for pets with liver disease can be found in Appendix C.

Nutritional and Herbal Supplementation

- **Whole-food supplementation:** Providing whole-food supplements such as Canine (or Feline) Hepatic Support made by Standard Process helps provide supportive nutrients to a stressed or damaged liver.

- **Milk thistle:** Extracts of milk thistle seeds have been shown to both protect liver cells and promote growth of new liver cells.[21] The whole seeds themselves are not biologically active if ingested; only the extracted compounds such as silymarin are effective.[22] Combinations of milk thistle extracts and SAM-e (below) are widely used in veterinary medicine for pets with liver conditions.

- **S-adenosylmethionine:** Better known as SAM-e, this supplement promotes the formation of the antioxidant glutathione within the liver, which is known to be highly protective of the liver.[23] Combinations of SAM-e and milk thistle extracts are widely used in veterinary medicine for pets with liver conditions.

- **B vitamins:** The spectrum of B vitamins, including folic acid and choline, are highly supportive of liver function and help protect against liver damage.

- **Antioxidants:** A variety of antioxidants—including vitamins C and E, coenzyme Q10 (CoQ10), and alpha lipoic acid—are known to protect the liver from damage and prevent liver scarring.[24, 25, 26]

- **Curcumin:** The active compound in the herb turmeric, curcumin has been shown to have both anti-inflammatory and antioxidant activities within the liver.[27]

Hyperbaric Oxygen Therapy

The use of hyperbaric oxygen therapy has been shown to improve liver function and facilitate healing after toxic exposure or liver/gallbladder injury.[28, 29]

Traditional Chinese Veterinary Medicine

Acupuncture and herbal therapy can be good adjunctive treatments for pets with liver disease. They may improve pets' overall well-being, and some herbs work in the same ways as those discussed above. That said, Chinese medicine should not act as a substitute for Western medical care.

Integrative Treatment Plan

Despite being a very forgiving organ, the liver must be treated with care. The best thing to do with regard to liver disease is to prevent it. Feeding high-quality foods and limiting the amounts of drugs, pesticides, and other toxins your pet is exposed to will save their liver a lot of heartache. The less that goes in, the better.

Acute Liver Disease

Acute liver conditions due to infection, toxicity, or a sudden interruption of bile flow are largely the purview of Western medicine. Appropriate use of antibiotics, anti-inflammatory drugs, supportive care, and occasionally surgery is necessary to successfully treat acute liver disease. Follow your veterinarian's recommendations with regard to diagnostic testing and treatment for these pets.

You can use liver-supportive supplements in acute cases where the dog or cat is eating, particularly the combination of milk thistle extract and SAM-e. The other vitamins and antioxidants noted above may be of benefit. Be cautious in your use of supplements; attempting to feed too many medications and supplements can lead to upset tummies and vomiting.

If it is available, hyperbaric oxygen therapy is an excellent treatment modality for inflamed and/or damaged livers. Treatment with HBOT, in conjunction with conventional Western therapy, will often help your pet get better faster.

Chronic Liver Disease

Western medicine is a little short on treatment options for chronic liver conditions. The first step of treatment should be to avoid any drugs that are not absolutely necessary, including flea, tick, and heartworm products, as they all eventually have to be processed by the liver. Anti-inflammatory drugs used for arthritis, especially NSAIDs, are to be avoided in particular. Prednisone or similar steroids may be of benefit in decreasing inflammation but may also have long-term side effects, so keep the dose as low as possible. (This can often be achieved through integrative care.)

Use both food and supplements to support a chronically inflamed liver. A liver-supportive diet minimizes the toxic load on a damaged liver, and appropriate supplementation keeps inflammation and scarring to a minimum.

Chronic liver disease is a condition for which multiple supplements will likely be of benefit. Excellent combination products for liver support are available for dogs and cats.

Hyperbaric oxygen therapy may be of benefit, although the effects are likely to be less dramatic compared to acute liver issues. Therapy will, however, often improve quality of life for these pets if they are experiencing symptoms related to CAH.

CHAPTER 19

RENAL DISEASE

The kidney is the organ of water and fire, the abode of yin and yang, the sea of essence, and it determines life and death.

— Zhang Jie-Bin, Famous Chinese Doctor (1563–1640)

In traditional Chinese medicine, the kidneys house *jing*, or the essence of qi. As the repository of life energy, the kidneys are among the most important organs from a Chinese medical perspective. In Western medicine, the kidneys are viewed in equally high regard, albeit for different reasons.

The Kidneys: Form and Function

The kidneys are a pair of organs within the abdomen, just behind the ribcage and one on either side of the spine. They play a part in the production of red blood cells, maintain water balance (hydration), and excrete waste through the urine.[1, 2] In addition, the kidneys play a vital role in regulating body pH, electrolytes, and blood pressure. Regardless of the medical philosophy, kidney health and overall health are inexorably linked.

The kidneys function primarily as a filter. Blood flows into the kidney, where waste products and some fluids are removed. In a complex process of active and passive filtration, the kidneys remove waste products and excrete (or reabsorb) electrolytes in order to maintain the proper balance in the blood. When all is said and done, clean, pH- and electrolyte-balanced blood reenters the body, while the material removed from the blood (urine) passes into the urinary bladder. Like many other functions within the body, this incredibly complex process carries on every second of every day.

Regardless of the nature of the kidney problem, there are two vital constants to remember:

- The number of kidney cells our pets are born with is the most they ever have. The body cannot make new kidney cells, and medical science has not perfected the means to grow more cells. Preserving kidney cells (nephrons) is of paramount importance, as any cell that dies is lost forever.

- The two major indicators of kidney function measured with blood tests are blood urea nitrogen (BUN) and creatinine; elevated levels are called azotemia. When azotemia of any degree is caused by kidney dysfunction, it means that at least 75 percent of the kidney cells are not functioning. Even mild azotemia can be a sign of severe loss of kidney function.

When Things Go Wrong

As elegantly designed as biology may be, things can go wrong. In the case of the kidneys, an injury or malfunction may lead to renal insufficiency or failure. The more commonly seen causes of kidney damage are toxicity, loss of blood supply, infection, inflammation, and acute or chronic dehydration.

Renal Toxicity

Toxicity refers to the kidneys being exposed to compounds that either damage or kill kidney cells. The kidneys may sustain varying levels of damage based on the type and amount of toxin they are exposed to. In many cases, toxins lead to relatively minor damage that may or may not contribute to chronic kidney disease later in life. There are circumstances, however, in which renal toxicity can be fatal. The most common (and potentially serious) renal toxic substances for dogs and cats are:

- Antifreeze (ethylene glycol)

- Pharmaceuticals, including ibuprofen and other nonsteroidal anti-inflammatory drugs (NSAIDs)

- Excess vitamin D (This is most frequently caused by rat/mouse poison.)

- Grapes and raisins (The exact nature of grape toxicity is unclear, and only a minority of pets are affected. When it occurs, however, the toxicity is severe and there is no way to predict which pet will get sick.)

If a pet ingests any of the above toxins, they require immediate and aggressive medical therapy even if they are acting and feeling fine. In most cases, hospitalization (often for days), IV fluid therapy, and specific treatment for the toxicity is necessary. Acute renal toxicity may lead to acute renal failure; not all patients survive.

Loss of Blood Supply

Loss of blood supply, or ischemia, to the kidneys can occur because of severe dehydration. In these cases, the kidneys may shut down and cease to function altogether. More commonly, however, the kidneys suffer a focal infarct, meaning the death of cells or tissue because of the loss of blood supply.

Small renal infarcts are often not recognized at the time they occur. Commonly, they are incidental findings picked up during ultrasound evaluation of the kidney of an older animal (cats in particular). Because infarcts represent the loss of kidney cells, they may contribute to renal insufficiency or failure in pets whose kidney function is otherwise compromised.

Infection

While bladder infections are seen in female dogs and cats, kidney infections are rare. The severity of kidney damage caused by a kidney infection can vary from minor to severe, depending on the type of bacteria, severity of infection, length of infection, and the relative level of kidney function when the infection occurs. Infections are occasionally acquired through bacteria in the blood, but usually occur when the bacteria from a bladder infection travels upstream through the ureter and into the kidney. When this occurs, a potentially serious medical condition can arise from a simple urinary tract infection. Pets with a kidney infection may strain to urinate, dribble urine, show blood in the urine, lick their urogenital area, or act generally sick.

One particularly serious blood-borne infection of the kidneys is called leptospirosis. Contracted through drinking water contaminated with urine from infected animals, leptospirosis can cause liver and/or kidney failure. While very rare in cats, leptospirosis in dogs can be fatal.

Inflammation (Glomerulonephritis)

A structure within the kidney called the glomerulus acts as a filter for the blood. Occasionally this filter becomes inflamed, clogged, and unable to function properly. Glomerular inflammation, known as glomerulonephritis, can damage the entire kidney and may lead to kidney failure. Pets with glomerulonephritis may show no symptoms until the condition progresses to kidney failure.

Dehydration

Of all possible insults to kidney cells, dehydration is the most common culprit, causing long-term damage. Severe dehydration arising when an animal has no access to water for days or weeks can be lethal, but is relatively uncommon. The bigger concern is long-term, low-level dehydration that often occurs when animals are eating very low-moisture-content foods such as kibble and are not drinking enough water. Mild dehydration has no real symptoms but has the potential to put excessive strain on the kidneys. Subclinical (no symptoms) dehydration may lead to several kidney-related problems.

When a dog or cat is in a dehydrated state, their kidneys may not receive an adequate blood supply. The effect can be the loss of function and/or death of kidney cells. The slow loss of kidney cells over a long period of time (usually years) is most commonly how pets find themselves in a state of renal compromise rather than there being a single event that causes massive kidney damage.

There is some debate over whether feeding a pet (cats in particular) food that is very low in moisture, such as kibble, contributes to the onset of kidney disease. While plenty of cats eat dry food and live long lives, there is no question that cats with renal disease should be on high-moisture-content diets.

Kidney Failure

Kidney failure is when your pet's kidneys are no longer able to maintain the body in a normal state. Not all kidney failure is permanent, though. If kidney cells are sick, they may be able to come back and return to function. Kidney cells that have died, however, cannot be replaced.

- **Acute renal failure:** Acute renal failure (ARF) describes a process in which the kidneys of a dog or a cat shut down suddenly. Pets with ARF act sick and may be lethargic, not eating, and/or vomiting. ARF is relatively uncommon and usually the result of a toxic or infectious insult to the kidneys. It is a medical emergency and requires intensive care. Prognosis for these patients varies and is based on the degree of toxicity and how quickly treatment was initiated.[3]

- **Chronic renal failure:** The vast majority of kidney problems in pets are related to chronic renal failure (CRF). While CRF occurs in dogs, it is much more frequently encountered in cats.

  The first sign of CRF in pets is usually an increase in water consumption or urinary output. As the kidneys fail, they lose their ability to conserve body water by concentrating the urine, so they produce large volumes of dilute urine instead. To compensate for the fluid loss, these pets will drink more water.

In veterinary medicine, the term for increased urination is polyuria (PU) and increased water intake is polydipsia (PD). When veterinarians describe these symptoms, they are often referred to as PU/PD. There are numerous medical conditions that cause PU/PD; CRF is one of the most common.

In addition to PU/PD, pets with chronic kidney disease often experience weight loss, decreased appetite, and dehydration. As the condition progresses and dehydration becomes more severe, pets will often stop drinking water because they feel sick, worsening their state. The prognosis for pets with CRF can be good in the short to medium term (months to years) if they receive appropriate care. For most pets, however, CRF will continue to progress over time, and quality of life becomes an issue.

Diagnosis of Kidney Disease and Therapeutic Monitoring

Diagnosing kidney disease is primarily accomplished through blood and urine analysis as detailed below. Once treatment is initiated, progression of kidney disease is monitored in the same way, so treatment recommendations can be based on the type and relative severity of the kidney problem. (CRF therapy, in particular, can be determined through staging, as described below.)

Blood Work

- **Creatinine:** Creatinine is a by-product of muscle metabolism and is normally filtered by the kidneys. Elevations in creatinine indicate either loss of kidney function or dehydration (or both). When the kidneys are not functioning optimally, blood creatinine becomes elevated and can ultimately make the patient feel sick.

- **Blood urea nitrogen:** Blood urea nitrogen (BUN) is a by-product of protein digestion. Because of this, pets eating high-protein diets or those with a bleeding ulcer may have elevated BUN levels. An elevated BUN with a normal creatinine level may be normal in pets eating a raw or other high-protein diet. BUN levels must be interpreted within the context of other lab results and the symptoms present.

- **Symmetric dimethylarginine:** Symmetric dimethylarginine (SDMA) is a relatively new parameter used to evaluate kidney function. Whereas elevations in BUN and creatinine indicate compromise of 75 percent of kidney function, SDMA begins to elevate when 40 percent of function is lost. SDMA allows for much earlier detection of kidney disease—even before outward symptoms arise.

- **Electrolytes:** Pets with abnormal kidney function often have abnormal levels of potassium and/or phosphorus. Maintaining appropriate levels of both improves quality of life for pets with kidney disease.

- **Hematocrit:** Hematocrit (HCT), also known as packed cell volume (PCV), is a measure of the percentage of the blood that is made up of red blood cells. In other words, HCT is a measure of whether a pet is anemic. Pets with CRF are frequently anemic, as their kidneys are not producing a hormone called erythropoietin, which stimulates the bone marrow to make red blood cells.

Urinalysis

Evaluation of urine is important for the diagnosis of kidney problems. In particular, three parameters are commonly evaluated:

- The presence (or absence) of bacteria

- Urine specific gravity, or urine concentration

- Levels of protein in the urine (High levels may be indicative of glomerulonephritis. A secondary test, a urine protein-to-creatinine ratio, may be run to make this determination.)

Blood Pressure

Pets with CRF frequently have high blood pressure. Controlling blood pressure through medication can help pets feel better and slow the progression of the kidney disease.

Ultrasound Imaging

While not always part of the diagnostic pathway for pets with kidney disease, ultrasound can be a valuable tool. Ultrasonic evaluation of the kidneys can help diagnose kidney infections, kidney damage such as infarcts, or genetic anomalies that may predispose a pet to kidney disease later in life.

IRIS and Evaluating Stages of Kidney Disease

The International Renal Interest Society (IRIS) has developed a four-stage system describing the severity levels of renal insufficiency or failure. Pets with kidney disease are often evaluated, or staged, based on IRIS guidelines. This allows a veterinarian to more easily determine treatment guidelines and prognosis.

IRIS stages of kidney disease range from mild (Stage 1) to severe, end-stage kidney failure (Stage 4). Staging is determined by evaluating creatinine, urine protein, and blood pressure. Specifics of IRIS staging and their accompanying treatment recommendations are laid out in great detail on the IRIS website: www.iris-kidney.com.

Not all veterinarians strictly follow the IRIS system for staging and treatment recommendations. Renal insufficiency or failure can be successfully managed without determining IRIS staging. However, the system is an excellent guideline for diagnosis and conventional medical treatment recommendations.

Conventional Medical Treatment

Acute Renal Failure

Therapy for ARF centers on inpatient hospitalization. Pets with ARF require fluid therapy, antibiotics, medications to regulate urination and blood flow to the kidneys, and careful monitoring. Prognosis for these pets is variable depending on the underlying cause of the kidney damage. Once stabilized, long-term conventional and/or complementary therapy may be necessary to manage any lasting kidney damage.

Chronic Renal Failure

Once a pet is diagnosed with CRF, there are many treatment options, mostly centering on hydration, maintaining blood flow to the kidneys, and supporting quality of life by normalizing parameters such as electrolytes and hematocrit. The intensity of treatment is directly proportional to the severity of the kidney failure.

Following is an outline of therapeutic options. Detailed treatment protocols organized by species and IRIS staging can be found at the IRIS website: www.iris-kidney.com.

- **Antibiotics:** Any underlying urinary tract infection should be treated to help preserve remaining kidney function.

- **Remove potential toxins:** Most drugs and chemicals are processed in the body by the kidneys and/or the liver; therefore, when either organ is compromised, all nonessential drugs should be stopped to preserve organ function. This includes NSAIDs and flea and tick medication. (Flea control can be used on an as-needed basis if necessary.)

- **Fluid therapy and hydration:** Pets with CRF always tend toward dehydration. When they are sick or in an advanced stage of CRF, hospitalization and IV fluid therapy may be necessary. For home care of stable pets, increasing water consumption is the first goal. (Please see Chapter 2 for detailed advice on increasing your pet's water intake.)

- **Supplemental fluids:** When pets are urinating more fluid than they are ingesting daily, they are dehydrating. In these instances, subcutaneous fluids are literally a lifesaver. Fluids are injected under the skin on a regular basis to make up for daily fluid deficits. Your veterinarian can show you how to do this.

- **Lower blood pressure:** Normalizing the high blood pressure that is common in pets with CRF helps preserve kidney function and maintain quality of life. Renal diets are restricted in sodium in order to keep blood pressure low. The most commonly used medications to control blood pressure in pets are benazepril or enalapril in dogs and amlodipine (Norvasc) in cats.[4, 5, 6]

- **ACE inhibitors:** The presence of excessive protein in the urine (proteinuria) is an indication of glomerular dysfunction. A class of drugs called ACE inhibitors decreases the blood pressure as it enters the kidney, thus decreasing the amount of protein pushed through the glomerulus. The most commonly used ACE inhibitors in pets are benazepril and enalapril.[7, 8]

- **Phosphate binders:** Phosphorus is a vital mineral; however, problems arise when failing kidneys are unable to excrete it as normal. Two options to lower phosphorus are to restrict it in the diet and to prevent ingested phosphorus from being absorbed. Since most dietary phosphorus is found in protein, phosphorus (and protein) restriction is one of the main parameters of a renal diet. In addition to diet, phosphate binders, such as aluminum hydroxide and calcium carbonate, are used to bind phosphorus and prevent it from being absorbed. Phosphate binders are effective, but only work when mixed in with food.[9, 10]

- **Potassium supplements**: Potassium supplements can be valuable even in patients whose levels appear normal. It is possible (and probably quite common) for patients in kidney failure to still have normal blood potassium levels while being low in total body potassium. Too little potassium can cause malaise, weakness, and in extreme circumstances, death.[11]

- **Iron supplements:** Animals with kidney failure are frequently anemic due to the kidneys not producing the hormone erythropoietin (EPO), which stimulates red blood cell production in the bone marrow. Injectable EPO along with iron supplementation can be given to stimulate red blood cell production.[12]

- **Nutrition:** Kidney disease represents perhaps the greatest use of veterinary prescription diets. Many Western veterinarians recommend these diets for all their patients with renal disease. They are designed to be highly digestible and have lower levels of protein, phosphorus, and sodium as a means of limiting BUN and phosphorus and reducing high blood pressure. These diets frequently contain extra omega fatty acids, as there is evidence that EFAs help these pets live longer.

However, these diets have several shortcomings: (1) many pets don't like the renal diets, resulting in weight loss and malaise, (2) the ingredients and amount of processing in most prescription diets are far from ideal, and (3) many veterinarians reach for a renal diet too early. (IRIS recommends starting these diets at Stage 2 for cats and Stage 3 for dogs. Even that may be too soon, as is explained in the nutrition section of complementary care below.) Restricting protein in these pets too early may do more harm than good.

Complementary and Alternative Medical Therapy

When it comes to acute renal failure, intensive Western medical therapy is primarily what is required. That said, acupuncture is a valuable adjunctive therapy for hospitalized pets. A trained acupuncturist can help with nausea and appetite, and possibly support kidney function in these patients. Most veterinarians are open to allowing hospitalized pets to receive acupuncture as long as it does not interfere with the pet's conventional medical treatments.

When it comes to chronic renal failure, complementary and alternative medicine has a lot to offer. Therapy begins with nutrition and expands from there. The discussion below includes a lengthy list of herbs and supplements that have potential to benefit these dogs and cats. You don't have to give all of them to have a positive effect. However, it is possible to give many of them by using high-quality combination supplements specifically formulated for dogs and cats. Because of the ever-changing landscape of supplements, consult with a veterinarian or a nutritionist regarding which combination products are the best currently available.

Nutrition

The basic philosophy regarding an optimal diet for a dog or cat with renal disease is more or less the same as for the prescription diets: a highly digestible diet with restricted levels of protein, phosphorus, and sodium as a means of limiting BUN, phosphorus, and high blood pressure. The most significant advantage a fresh, whole-food renal diet has over its commercially prepared counterparts is palatability. Dogs and especially cats love their protein, and diets restricted in protein may not be as tasty, leading to less food intake and unwanted weight loss.

There is some debate regarding the relative benefits of plant versus animal protein in renal diets. Despite some possible benefits of plant proteins, the greater bioavailability and palatability of animal proteins make them more desirable.[13]

When it comes to renal diets, the biggest question is: When do you start feeding a renal diet? One of the reasons IRIS recommends starting renal diets when it does is to get your pet used to eating a lower-protein diet while they still feel good. Thus, when they are in the later stages of kidney failure and don't feel great, they are already accustomed to the lower-protein food. Since home-prepared diets are more palatable in general, pets may be able to start a renal diet later in the progression of their renal disease.

Whole-Food Supplementation

Whole-food supplements for kidney support such as Canine Renal Support and Feline Renal Support from Standard Process are great foundational supplements. Along with a whole-food diet, providing these pets with the nutritional elements needed to support the kidneys is an excellent way to further their nutritional advantage in the face of kidney problems.

Essential Fatty Acids

The benefits of supplementing EPA and DHA in the form of fish oil or other marine oils are well documented. Not surprisingly, there is evidence to show these beneficial fats support kidney function as well.[14, 15]

Probiotics

Probiotics are advantageous for any pet, given how effectively they support the GI tract and the immune system. There are, however, specific probiotics designed for pets with renal disease. The goal of these products is to trap toxins in the GI tract so they won't need to be filtered by the kidneys. The most widely used product in the veterinary world is Azodyl. (One important note about Azodyl is it must be administered as an intact capsule. Opening the capsule and putting it on food diminishes its efficacy.)

Herbal, Vitamin, and Amino Acid Therapy

- **Astragalus:** A traditional Chinese herb, astragalus is commonly used in pets and humans with kidney disease. Studies suggest there may be benefit, although the research is not definitive.[16, 17]

- **Arginine:** The amino acid arginine has been shown to increase blood flow to the kidney as well as the rate at which blood is filtered through the glomerulus.[18] These effects should be beneficial for pets with CRF, although caution is advised in pets with glomerulonephritis. When excessive protein is in the urine, pushing more fluid through the glomerulus may exacerbate the problem.

- **Cordyceps:** A mushroom commonly used in Chinese medicine, Cordyceps has been shown to decrease renal scarring and improve function in patients with kidney disease.[19, 20]

- **Dong quai:** This Chinese herb also known as *Angelica sinensis* has been used to treat patients with chronic kidney disease. Dong quai is frequently used along with astragalus.[21]

- **Ginkgo:** A well-known herb used for memory support, ginkgo has been shown to protect the kidneys from damage and support healing of damaged kidney cells.[22, 23]

- **Glutamine:** The amino acid glutamine has been shown to increase production of arginine, which supports the kidneys.[24]

- **Green tea**: Research indicates that the polyphenol antioxidants in green tea protect the kidneys against free radical (oxidative) damage.[25, 26]

- **Melatonin:** This hormone that is naturally secreted by the pineal gland is mostly known for its ability to help regulate sleep, but it also protects the kidneys against damage from free radicals.[27]

- **Milk thistle:** Milk thistle protects kidney cells from damage, and extracts of milk thistle such as silymarin are known to be very supportive of the liver.[28] Adding liver support for a patient with kidney disease is always advisable given that the liver may have to pick up the slack as the other major detoxifying organ in the body.

- **N-acetylcysteine:** N-acetylcysteine has many uses in Western medicine, including a proven ability to support the kidneys and slow the progression of renal failure.[29]

- **Rehmannia:** Another traditional Chinese herb, Rehmannia has been shown to be highly protective of the kidneys after injury or loss of blood supply (ischemia).[30, 31]

- **Rhubarb:** Also commonly used in Chinese medicine, rhubarb has been shown to protect the kidneys and overall to "improve the therapeutic effect of conservative management" in patients with advanced kidney disease.[32]

- **Vitamins B and C:** Pets with kidney disease are at risk for a deficiency of the water-soluble vitamins B and C due to increased urinary loss. (Low levels of vitamin B are associated with malaise and poor appetite, which may hasten the progression of kidney failure.)

Traditional Chinese Veterinary Medicine

Acupuncture and herbal therapy are excellent adjunctive treatments for pets with kidney disease. As noted above, quite a few traditional Chinese herbs have been studied and shown to positively affect kidney function. In addition, acupuncture itself has been shown to improve kidney function.[33, 34] That said, Chinese medicine should not be used as a substitute for fluid therapy and pharmaceuticals for kidney support when they are clinically indicated.

Stem Cell Therapy

The use of stem cells in veterinary medicine began with dogs and cats with arthritis. In the past several years, however, stem cells have been successfully used in the treatment of cats with chronic renal failure. I have personally performed the procedure on multiple cats, with overall positive results. Not surprisingly, the earlier these pets are treated, the better they seem to do.

Integrative Treatment Plan

As with so many other medical challenges, the key to success with kidney failure is early diagnosis and treatment. Veterinarians frequently recommend routine annual blood testing as pets get a little older. There is no better way to diagnose kidney disease (and many other conditions) in its earliest stages. A short-term decision made for financial reasons could literally delay treatment for a year or more. When diagnosed relatively early, pets frequently live for years with appropriate integrative therapy.

Acute Renal Failure

Treat your pet with ARF primarily with Western medicine. Consider acupuncture for hospitalized pets, as it can be of great benefit for nausea and appetite, and potentially support kidney function. Once pets are discharged and back home, continue acupuncture and start an herbal therapy regimen. The best herbal supplements for these pets will depend on the condition of their kidneys, so a consultation with a veterinarian experienced with herbal therapy is recommended.

Chronic Renal Failure

This is the condition for which integrative care provides the most benefit. As seen above, there is no shortage of herbs and supplements with scientifically proven ability to support the kidneys.

With regard to Western medicine, the guidelines for treatment of dogs and cats with kidney disease are laid out in exquisite detail on the IRIS website: www.iris-kidney.com. Work with your veterinarian and use the IRIS recommendations to determine the most effective therapy. That said, not every drug that is recommended is absolutely necessary. Unless there is a crisis, the best plan is to add one drug at a time and monitor for effect.

In concert with appropriate therapy and monitoring from the Western medical perspective, integrating complementary care is strongly recommended. In particular, consider the following:

- All pets with kidney disease should be on a fresh, whole-food diet. Do not feed dry food of any kind. A renal-specific diet may not be necessary until BUN and creatinine are high enough to make pets feel ill.

- Encourage water consumption and add water to food if possible.

- Begin acupuncture and herbal therapy as described above.

- Combination nutritional and herbal supplements are an excellent way to give multiple supplements at once.

- Investigate for availability of stem cell therapy for cats with renal disease.

CHAPTER 20

CANCER

You never know how strong you are until being strong is your only choice.

– BOB MARLEY

Within the realm of medicine, few terms elicit the visceral response that arises when *cancer* is discussed. By the time we reach adulthood, most of us have been personally affected by cancer. The dreaded disease strikes unexpectedly and threatens to claim life and limb from our friends, family, and beloved pets.

Treating pets with cancer is a challenging medical problem and an emotionally taxing experience. As we all know, in many cases cancer is fatal. While dogs and cats can live years longer than expected with aggressive integrative care, many of these pets will ultimately lose the battle.

There is, however, a wonderful lesson to be learned from the veterinary cancer patient. Animals live in the moment every day. They have no self-pity; they don't think, *Why me?* They live every day without fear of death or disease. As long as they are not in pain, every day is a blessing. This is the most valuable piece of wisdom I have ever received from my patients. A good example is Tyler the golden retriever.

Success Story: Tyler

At our first meeting, Tyler was 10 years old and diagnosed with a tumor called an osteosarcoma on his right hind leg. Osteosarcomas are painful tumors with a high rate of metastasis to other parts of the body. Given the nature of the tumor, conventional medical options were limited, and Tyler's quality of life was of great concern. He was limping and in great pain, and his regular veterinarian and an oncologist both recommended amputation and chemotherapy.

Although the thought of amputation is upsetting to pet owners, it is sometimes the best way to eliminate a source of cancer pain and possibly prevent metastasis. Given Tyler's age, however, the owner elected to delay the amputation as long as possible and see if we would be able to keep Tyler comfortable through alternative medicine.

We began by changing Tyler's diet from a good-quality kibble to a fresh, raw-food diet. We also began a spectrum of nutritional and herbal supplements with the goal of supporting optimal body and immune system function while providing anticancer effects. Three months into his treatment, Tyler's tumor had not changed much in size, but he was much more comfortable.

By month four, however, Tyler's pain was increasing, so the owner elected to amputate the leg with the bone tumor. After a few days of recovery, the dog was up and around and happy. In fact, he was notably more energetic than he was before the surgery because the source of his pain was gone. Tyler continued to do great for another 14 months with a combination of complementary medicine and chemotherapy.

One day Tyler started coughing and an X-ray showed tumors in his lungs. Tyler's quality of life deteriorated quickly, and he was euthanized not long after the discovery of the lung tumors.

Although Tyler eventually succumbed to the cancer, he lived far longer and with better quality of life than anyone would have expected. This was accomplished by successfully changing the conditions within his body to optimize health and create an inhospitable environment for cancer cells.

In the medical sense, animals like Tyler embody the powerful biological drive to survive. A biological system never gives up and will work to the very end to stay alive and get healthy. Holistic medicine relies on this innate programming. Even in cases where the prognosis is poor, we can optimize the immune system to help fight cancer, use anticancer herbs to slow or stop the progression of disease, and leverage nutrition in a way that feeds the body and not the tumor.

When Things Go Wrong: What Is Cancer?

Cancer takes many forms and affects pets and people in many ways. Cancer is described as a disease in which cells reproduce inappropriately, leading to tumor formation. Under normal conditions, the body replaces old or damaged cells through mitosis, or division of cells. Cellular division is kept in check by certain body processes, including a mechanism called contact inhibition that turns off mitosis and prevents overcrowding when cells are touching one another. Mutations that turn off contact inhibition cause unregulated cell growth, or cancer.

The origins of cancer are less clear. Cancer may arise from a host of sources including exposure to toxins, viruses, chronic inflammation, and genetic influence. Much of cancer research focuses on discovering specific abnormalities occurring within cancer cells. There are two main competing theories regarding the nature of these abnormalities.

Most current research is founded on the premise that errors in DNA and gene replication lead to cellular malfunction and cancer.[1, 2] An alternative view of cancer is that it is a malfunction of a cell's ability to generate energy. In 1931, Dr. Otto Warburg evaluated cancer cells and theorized that the primary malfunction is within the mitochondria rather than the DNA. Changes within the cell as a response to the damaged mitochondria lead to secondary changes in DNA and gene expression and ultimately to cancer.[3] This process is known as the Warburg effect.

Regardless of the cause, in its earliest stages cancer occurs at the microscopic level. Although the exact figures are unknown, it is theorized that people (and presumably pets) develop cancer many times in their lives but the cancerous cell(s) are either destroyed or held in check by a process called immune surveillance. It is only when the cancerous cells evade immune surveillance that the cells replicate and cancer as a clinical disease occurs.[4, 5]

Many of the complementary and alternative therapies discussed in the sections below focus on supporting the immune system and immune surveillance. By the time cancer is diagnosed, however, more definitive measures are frequently needed to return pets to health.

Types of Cancer

Cancer is more than a single disease. There are many different cancers, each with its own pattern of behavior and susceptibility to treatment. While determining the specific type of cancer is paramount to Western medical therapy, it is not as important in the development of a holistic treatment protocol. Despite this, there are a couple of distinctions regarding cancer that are important to make.

Frequently, *benign* is thought of as "good" and *malignant* as "bad"; that is about 75 percent correct. Medically speaking, the term *benign* is used in several ways.

Benign can be used to describe a noncancerous growth like a skin tag, and it can also be used to describe certain cancerous masses. The distinction of a benign cancer is that it is not expected to metastasize (spread) to distant sites in the body.

Clearly, not metastasizing is a good thing. Unfortunately, this does not make a benign tumor harmless. If a tumor grows large enough or occurs in a very sensitive part of the body, its mere presence can lead to major complications. For example, a benign cancer growing in the brain may not metastasize, but its mere location can cause a massive problem. Additionally, benign tumors arising from glandular tissue may secrete hormones affecting the body.

In contrast to benign tumors, malignant masses tend to metastasize. They don't always do so, but the risk is ever present; treatment decisions are frequently made based on a tumor's metastatic potential. Even a small malignant mass that may not be causing any immediate danger should be removed (if possible) if there is a high metastatic potential. This would not be the case for a benign tumor in the same location. Once the tumor has spread, the horses are out of the barn (so to speak), and the hopes of achieving a cure drop dramatically.

The other major differentiator of cancer is whether it is a solid mass or is disseminated.

Solid tumors are growths that occur either on the surface or within the body. Solid tumors can be either benign or malignant.

Disseminated cancer describes cancer of various blood cells, such as lymphoma and leukemia. Because these cancers affect the blood, they do not occur in one place such as with a solid tumor. Disseminated cancers live in the blood, lymph nodes, bone marrow, and, sometimes, vital organs. These cancers are, by definition, malignant, as they are not localized in a single location or lump. Some are more aggressive than others, but all present a big challenge, medically speaking.

Diagnosis of Cancer

Like many diseases, in its early stages cancer often shows no symptoms. Pets often act and feel fine even if they have a visible tumor growing. The initial diagnosis of cancer generally starts either with a visible mass or some change in behavior that leads to a veterinary evaluation and further testing.

Solid Cancer

Most growths or masses occurring on dogs and cats are noncancerous or very low-grade benign tumors. Even for the trained eye, however, it is difficult to determine what is no big deal and what needs to be addressed immediately. Take your pet to the veterinarian for any new growth, ones that are changing, or if a growth bothers your pet.

Pets with cancer occurring within the body (rather than on the surface) are frequently diagnosed later in the course of the disease. Internal tumors can occur anywhere in the body, including the chest, abdomen, and head. Tumors within the abdomen can sometimes be palpated during a veterinary exam. Often, however, discovery requires some kind of imaging.

Disseminated Cancer

For cancers of the blood like lymphoma and leukemia, there is not a discrete mass to look for and evaluate. In the case of lymphoma, one or more lymph nodes are frequently enlarged. These enlarged lymph nodes may be peripheral, meaning they are just under the skin and can be palpated by hand. In other cases, the enlarged nodes are internal and require imaging to diagnose. By contrast, leukemia is most frequently diagnosed through the presence of abnormal cells noted on a blood panel.

Diagnostic Testing

- **Physical exam:** As with most diseases, the diagnostic pathway for cancer begins with a thorough history and physical examination. Your veterinarian will conduct a comprehensive exam, including lymph node palpation, abdominal palpation, and a rectal exam. Anything suspicious should be evaluated further as detailed below.

- **Blood work:** Many believe that cancer can be diagnosed via a blood panel; however, this is only the case with leukemia, which causes very high levels of white blood cells. The vast majority of pets with cancer have completely normal blood work. In these cases, the value in the blood work is determining your pet's overall health as part of the diagnostic pathway and development of a cancer treatment plan.

- **Imaging:** Imaging is used for diagnosing and staging cancer as well as to screen for metastasis and help surgeons determine whether a tumor can be removed safely. The most common types of imaging in veterinary medicine are X-rays and abdominal ultrasound. Between these two modalities, the chest and abdomen can be very thoroughly evaluated. If there is a tumor to be found, chest X-rays and/or an abdominal ultrasound will very likely find it.

  Some conditions, such as those involving the head and spine, are beyond the reach of ultrasound and X-rays. In these cases, imaging such as MRI or CT scanning may be necessary. Fortunately, advanced imaging is readily available at many veterinary specialty facilities.

- **Fine needle aspiration and cytology:** When a pet has a growth or swelling, the first test performed is often a fine needle aspirate (FNA). During an FNA, a needle is inserted into the mass, and cells are extracted and placed on a microscope slide. Evaluating material on a slide is known as cytology. FNAs and cytology can be performed on superficial lumps, palpable lymph nodes, and internal masses with the help of ultrasound guidance.

  Cytology is a highly attractive diagnostic option because it is noninvasive. Only a very small needle is used, and no sedation or anesthesia is required. The limitation is the relatively small sample size. A lot can be determined from looking at cells on a slide, but sometimes a definitive diagnosis requires a larger sample such as one obtained through a biopsy.

- **Biopsy and histopathology:** When cytology does not provide enough information, biopsy is the next step. Rather than collecting small amounts of cells with a needle through an FNA, a biopsy removes a piece of tissue. The preparation and evaluation of tissue samples is called histopathology. Depending on the nature of the biopsy, tissue samples can be as small as a pencil point or as large as an entire organ.

  Depending on your pet and the location of the mass, a biopsy can sometimes be done with sedation and a local anesthetic; other times general anesthesia is required. Options for sampling internal masses include ultrasound-guided biopsies, biopsies of the GI tract via an endoscope (flexible fiber-optic camera), or biopsies collected during surgery.

  When a pet needs immediate surgery for cancer, such as with a bleeding splenic mass, diagnosis and treatment become one. When the organ or tissue in question is removed, it is submitted whole for histopathology.

- **Special staining:** In recent years, advanced techniques in cytology and histopathology have become available. One technique called special staining allows pathologists to diagnose more conditions with small samples such as through cytology or small biopsies. The special stains used allow pathologists to identify biomarkers specific to certain types of cancer. This process allows for easier diagnosis and more effective treatment.

Philosophy of Cancer Therapy in Pets

Prior to discussing the various methods of how to treat cancer in pets, let's take a moment to look at the why: *Why* are we treating cancer in pets?

Answer: To preserve the quality of life for our pet for as long as possible. There is a very important distinction to make in comparison to the why of human oncology. The goal of cancer care for humans is often to preserve life for as long as possible (less emphasis on quality).

Because of the differences in objectives between human and veterinary oncology, treatment strategies differ. Veterinary oncologists do not always strive for a "cure." In many cases, the goal of treatment is to slow the progression of disease so pets can live happily for longer, even though they may succumb to cancer in time. Veterinarians don't push their patients as hard with treatment, and thus pets rarely have dramatic or prolonged negative responses to cancer therapy. When they do have strong negative reactions to therapy, veterinarians either change therapy or stop altogether. No one wants to torture a pet through medicine.

Conventional Medical Treatment

In veterinary medicine, the majority of Western cancer treatment can be classified into three groups: surgery, radiation, and chemotherapy. The course to take is determined by the specific diagnosis and stage of the cancer as well as the age and overall health of your pet. In deciding whether to choose one or more of these therapies, please consult with a board-certified veterinary oncologist. Even if you ultimately decide against Western cancer therapy, having all of your questions and concerns addressed by a highly trained specialist is time (and money) well spent.

Surgery

The ideal treatment for cancer is to just make it go away, and there is no quicker way to do this than with surgery. For benign masses or malignancies that have yet to metastasize, surgery can fully remove and thus cure the cancer. At times, however, surgery to remove as much of the cancer as possible is only the first step of treatment.

Although the primary goal of surgery is removing cancer, it is also used to resolve a life-threatening condition, such as a bleeding tumor in the spleen, or to relieve pain, such as amputating a limb with a bone tumor. If there is knowledge (or suspicion) of cancer cells left behind after surgery, the next step is chemotherapy and/or radiation.

Chemotherapy

Chemotherapy is a term used to describe any pharmaceuticals used for the control of cancer. With solid tumors, chemotherapy is ideally used as a secondary therapy to "clean up" microscopic disease after a mass has been removed with surgery. For disseminated cancers like lymphoma and leukemia, chemotherapy is the primary treatment.

Possible side effects of chemotherapy are usually restricted to GI upset, although infections may occur due to suppression of the immune system. Both are frequently controlled with a combination of Western and complementary care.

Electrochemotherapy

In recent years, electrochemotherapy (ECT) has become available in veterinary medicine. In contrast to traditional chemo, which is given orally or by systemic injection, ECT delivers chemotherapy drugs directly into a tumor through an electrical current. The goal is to achieve higher doses of chemotherapy where it is needed while minimizing systemic side effects.[6] Consultation with a veterinary oncologist is a must when considering ECT.

Melanoma Vaccine

Described in detail in Chapter 10, the melanoma vaccine is a unique form of chemotherapy. The melanoma vaccine is designed to simulate the dog's own immune system to recognize and destroy melanoma cells. The vaccine has been shown to have a significant effect on the progression of malignant melanomas in dogs and has extended the life span and quality of life in many pets.[7, 8]

Radiation Therapy

Similar to chemotherapy, radiation therapy is used to clean up residual microscopic disease after a tumor has been removed surgically. Radiation is becoming more effective as better technology allows oncologists to use higher doses of radiation while minimizing collateral damage.

Because radiation patients have to be completely still during therapy, pets are briefly anesthetized for each session. Side effects are almost exclusively limited to tissue burns, which are similar to a bad sunburn. Hyperbaric oxygen therapy is very effective at treating these burns.

Nutrition

From a Western medical perspective, nutrition is not generally part of the conversation about cancer therapy in pets. The most important goal is to make sure pets are eating and maintaining their weight.

There is a prescription diet for pets with cancer. Its high-protein, high-fat, and low-carbohydrate content makes it very similar to diets suggested for cancer treatment based on the Warburg effect. However, the diet is not very palatable and sometimes causes GI upset.

Complementary and Alternative Medical Therapy

From a holistic perspective, cancer therapy is a three-pronged approach. First, we provide your pet with optimal nutrition, creating an environment that is inhospitable to cancer cells and supports ideal function of body systems. The next facet is to further optimize body and immune function through herbs and supplements. Last, herbs and supplements can also be used for their natural cancer-fighting abilities.

Nutrition for the Cancer Patient

Feeding a pet with cancer is a balancing act. The goal is to provide optimal nutrition to support the immune system while restricting nutrient access by cancer cells. Designing a nutritional plan to achieve this goal requires understanding the differences between cancer cells and normal cells. With this, we can exploit the cancer's weaknesses.

According to the Warburg effect, cancer cells have an altered metabolism due to a defect in their mitochondria. The mitochondrial defect means cancer cells produce relatively little energy per molecule of glucose (fuel). The cancer cells' increased requirement for fuel can be leveraged to your pet's benefit.[9]

If cancer cells need excessive amounts of glucose to survive and multiply, the obvious nutritional solution is restricting your pet's glucose intake. It's not quite that simple, but close. Since pets generally don't consume sugar like we humans do, the glucose in their body largely comes from carbohydrates and, to a lesser extent, protein. "Cancer diets" frequently are high protein, moderate to high fat, and low carbohydrate.

Certain fats also have the potential to benefit the cancer patient through even more direct cancer-fighting effects. Omega-3 fatty acids such as those found in fish oil have been shown to decrease inflammation and improve survival times in certain cancer patients.[10, 11, 12] Conversely, diets high in omega-6 fatty acids (often found in grains) may actually increase the rate of cancer progression due to their pro-inflammatory nature.[13]

To be clear, a certain amount of blood glucose is necessary for pets to live. That said, animals are able to generate what they need from a small amount of dietary carbohydrates and protein. Anything beyond the necessary amount of glucose is potentially feeding the cancer. Remember that old saying, "Feed a cold, starve a fever"? Let's rephrase that as "Feed the pet, starve the cancer." Diets to support canine and feline cancer patients can be found in Appendix C.

When it comes to nutrition for cancer patients, there is a lot of discussion about the ketogenic diet. These diets have nearly zero carbohydrates and rely on fat and protein as energy sources to put the body in a state of nutritional ketosis. Very low carbohydrate intake results in low blood glucose and the production of ketones as fat is metabolized for fuel. Because cancer cells are unable to use ketones for fuel, and there is no glucose available for them either, the cancer cells starve.

While there is promise when it comes to ketogenic diets for human cancer patients, it is very difficult to put a dog or cat into a state of nutritional ketosis. A certain level of ketosis, however, may be achievable through the addition of the fat caprylic acid (see the next section on nutritional supplementation). The only way to accomplish ketosis in pets is with a diet that is very high in fat (50 percent or more), which is not palatable and is likely to cause diarrhea and possibly pancreatitis. For these reasons, truly ketogenic diets are *not* recommended for pets.

Nutritional approaches to cancer are powerful tools. These diets can help fight cancer and slow its growth, and are most valuable when used in conjunction with other cancer therapies. Cancer diets not only limit the debilitating effects of cancer and restrict energy to tumor cells but also have the potential to improve how a pet responds to chemotherapy and mitigate the adverse effects of radiation therapy.[14]

One final note regarding nutrition in cancer patients: The most important thing is that your dog or cat is getting *enough* nutrition. If they are running a calorie deficit and losing weight, their body's natural cancer-fighting abilities cannot be optimized. It is more important that your pet eat and maintain their body weight than that you try to force them to eat the "best" food.

Nutritional and Herbal Supplementation for Pets with Cancer

A professor of mine once said that if a medical condition has a lot of different treatment options, it means nothing works consistently. If you do an Internet search for the term "treatments for cancer," you get more than 200 million hits. That speaks volumes.

The following section outlines categories of supplements and specific compounds that I have used successfully in cancer patients or that are scientifically proven to have anticancer activity. There are many more supplements that may benefit pets with cancer; however, when considering a supplement not listed below, it is important to know whether the product is truly safe and effective. Always consult with a trained veterinarian before starting any supplement. Caveat emptor: Let the buyer beware.

- **Whole-food supplementation:** Immune system support is a cornerstone of holistic cancer care. Whole-food supplements help provide nutrition above and beyond what is possible through diet alone. The easiest products to use for pets with cancer are Canine Immune Support and Feline Immune Support by Standard Process. A health practitioner with experience using Standard Process may be able to further fine-tune a supplement protocol using whole-food nutrition.

- **Probiotics:** If a well-functioning immune system matters, then probiotics are a must. As previously discussed in Chapter 6, probiotics have significant positive effects on the immune system. Remember, 70 percent of the immune system resides in the GI tract.

- **Caprylic acid:** Caprylic acid is a medium-chain triglyceride (MCT), which are specific fats that have anticancer properties. When the body is in a state of ketosis, the combination of a low-carbohydrate diet with caprylic acid may create an environment where cellular food is preferentially provided to normal cells and restricted to cancer cells. Furthermore, research has shown caprylic acid to have specific anticancer properties.[15] One of the most readily available sources of caprylic acid is refined coconut oil. The supplement Brain Octane made by Bulletproof is distilled from coconut oil to have a much higher concentration of caprylic acid.

- **Essential fatty acids:** In addition to overall body support and immune system support, omega-3s have been shown to prevent cancer and improve survival times in pets with cancer.[16, 17, 18] Studies also suggest that the combination of fish oil and the amino acid arginine may have a synergistic effect in pets with cancer.[19]

- **Mushrooms:** A mountain of scientific evidence has been published on the medical benefits of mushrooms. Mushrooms and other fungal organisms contain compounds called beta glucans, which have profound immune-supportive and anticancer effects.[20, 21] A wide variety of mushrooms are currently being utilized in the treatment of pets with cancer, including Cordyceps, Agaricus, coriolus, maitake, shiitake, and reishi. Coriolus versicolor (turkey tail mushrooms) in particular have been shown to increase survival time in dogs with a severe cancer called splenic hemangiosarcoma.[22] The beneficial effects of mushrooms are a robust area of study, and undoubtedly more species and benefits will be discovered in the future.

Appropriate levels of dietary vitamins, minerals, and amino acids are necessary for optimal health. In certain instances, the use of specific vitamins, minerals, and amino acids in levels exceeding normal nutritional requirements has been shown to have immune-supportive and anticancer effects. Consult with a veterinarian for appropriate dosage and monitoring before starting supplementation with the following.

- **Vitamins A and D:** Supplementing with high doses of Vitamins A and D leads to apoptosis, or programmed cell death, of cancer cells.[23, 24, 25] Caution is required as toxicity is possible with excessive A and D supplementation.

  Caution: To avoid overdose, watch out for other supplements, such as fish oil, that also contain vitamin A.

- **Vitamin E:** In addition to being an antioxidant that helps support good health and immunity, vitamin E kills tumor cells.[26]

- **Vitamin C:** A well-known antioxidant, vitamin C is commonly supplemented for immune support and general well-being. In the field of cancer therapy, administering orthomolecular (megadoses given intravenously) vitamin C is reported by some to have significant anticancer effects. There is evidence of this in the scientific literature, although with inconsistent results.[27] Unlike with vitamins A and D, the kidneys readily excrete vitamin C and therefore toxicity is not a major concern.

- **Minerals:** The minerals selenium and zinc can kill cancer cells and inhibit metastasis.[28, 29] Caution is required when supplementing with these minerals, as toxicity is possible.

- **Amino acids:** As the building blocks of protein, dietary amino acids are critical to supporting normal body processes. In pets with cancer, maintaining muscle mass is of particular concern. Beyond this, the amino acids arginine and glutamine are particularly important.

  Arginine decreases both tumor growth and metastatic rates. When combined with omega fatty acids, it improves symptoms, quality of life, and survival times for pets with cancer.[30]

  Glutamine has known health benefits to the liver, GI tract, muscle support, and general support for pets undergoing chemotherapy. While cancer cells can use glutamine as an energy source in addition to glucose, current research indicates that supplementing glutamine does not promote tumor growth. Ultimately, the benefits of supplementation definitively outweigh the concerns.[31]

Below is a list herbs and supplements with known anticancer properties. These are not the only ones; they are the ones I have had the most positive experiences with in treating pets with cancer.

The following herbs inhibit cancer progression by slowing growth, stopping metastasis, and/or inducing apoptosis (cell death) of cancer cells:

- Ashwagandha[32]
- Astragalus[33]
- Boswellia (frankincense)[34]
- Curcumin[35]
- Green tea extract (EGCG)[36]
- Inositol hexaphosphate(IP-6)[37]
- Quercetin[38]
- Resveratrol[39]
- Superoxide dismutase[40]

Cannabis

This particular herb deserves special mention. Until recently, the use of medical cannabis has been kept in the shadows. The current changes in public perception and medical marijuana laws have finally created an environment where cancer patients and owners of pets with cancer can finally speak with their health care providers about using this versatile herb.

There are more than 100 published scientific studies proving anticancer benefits provided by cannabis. Studies indicate that cannabis's efficacy stems from multiple different metabolic pathways and that it enhances the effects of chemotherapy.[41] There are no known specific interactions with conventional chemotherapy or radiation. The use of medical cannabis should be part of the treatment planning for every pet with cancer. (Chapter 9 reviews how and why medical cannabis works and provides an outline for dosing.)

Traditional Chinese Veterinary Medicine

With its aim of treating cancer while helping to maintain quality of life, Chinese medicine is an excellent therapy for pets with cancer. Acupuncture helps maintain a feeling of well-being, suppresses nausea, supports appetite, and helps control pain.[42, 43] Herbal therapy addresses these issues as well, while also possessing definitive anticancer effects.[44, 45]

Most herbal therapy for cancer is patient-specific and based on a Chinese medical diagnosis. However, in the case of pets with bleeding tumors, the herbal preparation Yunnan Baiyao is so consistently effective that many Western veterinarians have embraced it. Yunnan Baiyao is frequently given to pets with internal tumors of the spleen, liver, or heart that are at risk for spontaneous bleeding. It is also used to help stabilize pets whose tumors are already bleeding.

Hyperbaric Oxygen Therapy

While there are those who promote hyperbaric oxygen therapy (HBOT) as part of a treatment for cancer, the research is equivocal. Benefits have not been proven, although there is no evidence of any harm done either. I have treated pets with cancer using HBOT as part of a larger treatment plan, and they do seem to feel better overall. Whether it changed the course of their cancer progression is more difficult to assess.

One well-accepted use of HBOT in oncology is in the treatment of the side effects of radiation therapy.[46] HBOT is an excellent way to speed the course of healing for these pets.

Integrative Treatment Plan

In a perfect world, the best therapy for pets with cancer is an aggressive integrative treatment plan that takes advantage of the best that both sides have to offer. In the real world, mitigating factors tend to get in the way. Availability of high-end Western and alternative oncology varies by geographic location. In addition, the age and overall health condition of your pet must be considered. Last, financial concerns frequently play a part in treatment decisions.

The integrative outline below represents what is possible when all the stars align. For many pets, some modification will be necessary for one or more of the reasons listed above. Your veterinarian can help you prioritize the most important aspects of your pet's care.

Diagnostics

In a perfect world, a definitive diagnosis provides a clear treatment path. This is particularly true when it comes to Western care. Getting *to* the diagnosis, however, could require multiple tests, and sometimes the risk to your pet or the financial burden is too great.

When deciding whether to move forward with a particular test, weigh the risks of the procedure against the benefits of having additional information. When you consider the potential risks and benefits of a test, ask your veterinarian this one very important question: Are the results of the test likely to change the recommended treatment plan?

If the answer is yes, move forward if you can. If the test is not likely to provide additional treatment options or if the options available are financially out of reach or otherwise not acceptable to you, the test is not necessary. It is always better to spend limited funds on treatment.

Treatment

—**Surgery:** When it comes to cancer, if a tumor can be removed safely, it probably should be. While there are extenuating circumstances in which the risks are too great or the prognosis is grave, overall it's best to get rid of as much cancer as you can up front. Regardless of what comes after surgery, the fewer cancer cells left behind, the better.

—**Chemotherapy and radiation:** If chemotherapy and/or radiation is recommended, it is worth considering. Ask the oncologist what the average survival times are with and without this treatment, and then find out what the expected side effects are. Short-term side effects are an acceptable price to pay for long-term gain. If the math doesn't work in your favor, chemo or radiation may not be the best way to go.

—**Complementary and alternative care:** Alternative care is beneficial with or without Western therapy. Ideally, they are combined, but every situation is unique; I have treated plenty of pets with complementary therapy alone. A good combination complementary and alternative regimen looks something like this:

- Transition to a fresh, whole-food diet that is low in carbohydrates.
- Supplement with probiotics, whole-food supplements, caprylic acid, and fish oil. Consider combination supplements for pets with cancer. Reference ingredient lists for the mushrooms, herbs, and supplements listed previously, and consult

with a veterinarian experienced with herbal therapy to determine the best combinations for your pet.

- If at all possible, use medical cannabis as part of the treatment. If you live in a state where this is available, consult with your veterinarian and use the information in Chapter 9 as a guide. If medical cannabis is not available to you, be aware that CBD oils from hemp are legal in all 50 states.

- Consult with your veterinarian about the potential benefits of high-dose therapy of vitamins A, D, and/or C. (Megadose treatments should be done only under veterinary supervision.)

CHAPTER 21

THYROID DISEASE

The good physician treats the disease; the great physician
treats the patient who has disease.

– WILLIAM OSLER

Near the base of the neck on either side of the trachea (windpipe) is a small, unassuming piece of tissue shaped vaguely like a butterfly. You wouldn't know it just to look at it, but that piece of tissue is in the driver's seat of metabolic control for the entire body. When it malfunctions, nearly every body system can be affected.

The Thyroid: Form and Function

In truth, the tissue described above is actually two glands. The lion's share is the thyroid gland, which is the focus of this chapter. Within the thyroid lie the parathyroid glands, which control calcium levels in the body. (While parathyroid problems do occur, they are relatively rare.)

Primary thyroid disease in dogs and cats is the most prevalent cause of endocrine (hormone) disturbance in pets. To put it simply, the thyroid gland controls the body's metabolic rate. It also affects heart rate, respiratory rate, and organ function.[1] The interactions among the thyroid gland, target organs, and other endocrine organs are incredibly complex, so for the purposes of this chapter, we are going to focus on thyroid gland function.

The thyroid gland has one purpose, which is to utilize iodine from food to create thyroid hormones called T3 and T4. Levels of thyroid hormone in the bloodstream are controlled through negative feedback. In other words, when there is a lot of a hormone in the blood, the thyroid gland slows production. When more is needed, production is ramped up.

The mechanics of how this is accomplished involve secondary hormones called thyroid stimulating hormone (TSH) and growth hormone (GH). (Other hormones, in turn, control these hormones, but we're not going down that rabbit hole. TSH and GH are as far as we need to go.)

When Things Go Wrong

There are relatively few things that can go wrong with the thyroid gland; most problems are associated with the loss of normal regulatory controls. Most commonly, a malfunctioning thyroid will either underproduce or overproduce thyroid hormones. In other cases, the thyroid gland may become cancerous or inflamed due to autoimmune disease.

Dogs

- **Hypothyroidism:** When dogs develop thyroid disease, it is almost always due to the gland underproducing thyroid hormone. This condition, known as hypothyroidism, may present with symptoms ranging from mild to quite severe.

  Symptoms commonly seen in hypothyroid dogs are: weight gain; poor-quality hair coat; greasy, flaky, or infected skin; mental dullness; mood swings; seizures; and infertility.[2] Most hypothyroid dogs will not display all of these symptoms. From a veterinary perspective, suspicion of low thyroid may begin with an offhanded remark about decreased energy or unexplained weight gain.

- **Thyroiditis:** Inflammation of the thyroid gland, known as thyroiditis, is caused by a hereditary autoimmune condition. The immune system mistakenly identifies the thyroid gland as "foreign," so white blood cells attack it, leading to inflammation and destruction of the thyroid tissue. Up to 90 percent of hypothyroidism in dogs is caused by thyroiditis.[3]

  In early stages of the condition, dogs with thyroiditis are still producing thyroid hormone and do not display symptoms of hypothyroidism. Later stages of the condition can lead to seizures and behavioral changes such as unexplained aggression. As thyroiditis progresses, however, the thyroid gland is slowly destroyed and signs of hypothyroidism become apparent.

- **Nonthyroidal illness:** Nonthyroidal illness (NTI), also known as euthyroid sick syndrome, is not a form of thyroid disease, but understanding it is important because it can muddy the waters when diagnosing hypothyroidism.

  On any given day, the thyroid gland regulates thyroid hormone levels to optimize body function. Under certain circumstances, such as illness or injury, the body may downregulate production. Drugs such as prednisone (a steroid) and phenobarbital (an antiseizure medication) can also cause this.

- **Thyroid carcinoma:** Thyroid cancer in dogs is uncommon. When it occurs, dogs may have a palpable lump in the area of the thyroid gland. Thyroid carcinomas are frequently productive tumors, meaning they secrete thyroid hormones. Without normal negative feedback controls, these dogs become hyperthyroid. Signs of hyperthyroidism in dogs include weight loss, hyperactivity or hyperexcitability, mood changes, and unexplained aggression.

Cats

- **Hyperthyroidism:** Thyroid disease in felines is usually the opposite of what we see in dogs. Overproduction of thyroid hormone, or hyperthyroidism, is common in cats as they get older; an estimated 10 percent of geriatric cats will become hyperthyroid.[4] The condition occurs when a nodule on the thyroid gland overproduces thyroid hormone. While the nodule is benign, it still has profound health effects. Research suggests underlying causes may be due to environmental toxins, including fire retardants, canned cat food, and cat litter.[5, 6]

  Symptoms of hyperthyroidism in cats include: ravenous appetite, weight loss, increased activity level, hyperexcitability and/or excessive vocalization, sudden blindness (due to high blood pressure), and signs of heart disease due to secondary hypertrophic cardiomyopathy. Most hyperthyroid cats will not display all the symptoms. Cats who are middle-aged and older with unexplained weight loss, particularly in the face of a good appetite, are always suspect for hyperthyroidism.

- **Iatrogenic hypothyroidism:** The term *iatrogenic* refers to a condition caused by medical treatment. In this case, cats occasionally become hypothyroid after being treated for hyperthyroidism. Hypothyroid cats may be sluggish and have a tendency to put on weight. They do not, however, display the constellation of symptoms described above for hypothyroid dogs.

Diagnosis of Thyroid Disease

Diagnosing a dog or cat with thyroid disease frequently begins with the owner noticing unusual behavior in their pet at home, and then bringing them to the veterinarian for a physical examination. Pets displaying any of the physical symptoms or behaviors listed above should be tested for thyroid dysfunction.

THE ULTIMATE PET HEALTH GUIDE

Blood Parameters for Thyroid Function

Thyroid function is evaluated based on levels of thyroid hormones and antibodies in the bloodstream. The following parameters are commonly used in determining thyroid function:

- **Total T4 (or T4):** This represents the total amount of T4 hormone in the bloodstream. Much of the T4 in the blood is bound to proteins and is not active.

- **Free T4 (or FT4):** Free T4 is the active form of the hormone. FT4 represents the fraction of the total T4 that is not protein bound.

- **Total T3 (or T3):** This represents the total amount of T3 hormone in the bloodstream. Much of the T3 in the blood is bound to proteins and is not active.

- **Free T3 (or FT3):** Free T3 is the active form of the hormone. FT3 represents the fraction of the total T3 that is not protein bound.

- **Thyroglobulin autoantibody (TgAA):** TgAA levels measure the level of autoimmune disease present in dogs with thyroiditis.

- **Thyroid stimulating hormone (TSH):** TSH is the hormone that signals the thyroid to produce thyroid hormone. In dogs, growth hormone also sends that signal, so TSH levels are not very useful indicators of thyroid function. TSH does have diagnostic value in cats.

Canine Hypothyroidism

Depending on the blood panel your veterinarian chooses, the thyroid parameters measured could be T4 alone, T4 and FT4, or the entire list above. Unless he or she is specifically running a thyroid panel, however, most routine blood screenings evaluate only T4. This can be problematic, as hypothyroidism cannot be diagnosed based on T4 alone. At the least, a concurrently low FT4 is needed to confirm the suspicion of hypothyroidism. (When FT4 is normal and T4 is low, the dog has nonthyroidal illness.)

The FT4 test isn't automatically ordered because it costs double the amount of a total T4. So if the total T4 comes back normal, there is no need to spend money on the more expensive test.

Canine Thyroiditis

A diagnosis of thyroiditis is made when TgAA levels are elevated, indicating the presence of antibodies attacking the thyroid gland. Dogs with thyroiditis frequently go undiagnosed because checking a TgAA level is not commonplace in most veterinary practices. Usually a full thyroid panel is necessary to obtain this information.

Thyroid levels (other than TgAA) in these dogs may vary from normal to low, depending on the level of thyroid destruction at the time of the blood test. In some cases, the levels can be elevated, as the presence of TgAA can falsely raise levels on the testing. Dogs with elevated TgAA levels must be treated to stop the immune-mediated destruction of the thyroid gland.

In these dogs, a comprehensive thyroid panel (T4, FT4, T3, FT3, TgAA) is valuable as it provides a more detailed view of overall thyroid function, the presence of thyroiditis, and the extent of nonthyroidal illness. This information helps guide treatment in dogs with borderline hypothyroidism.

Thyroid Carcinoma in Dogs

Thyroid cancer is rare. Dogs with a productive thyroid carcinoma will commonly have significantly elevated T4 and/or FT4 levels. Dogs suspected of a thyroid carcinoma should have an ultrasound of their thyroid gland to determine the size and extent of the mass.

Feline Hyperthyroidism

Just as with dogs, thyroid disease in cats is diagnosed via blood work, and most standard blood panels evaluate T4 as the only parameter of thyroid function. T4 alone may or may not be sufficient to diagnose hyperthyroidism.

When the T4 level is elevated, the cat is hyperthyroid and treatment can be initiated. When it is in the normal range, however, hyperthyroidism is still possible. Older cats may have T4 values in the mid- to upper levels of the normal range. This is sometimes called the gray zone. Cats whose symptoms suggest hyperthyroidism and/or are in the gray zone should have an FT4 run as well. An elevated FT4 is diagnostic for hyperthyroidism regardless of the T4 level.

You may wonder why your veterinarian didn't just run an FT4 test to begin with. The FT4 test costs double the amount of a total T4, so if the total T4 comes back normal, there is no need to spend money on the more expensive test.

Iatrogenic Feline Hypothyroidism

Low thyroid function due to previous treatment for hyperthyroidism does happen occasionally. Given that many of these pets are older, differentiating hypothyroidism from nonthyroidal illness is crucial in deciding treatment.

Cats suspected of iatrogenic hypothyroidism should have a full thyroid panel run, including T4, FT4, T3, FT3, and TSH. The FT4 and FT3 help distinguish hypothyroidism from NTI, as does the TSH. Cats with nonthyroidal illness will have normal TSH levels, as the body has intentionally downregulated thyroid function. By contrast, if thyroid hormone is being underproduced, TSH will be elevated in an attempt to kick the gland into gear.

Conventional Medical Treatment and Therapeutic Monitoring

Canine Hypothyroidism

Canine hypothyroidism is treated with hormone replacement therapy for the life of your pet. In most cases, the dog is supplemented with thyroxine, a synthetic form of T4.[7] However, some pet owners and veterinarians choose to use natural thyroid products instead, such as Armour Thyroid by Forest Pharmaceuticals, that are made from desiccated porcine (pig) thyroid gland and contain both T4 and T3.[8] This may be beneficial for pets with a compromised liver, as that is the organ where conversion of T4 to T3 normally occurs.

Thyroid supplements, regardless of the type, should be administered at least one hour before or two hours after eating. Dietary calcium and soy can bind thyroid hormones and prevent them from being absorbed.

Therapeutic monitoring of hypothyroid dogs includes evaluating symptoms as well as improvements in thyroid levels. For pets on synthetic thyroxine, a minimum of a T4 and an FT4 test are recommended. Dogs on natural, desiccated thyroid should be evaluated for T3 and FT3 as well. For the most accurate results, blood should be tested two months after starting (or changing) the supplement, and the sample should be drawn four to six hours after the dose was given.[9]

Canine Thyroiditis

Thyroid hormone supplementation for dogs with thyroiditis uses the same protocols as for hypothyroidism. While on supplementation, negative feedback causes thyroid hormone production to shut down. When the gland becomes dormant, the autoimmune process quiets down as well.

Thyroid supplements, regardless of the type, should be administered at least one hour before or two hours after eating. Dietary calcium and soy can bind thyroid hormones and prevent them from being absorbed.

Therapeutic monitoring of thyroiditis requires a full thyroid panel, including T4, FT4, T3, FT3, and TgAA levels. The hope is that TgAA levels will decline over time.[10]

Thyroid Carcinoma in Dogs

Therapy for thyroid carcinomas may involve surgery and/or radiation. Not all of these tumors are treatable, but many are. I have a patient in my practice that was treated for a thyroid carcinoma more than 10 years ago and is doing great!

Feline Hyperthyroidism

There are several effective therapies for hyperthyroidism in cats. Your veterinarian will help you choose an option based on the age, health, and disposition of your cat. Regardless of the ultimate choice of therapy, nearly all cats begin treatment with methimazole.

- **Methimazole:** Methimazole does not cure the disease, but it interferes with the thyroid gland's ability to create thyroid hormone as long as the drug is given. By administering methimazole to cats, we are able to lower thyroid hormone production to appropriate levels.[11]

  Methimazole is generally made as tablets, but can be ordered "compounded" as a flavored liquid or chewable treats. Transdermal preparations, which are absorbed through the skin, are also available, but efficacy is not consistent. Transdermals should be reserved as a last resort for cats that cannot be medicated in any other way.

- **I-131 therapy:** I-131 (radioactive iodine) is frequently used in both human and veterinary medicine to permanently resolve hyperthyroidism. The procedure involves a single injection of a radioactively tagged iodine compound, which concentrates in the gland and inactivates the nodule that is overproducing hormone.

  By law, pets receiving I-131 are hospitalized in isolation until the radiation has left their system, which takes up to a week. Most pets are cured with one treatment and require no further therapy other than periodic blood monitoring for thyroid function.

  I-131 therapy is generally very effective, although some cats may become hypothyroid after treatment. This state is sometimes transient as the thyroid gland slowly regains function, but approximately 2 percent of cats remain hypothyroid for the long term and need lifelong thyroid hormone supplementation.[12] Depending on their particular thyroid values, some cats need supplementation with T4 only, some need T3 only, and some need both. Your veterinarian can help you determine the best supplement in these situations.

- **Nutrition:** There is a prescription diet available designed to treat hyperthyroid cats that is very low in iodine, the key component to thyroid hormone, which leads to decreased thyroid hormone production. The catch is that the cat cannot be allowed to eat anything else; even a mouthful of another food or treat will provide enough iodine for thyroid hormone production.

Beyond keeping an eye on thyroid hormone levels, hyperthyroid cats should be monitored for blood pressure as well as kidney, liver, and cardiac function.

- **Blood pressure:** Uncontrolled thyroid disease can cause blood pressure to rise so high that it causes retinal detachment and blindness. Therefore, monitoring blood pressure in these cats is vital. As hyperthyroidism comes under control, blood pressure will go down, although not always back to normal levels. Cats may need medicine to control their blood pressure for the short term, or potentially the long term. The most commonly used medicine to control blood pressure in cats is called amlodipine.[13]

- **Kidney function:** The systemic high blood pressure caused by hyperthyroidism also increases the pressure with which blood flows into the kidneys. Since many hyperthyroid cats are older, they may have concurrent kidney disease. Normally, kidney function is monitored with kidney parameters in the blood (see Chapter 19). When blood flow to the kidneys is increased due to hyperthyroidism, it can mask elevations in the kidney parameter.

    Hyperthyroid cats with normal or near-normal kidney values can suddenly be in kidney failure as their thyroid function comes under control. This is why cats should always start treatment with methimazole before undergoing I-131 therapy. Methimazole doses can be adjusted as needed to support kidney function. Once I-131 has been done, however, its effects cannot be reversed.

- **Liver function:** The hyperthyroid state commonly leads to elevations in liver values such as ALT and ALP on blood work. As thyroid function comes under better control, the values often return to normal.

- **Cardiac function:** Cats with long-standing untreated hyperthyroidism can develop secondary hypertrophic cardiomyopathy (HCM). HCM causes a thickening of the heart muscle that may lead to blood clots and/or heart failure (see Chapter 17). Unlike other forms of HCM, however, the changes in the heart muscle will improve over time as thyroid levels are brought under control. If there are any signs suggestive of heart disease, a cardiac ultrasound is highly recommended.

Complementary and Alternative Therapy

Diseases defined by hormonal imbalances are among the most challenging to treat holistically (although it could be argued that supplementing with naturally occurring hormones *is* holistic). When it comes to hyperthyroid cats, Western therapy is necessary to lower thyroid levels. Complementary and alternative care for dogs and cats with thyroid dysfunction focuses on alleviating symptoms and improving quality of life.

Lifestyle and Nutrition

Given that exposure to environmental toxins is suspected to be a cause of feline hyperthyroidism, maintaining a "clean" lifestyle is advisable. Clearly there is a limit to what is possible, but feeding your pet a fresh, whole-food diet helps them avoid toxins associated with food processing and packaging. In addition, use food and water bowls made out of glass or stainless steel rather than plastic, and use all-natural cat litter without chemicals or fragrances.

Some pet owners feeding a home-prepared raw-food diet have inadvertently caused hyperthyroidism by feeding meat containing thyroid tissue. Meat from the gullet (throat) can contain thyroid, so be sure to cook it before feeding it to your pet in order to inactivate the thyroid hormones.

Whole-Food Supplementation

There are anecdotal reports of cats whose thyroid levels have improved on whole-food supplementation. The use of whole-food supplements such as those made by Standard Process have been helpful in some pets with thyroid disease. Canine Thyroid Support for dogs and Feline Whole Body and Hepatic Support for cats are the most commonly used.

Herbal Supplementation

- **Hypothyroidism:** There are *no* specific herbs successfully used to treat hypothyroidism. While some products containing kelp claim to treat low thyroid function due to their iodine content, the majority of hypothyroidism cases in dogs are due to autoimmune thyroiditis, not an iodine deficiency. Supplementing iodine in these pets may *worsen* the destruction of thyroid tissue.[14]

   Other herbal therapy for hypothyroidism focuses on supporting the body systems affected by low thyroid function. Herbs and supplements for skin support can be highly beneficial (see Chapter 11).

- **Hyperthyroidism:** The most commonly used herb for hyperthyroidism is bugleweed. Studies show that bugleweed decreases levels of thyroid hormones in rats. Bugleweed is frequently combined with a second herb, *Melissa officinalis* (lemon balm).[15] While preparations containing bugleweed and Melissa are marketed for use in hyperthyroid cats, I wouldn't rely on these (or any) herbs to control hyperthyroidism. If your cat is borderline high, however, it may be worth a try; but be prepared to fill that prescription of methimazole. You can also consult with your veterinarian about giving herbs with methimazole to keep the dose lower.

    Other herbal therapy for hyperthyroidism focuses on supporting the body systems affected by elevated thyroid function. In particular, herbs and supplements for heart (Chapter 17), liver (Chapter 18), and kidney (Chapter 19) support can be highly beneficial.

Traditional Chinese Veterinary Medicine

Chinese medicine does an excellent job with the ancillary issues associated with thyroid disease. Hypothyroid dogs with low energy and skin issues, and hyperthyroid cats with hypertension or kidney disease, will benefit from acupuncture and herbal therapy. The specific acupuncture regimen and recommended herbs vary based on the individual and must be assessed by a TCVM practitioner.

Integrative Treatment Plan

Thyroid disease in dogs and cats is common and can lead to serious complications if diagnosis or treatment is delayed. Blood work should be performed on any pet suspected of thyroid dysfunction as well as in older pets during their scheduled health checks.

Blood work sufficient to diagnose hypothyroidism in dogs and hyperthyroidism in cats is necessary for an accurate diagnosis. This may mean running additional tests if the first ones do not provide a definitive answer. Two critical points to remember are:

- A low T4 alone is not sufficient to diagnose hypothyroidism in dogs.

- A normal T4 alone is not sufficient to rule out hyperthyroidism in cats.

Once a diagnosis is made, begin Western therapy and utilize complementary and alternative methods to smooth out the edges and improve quality of life.

Hypothyroidism

Dogs with hypothyroidism and/or thyroiditis primarily require thyroid hormone supplementation. The decision to use synthetic thyroxine or natural desiccated thyroid is largely a personal preference, as it does not seem to make a huge difference in most pets. Dogs with compromised liver function may do better on the natural product.

In addition to thyroid hormone supplementation and a fresh, whole-food diet, whole-food supplements such as Canine Thyroid Support by Standard Process may be of benefit. Use supplements as needed that support the body systems, such as the skin, affected by low thyroid function. TCVM can help mitigate any persistent symptoms.

Hyperthyroidism

The decision of how to manage a hyperthyroid cat has a lot to do with the cat's tolerance toward being medicated. All things being equal, long-term methimazole is probably preferable to irradiating cats. However, methimazole therapy hinges on successfully medicating the cat twice daily for life. Even if you are going to try using an herbal preparation of bugleweed and Melissa, your cat has to be medicated every day. In cases where this is not possible, either due to the cat or the humans involved, I-131 therapy is a reasonable option.

Regardless of the primary method of treatment, most hyperthyroid cats are older and in need of integrative care. Whole-food nutrition and whole-food supplements such as those made by Standard Process are wonderful ways to support older kitties. Concurrent issues such as heart, liver, or kidney problems should also be managed through a combination of Western and alternative care. TCVM can help mitigate any persistent symptoms.

CHAPTER 22

ADRENAL DISEASE

Natural forces within us are the true healers of disease.

– HIPPOCRATES

It's fascinating how both in life and within the body, the smallest things can be the most powerful. Microscopic bacteria and viruses can bring down any living thing. The energy within atoms can power the world (or destroy it).

Within the body, some of the smallest pieces of tissue are in control of nearly every physiologic function. Endocrine glands such as the thyroid, parathyroid, pancreas, and pituitary glands play an active role in controlling every aspect of physical, emotional, and cognitive body function. The adrenal glands, in particular, wield awesome power.

The Adrenals: Form and Function

A pair of glands about the size and shape of a small peanut, the adrenal glands live deep within the abdomen near the spine and not far from the kidneys. These tiny structures secrete some of the most potent hormones in the body. Epinephrine (adrenaline), testosterone, estrogen, and cortisol are only a portion of the hormones produced and secreted by the adrenals. These hormones play a major role in our physical and emotional responses to stress, illness, and injury. In many ways, adrenal gland function shapes who we are as individuals.

You know how when you are startled or scared, your heart rate goes up and pounds in your chest, as your whole body seems to tingle? That's your adrenal gland secreting epinephrine into your bloodstream. It's an evolutionary "fight or flight" response and an excellent example of how quickly and profoundly the adrenal gland can alter body functions.

Like the other endocrine organs, the adrenal glands do not function as an independent system. Communication with other glands using chemical signals, neurologic input, and feedback loops provides the adrenal glands with status updates and determines which hormones should be released into the body. Not surprisingly, the communication network is incredibly complex. For the purposes of this chapter, the important thing to remember is that the pituitary gland sends chemical signals to the adrenal gland, telling it what to do.

When Things Go Wrong

Any type of adrenal disease in cats is exceptionally rare. Nearly all adrenal diseases are found in dogs and are related to the underproduction or overproduction of various types of steroids. The remaining adrenal diseases are rarely seen and are caused by overproduction of specific hormones due to an adrenal tumor.

Addison's Disease

When the adrenal glands are underproducing steroids, the resulting condition is called Addison's disease, or hypoadrenocorticism. The underlying cause of Addison's is not fully understood, although there appears to be a genetic and autoimmune component.

Addison's disease is sometimes called the "Great Masquerader" because the disease's vague and shifting symptoms can make it difficult to diagnose. Some of the classic symptoms of Addison's disease are lethargy, diarrhea (often with blood), dehydration, regurgitation of food, and general malaise. In extreme cases, a dog may collapse in what is termed an Addisonian crisis, which can be fatal without immediate medical intervention.[1]

Cushing's Disease

When the adrenal glands are overproducing steroids, the resulting condition is Cushing's disease, or hyperadrenocorticism. Cushing's disease can be pituitary-dependent or adrenal-dependent, and treatment options for each vary.[2]

About 85 percent of Cushing's in dogs is pituitary-dependent. It is caused by a benign mass on the pituitary gland, which oversecretes the adrenocorticotropic hormone (ACTH), stimulating the adrenals to release cortisol. The other 15 percent of dogs have adrenal-dependent Cushing's disease. They have an adrenal tumor that is causing the overproduction of cortisone.

Unlike Addison's, Cushing's disease does not generally hide from diagnosis. Common symptoms of Cushing's disease are:

- Excessive appetite, thirst, and urination (In veterinary terminology, this set of symptoms is known as PU/PD/PP, which stands for polyuria [excessive urination], polydipsia [excessive thirst], and polyphagia [excessive appetite].)

- Panting and restlessness

- Weight gain

- Development of a potbelly

- Symmetrical thinning or loss of fur along the flanks

- Heat intolerance (The dog seeks out cooler temperatures.)

Not every dog will display all the symptoms listed above; however, *all* will be PU/PD/PP. Unlike with Addison's disease, there is no crisis with Cushing's; dogs can live this way for years. But the disease affects quality of life for both pets and their owners, and long-term use of steroids can cause excessive strain on vital organs, particularly the liver.

Iatrogenic Cushing's Disease

The term *iatrogenic* describes a disease caused by medical treatment. It is possible to make dogs "Cushingoid" (having the symptoms of excess cortisol) by giving them too much of the steroid prednisone. This used to be more common when steroids were the only treatment option for dogs with severe allergies. These days, nonsteroidal therapies are more commonly used so as to avoid these side effects. The symptoms of iatrogenic Cushing's disease are the same as those for Cushing's disease.

Diagnosis of Adrenal Disease

Diagnosing adrenal disease in dogs begins with a suspicion of either Addison's or Cushing's. Symptoms of Cushing's are usually pretty clear-cut, but Addison's can be tricky. Regardless, once the suspicion is there, either due to symptoms or something your veterinarian sees on a physical examination, the hunt is on.

Addison's Disease

A suspicion of Addison's disease may not even arise until a routine blood panel is performed. Typically, an Addisonian dog will have a decrease in sodium (Na) and an increase in potassium (K) in the blood. The levels are evaluated to determine the sodium-to-potassium ratio (Na:K). Some Addisonian dogs will also have elevated kidney values and low blood sugar. Blood work suspicious for Addison's disease requires further testing to confirm the diagnosis.

Atypical Addisonian dogs will have a normal Na:K ratio and generally normal blood work. This occurs when a dog is deficient in some (but not all) of the hormones normally affected by Addison's disease. If your dog's other symptoms still fit the diagnostic picture for Addison's disease, continue with further testing.

The definitive test for Addison's disease is called an ACTH stimulation test. The test begins with collecting blood to check a baseline blood cortisol level. ACTH is then given by injection, and cortisol levels are checked again. Normal dogs will produce more cortisol in response to the ACTH injection, but Addisonian dogs' adrenal glands are unable to respond to the ACTH, and thus there is little to no elevation in cortisol.

Cushing's Disease

Most affected dogs are practically screaming their Cushing's symptoms. The PU/PD/PP and restless, panting behavior is tough to miss once you know what you are looking for. Unlike Addison's disease, there is no such thing as atypical Cushing's; dogs with Cushing's all have symptoms and telltale signs on their lab work. (Dogs that have been administered steroids may show similar patterns.)

The most recognizable change is an elevation in one or more liver enzymes. The ALP, in particular, is always elevated in these dogs, sometimes by a lot. In addition, ALT and/or GGT may also be elevated. Other changes are frequently apparent in the blood as well, including a particular pattern of white blood cells called a stress leukogram. Your veterinarian will recognize this as a possible sign of Cushing's disease, steroid administration, or high cortisol levels due to stress or anxiety.

There are two definitive tests for Cushing's disease: the low-dose dexamethasone suppression test (LDDS) and the ACTH stimulation test. While either test can diagnose Cushing's, the LDDS is preferred as the ACTH stim is more likely to give an equivocal answer.

With the LDDS, a blood sample is first collected to get a baseline cortisol level, then a steroid called dexamethasone is administered. After four to eight hours, blood is collected and cortisol is measured again. While normal dogs will show decreases in cortisol after being given dexamethasone, Cushingoid dogs will continue to have elevations in cortisol. In many cases, an LDDS is sufficient to diagnose Cushing's disease and differentiate between the pituitary- and adrenal-dependent forms. If this is not the case, an abdominal ultrasound will answer the question.

A dog with pituitary-dependent Cushing's will have an ultrasound that shows both adrenal glands to be enlarged but otherwise normal. The ultrasound of a dog with adrenal-dependent Cushing's will show one enlarged adrenal gland (abnormal due to the tumor) and one that is small and atrophied, shut down due to the excess of cortisol in the system.

Conventional Medical Treatment and Therapeutic Monitoring

Addison's Disease

Home therapy for Addison's disease can begin when the dog is stable. For some dogs, this will be at the time of diagnosis. For dogs in an Addisonian crisis requiring hospitalization, this may be afterward.

Most Addison's dogs are deficient in cortisol and mineralocorticoids. It is the mineralocorticoids that cause the typical changes in sodium and potassium and are also responsible for the onset of an Addisonian crisis. Primary therapy for most Addisonian dogs involves mineralocorticoid replacement and sometimes cortisol replacement.

Mineralocorticoids are most frequently administered with a medication called DOCP (Percorten-V). DOCP is given via injection every 25 to 28 days.[3] Depending on the veterinary practice, these injections are sometimes given in the clinic and sometimes at home by the owner. In addition to DOCP, some Addisonian dogs will also need a low dose of cortisone (prednisone) supplementation, administered orally at home.

Dogs with atypical Addison's disease do not have a mineralocorticoid deficiency and thus do not need DOCP. They are managed, at least initially, with low doses of cortisone given orally. In time, some of these dogs will progress to requiring DOCP as well.

Monitoring dogs with Addison's disease is accomplished by checking their blood sodium and potassium levels. While atypical Addisonians have normal Na:K at the time of diagnosis, they should be monitored to make sure they have not developed a mineralocorticoid deficiency. Testing is recommended monthly for a couple of months to make sure dogs are stable, after which every six months is usually sufficient.

Cushing's Disease

Therapy for Cushing's disease centers on decreasing the amount of cortisol in the system. Depending on whether the condition is adrenal- or pituitary-dependent, therapy differs.

- **Adrenal-dependent Cushing's:** When a dog is diagnosed with an adrenal tumor causing Cushing's disease, it could be good or bad news. If the tumor is relatively small and is not invading neighboring structures, removal of the tumor may cure the dog.

  If the mass is malignant, the fight may not be over. To complicate things, the adrenal glands live right next to the inferior vena cava (the largest vein in the body), and tumors tend to wrap themselves around, and even potentially invade, its walls. When this happens, surgery is very risky, if not impossible.

  If surgery is not an option, treatment to control Cushing's disease is the same as for dogs with pituitary-dependent disease for as long as the tumor is not causing any other medical problems. Consult an oncologist to discuss possible chemotherapy.

- **Pituitary-dependent Cushing's:** The pituitary gland is smack dab in the middle of the head, making surgical access impossible. (While there is a procedure available for humans who need pituitary surgery, it is of a magnitude and complexity not available in veterinary medicine.)

  Since we can't get to the pituitary gland, the only other option is to suppress production of cortisol by the adrenals. There are two drugs up to the task: mitotane (Lysodren) and trilostane (Vetoryl).[4, 5] Although mitotane has been around for decades, trilostane is the preference due to lower incidence of complications.

  Caution: If dosed in excess, these drugs can cause severe complications due to adrenal gland shutdown.

  Even on trilostane, dogs with Cushing's disease must be monitored closely. Once treatment begins, PU/PD/PP, panting, and restlessness should improve dramatically. Although a low-dose dexamethasone suppression test is used to diagnose Cushing's, an ACTH stimulation is the test of choice for monitoring dogs on therapy. The goal of therapy is to get the dog's cortisol production in a range slightly higher than normal but low enough for symptoms to be minimized or resolved. Pushing the levels any lower risks adrenal toxicity and an Addisonian crisis.

Complementary and Alternative Therapy

Complementary and alternative options are limited for most endocrine conditions, and adrenal disease is no exception. However, there are a few strategies to support these pets in ways that may allow them to respond better to therapy and the stresses of the disease.

In both Addison's and Cushing's, the benefit of a fresh, whole-food diet is clear. Either condition is a stress on the dog's body, never mind the meds and frequent trips to the veterinarian. There are no specific diet formulations for dogs with adrenal disease, but fresh, whole foods supplemented with appropriate vitamins and minerals provide these pets with the nutrition they need under stressful conditions.

Addison's Disease

- **Whole-food supplementation and glandular therapy:** Low-functioning endocrine organs call for consideration of glandular therapy (see Chapter 7). In the case of Addison's disease, products made by Standard Process such as Canine Adrenal Support or Drenatrophin PMG may be beneficial in providing micronutrients to support normal adrenal gland function.

- **Licorice:** Licorice is sometimes recommended for Addisonian dogs due to its ability to increase cortisol levels and decrease high potassium levels. However, these potential benefits are overshadowed by potential negative interactions with the prednisone that most of these dogs receive as part of their treatment.[6] Pass on this supplement.

- **Traditional Chinese veterinary medicine:** The use of TCVM in Addisonian dogs can be beneficial in supporting their energy levels and overall feeling of well-being.

Cushing's Disease

- **Ginkgo:** This herb has been shown to reduce cortisol levels in the blood and thus may have benefit in dogs with Cushing's disease.[7] It is unknown if ginkgo could negate the need for pharmaceuticals in very mild or borderline cases of Cushing's disease, but it may help reduce the doses needed.

- **Traditional Chinese veterinary medicine:** TCVM is an excellent modality to use in the treatment of Cushing's disease. Signs of excess "heat" such as elevated water consumption, panting, and restlessness can be improved with acupuncture and herbs. In some borderline dogs, it is possible to maintain them for a while and delay the necessity of medical therapy. TCVM is also beneficial in mitigating residual symptoms in pets currently on therapy.

Integrative Treatment Plan

Adrenal gland disease requires treatment and regular monitoring, and integrative treatment protocols should always be tailored to the individual. While Western medication for borderline Cushing's disease could be delayed in favor of complementary therapy, definitive treatment of Addison's disease must start immediately upon diagnosis. With either condition, dogs on an appropriate regimen of medication, nutrition, and alternative therapy should live long and happy lives.

The protocols below are a starting point after a dog has been diagnosed. Consult with your veterinarian to determine the best course of action for your dog.

Addison's Disease

- DOCP injections and oral prednisone
- Routine monitoring of sodium and potassium levels
- Fresh, whole-food diet
- Glandular therapy
- Traditional Chinese veterinary medicine, if indicated

Cushing's Disease

- Mitotane (Lysodren) or trilostane (Vetoryl) per veterinary recommendation
- Routine monitoring (ACTH stimulation)
- Fresh, whole-food diet
- Traditional Chinese veterinary medicine
- Ginkgo

CHAPTER 23

AUTOIMMUNE DISEASE

A house divided against itself cannot stand.

– ABRAHAM LINCOLN

When our 13th president uttered the words in this chapter's epigraph, he was referring to the impending civil war rather than anything to do with health and well-being, yet his words ring true just the same. The immune system is a complex creation that specializes in protection from foreign invaders like bacteria and viruses. It heals the body when sick or injured. It participates in the removal and recycling of old or dead cells. The immune system is like the body's police, fire department, and ambulance all rolled into one. But what happens when it mistakes a friend for an enemy?

When Things Go Wrong

Any immune system malfunction leading to its attacking normal tissues within the body is termed an autoimmune disease. There are many types of autoimmune disease—some minor and some deadly. While each condition is individual with regard to its presentation, diagnosis, and treatment, there are some common threads that run through the group.

What causes the body to turn on itself? On some level the development of autoimmune disease is a mystery. We do know that genetics, exposure to environmental toxins, and certain viral infections play a role.[1, 2, 3] Other than making an effort toward clean living and feeding fresh foods that are low in contaminants and toxins, there is not much we can do to control these variables. We do, however, have control over the following contributing factors.

- **Vaccines:** A quick Internet search will reveal how many terrible things have been attributed to vaccination, ranging from autoimmune conditions to autism to bad taste in music. (Yes, people have actually made that last connection— look it up!) Clearly, vaccines are blamed for more problems than they actually cause. It bears repeating that vaccines are highly beneficial and many dogs and cats would not survive to reach adulthood without them. That said, vaccines are not completely benign substances, and complications can occur.

  The syndrome known as vaccinosis refers to complications associated with vaccines, including the onset of autoimmune conditions. (However, there is disagreement within the medical community regarding the exact parameters of vaccinosis, or whether it even exists.[4]) Hypersensitivity (allergic) reactions to vaccines are well documented, and connections have been made between vaccines and severe autoimmune conditions.[5] That said, research has not been able to draw a direct correlation between vaccines and many of the severe autoimmune and neurologic conditions often attributed to them.

- **Leaky gut syndrome and food sensitivity:** The onset of autoimmune disease may have origins in the gastrointestinal tract. Under normal conditions, food particles are digested and broken down into components small enough to pass through and between the cells of the intestinal wall and into the bloodstream. When chronic inflammation in the GI tract causes increased permeability of the gut wall, this is called leaky gut syndrome. This condition allows the passage of larger molecules into the blood, which causes an inflammatory immune response.

  Leaky gut syndrome is primarily caused by a poor diet or dietary sensitivities, but the effects of the inflammation can occur anywhere in the body, including the onset of autoimmune disease.[6] Although somewhat controversial in Western medicine, leaky gut syndrome is a well-recognized condition to practitioners of complementary and alternative medicine.

Autoimmune Conditions of the Blood

Conditions affecting blood cells are frequently the most serious autoimmune disorders seen in pets, and have been associated with exposure to chemicals, toxins, drugs, bacterial or viral infection, and vaccination. Once the initial crisis is weathered, these serious diseases will often abate with treatment over a period of months; many pets do not need lifelong medication. Early diagnosis and treatment are the keys to successful therapy.

- **Immune-mediated hemolytic anemia (IMHA):** Immune-mediated hemolytic anemia is a condition in which a pet's immune system attacks and destroys their own red blood cells. The result is severe anemia and an inability to transport oxygen through the blood. Mostly seen in dogs, IMHA is rare in cats. Pets with IMHA are frequently lethargic, have pale gums, and may also be icteric (jaundiced) and have a fever.

If a complete blood count (CBC) reveals a low red blood cell count in the absence of blood loss, kidney failure, or other known causes of anemia, IMHA is a prime suspect. Additional testing known as saline agglutination and Coombs testing is often used to confirm the diagnosis.[7]

- **Immune-mediated thrombocytopenia (ITP):** Immune-mediated thrombocytopenia is a condition in which platelets are attacked and destroyed by the immune system. Dogs with ITP (it's rare in cats) are frequently lethargic and may have bruising, nosebleeds, and bloody diarrhea. A CBC will show decreased platelets and possibly anemia due to blood loss from an inability to clot.[8]

- **Evans syndrome:** Evans syndrome describes IMHA and ITP occurring at the same time. Needless to say, aggressive treatment for Evans syndrome is critical to a dog's survival.

Autoimmune Conditions of the Skin

Autoimmune conditions affecting the skin often present as inflammation, crusting, scabbing, and/or ulceration of the affected tissues. Dogs are more frequently affected than cats. Lesions can occur anywhere but frequently are seen around the head and feet. Causes of these diseases are frequently unknown, although environmental toxins, viruses, nutritional factors, drugs, and vaccinations may be involved.[9, 10] The following conditions are among the most commonly seen autoimmune conditions of the skin.

- **Pemphigus:** This term describes several different autoimmune skin conditions in which the superficial layers of skin separate from the underlying tissues. Diagnosis is made via skin biopsy.

- **Discoid lupus erythematosus (DLE):** Pets with DLE commonly have ulcerated lesions around the nose. Diagnosis is made via skin biopsy.

- **Lupoid onychodystrophy:** Lupoid onychodystrophy affects the toenails of dogs, causing the nail beds to become inflamed and painful. In many cases, the nails actually fall off and leave the sensitive quick exposed. Diagnosis is usually made based on symptoms alone.

- **Vasculitis:** Vasculitis most frequently occurs in areas of the body with limited blood circulation, including the ear tips, tail tip, and paw pads. Pets frequently have scabbing of affected areas; bits of fur and skin come away as the scabs fall off. Diagnosis is made based on symptoms and a skin biopsy.

- **Masticatory muscle myositis:** Dogs with masticatory muscle myositis have inflammation of the muscles they use to chew. Affected dogs have pain upon opening their mouth and a decreased ability to fully open it. Diagnosis is made through symptoms and a blood test called a masticatory myositis autoantibody test.

Autoimmune Conditions of the Eyes

Autoimmune inflammation in and around the eyes can cause irritation and potentially impairment of vision. Underlying causes include drugs, infections, and UV exposure (in the case of pannus). These conditions most frequently occur in dogs, although autoimmune disease in the eyes of cats is possible.

- **Keratoconjunctivitis sicca (KCS):** KCS, or dry eye, results in a decrease of the production of tears. KCS causes dry, irritated eyes that can lose vision over time due to chronic irritation. KCS is diagnosed based on symptoms and measuring tear production through a Schirmer tear test.

- **Pannus:** Also known as chronic superficial keratitis, pannus is an immune-mediated inflammation of the cornea of dogs. The cornea (clear part of the eye) becomes raised and discolored red, brown, or gray. Although not painful, untreated pannus will affect vision. German shepherds are particularly susceptible.

Autoimmune Conditions Attributed to Vaccination

Although there is no doubt vaccines can lead to autoimmune conditions, how frequently they occur is up for debate. In addition, vaccinosis has been attributed to the onset of neurologic disease such as seizures, weakness, and paralysis. Research data to prove these connections is tough to come by; regardless, these medical crises do occur and require treatment.

Conventional Medical Treatment

Since autoimmune disease is an overresponse of the immune system, the Western medical approach is to modulate (suppress) the immune system. Depending on the severity of the condition, treatment is often successful, although not without side effects. Long-term use of high doses of immunosuppressive drugs can lead to susceptibility to infection, cancer, and strain on vital organs like the liver. Whether from the Western or complementary perspective, the goal with these very potent drugs is to limit long-term use or at least keep dosing as low as possible to avoid side effects. Long-term topical medication is much less of an issue.

Limitation of Exposure

Given what we know about autoimmune disease, limiting an affected pet's exposure to drugs and chemicals is a good idea. From a Western perspective, this means withholding all medications but those that are absolutely necessary. Flea, tick, and heartworm products should be avoided if possible. Vaccinations should be discontinued, although a rabies vaccine may still be legally required.

Systemic Therapy

The most severe autoimmune conditions like IMHA, ITP, and Evans syndrome require immediate and aggressive medical therapy. Many of these pets need hospitalization and blood transfusions during the initial stages of the disease. Once stabilized, pets can begin a regimen of oral immunosuppressive therapy. The following are three of the most commonly used medications.

- **Prednisone:** Due to its rapid onset, this steroid is the first line of defense against severe autoimmune disease. Prednisone is always used (at least initially) for systemic autoimmune disease and often for skin-related conditions. However, high doses of prednisone may lead to problems with the liver, heart (cats), diabetes (cats), and the onset of signs of Cushing's disease (see Chapter 22).[11]

- **Azathioprine:** Used in dogs, azathioprine suppresses the immune system. It is commonly used in conjunction with prednisone. The combination of the two allows for a lower dose of each drug.[12]

- **Doxycycline and niacinamide:** The combination of the antibiotic (doxycycline) and immunomodulating drug (niacinamide) is commonly used to control symptoms of a variety of autoimmune conditions, including pemphigus, lupus, and lupoid onychodystrophy.[13, 14]

- **Pentoxifylline:** This unique drug can help improve circulation in cases of vasculitis.[15]

Topical Therapy

Topical medication is commonly used to treat a variety of autoimmune diseases including pemphigus and lupus. Topical meds have an advantage over orally administered medication in that they do not cause systemic side effects.

- **Steroids:** A variety of steroids can be used in the topical treatment of autoimmune diseases of the skin, including pemphigus, lupus, and vasculitis. Ophthalmic prednisone is also commonly used in the treatment of pannus.[16]

- **Cyclosporine:** Used topically, cyclosporine is most frequently used as a treatment for KCS.[17]

- **Tacrolimus:** This immunomodulating drug can be used topically for pemphigus, lupus, or vasculitis. Eye drops or ointments are also available for the treatment of KCS.[18]

Complementary and Alternative Therapy

While there are complementary and alternative therapies recommended for autoimmune disease, the single greatest recommendation is to clean up the environment within your pet's body. Environmental toxins and poor diet can contribute to autoimmune disease, so step one has to be to remove as many of these compounds as possible.

Remove the Toxins

All nonessential medications and treatments should be discontinued in pets with autoimmune disease. This includes flea and tick control, heartworm preventive, and any medication that is not absolutely necessary.

Ideally, these pets should not be vaccinated anymore. While local laws may require a rabies vaccine, in some jurisdictions there may be an opportunity to get a legal exemption. Exposure to any other household, automotive, or industrial chemicals should also be restricted.

Nutrition

Pertaining to autoimmune disease, the concerns regarding nutrition are twofold. The first step is to remove all processed foods from the diet to eliminate the potential of exposure to bacterial and mold toxins. Converting pets to a fresh, whole-food diet is an excellent way to clean up their act.

In addition to the diet change to a fresh-food format, the possibility of leaky gut syndrome must be addressed. Converting to a fresh, whole-food diet is an excellent place to start. Many pets with leaky gut syndrome will have gastrointestinal signs, but not all. If there are further concerns regarding leaky gut or possibly a dietary sensitivity, pets can be tested easily using a NutriScan food sensitivity panel from Hemopet labs. A more detailed description of the NutriScan assay can be found in Chapter 14 or at www.hemopet.org.

Whole-Food Supplementation

Whole-food supplements, such as those made by Standard Process, can help provide micronutrients to pets suffering from autoimmune disease. These nutrients will contribute to proper function of the body and immune system and aid in healing. The ideal formulas are dependent on the type of condition present.

Nutritional Supplements and Herbal Therapy

The operative word on herbal therapy for autoimmune disease is *caution*. Many of the supplements frequently used in alternative medicine have effects on the immune system. When immunity is working correctly, we use these effects to our benefit. In the case of auto-immune disease, extreme care is indicated—the last thing we want to do is stimulate the immune system.

Working within these parameters, the following supplements are safe and supportive for pets with autoimmune conditions.

- **Milk thistle and SAM-e:** Frequently combined into one supplement, milk thistle and SAM-e are both highly supportive of liver function (see Chapter 18). Liver support is vital to these pets because of the stress on the liver from the disease and the medications they are taking.

- **Probiotics:** In addition to being generally supportive of the immune system, probiotics may help reduce the inflammatory process in autoimmune disease.[19] They are also helpful in the treatment of leaky gut syndrome.

- **Antioxidants:** Antioxidants may help reduce inflammation attributed to autoimmune disease.[20]

- **Omega fatty acids:** Diets high in omega-3 fatty acids such as those found in fish oil reduce severity of symptoms and increase survival times when autoimmune disease is present.[21] There is evidence of fish oil affecting platelet function, although it is unclear if this would present a problem to a dog with ITP.[22] Caution is advised in pets with ITP.

Traditional Chinese Veterinary Medicine

TCVM often excels with conditions Western medicine considers vague in origin, but as it turns out, autoimmune disease is a challenge regardless of medical philosophy. In addition to addressing the primary disease, acupuncture and herbal therapy can help make pets more comfortable, particularly given the levels of medication many of them are on.

The herbal combination Yunnan Baiyao is so effective in controlling bleeding, many Western veterinarians use it regularly. Pets with ITP and a propensity to bleed may benefit from Yunnan Baiyao while waiting for medication like prednisone to improve platelet numbers.[23]

Hyperbaric Oxygen Therapy

Hyperbaric oxygen therapy (HBOT) has been shown in multiple studies to suppress the autoimmune response in patients with autoimmune disease.[24, 25] Personally, I have used HBOT in several cases of IMHA and Evans syndrome with very good effect. If HBOT is available, it is an excellent treatment option for autoimmune patients.

Homeopathy

Homeopathy for autoimmune diseases is best left to a classically trained homeopath. In order for therapy to be at its most effective, a full constitutional analysis should be performed. However, there are several remedies that are commonly used in pets with autoimmune disease.

- **Thuja:** This homeopathic remedy is commonly given when vaccinosis is suspected.

- **Lyssin:** This homeopathic remedy is commonly given when vaccinosis is suspected to be due to a rabies vaccine.

- **Traumeel:** Topical Traumeel can be used to improve lesions for pets with vasculitis.

Cannabis

Research indicates that medical cannabis is valuable in limiting the immune response with autoimmune disease.[26] Although research regarding the use of cannabis in the treatment of autoimmune disease in pets is limited, it holds a lot of promise.[27]

Integrative Treatment Plan

Autoimmune disease is difficult to treat because the primary means by which the body normally heals—the immune system—is at the root of the problem. The best way to address autoimmune disease is to make sure it never happens. While a certain number of vaccines and medications are a necessary part of every pet's life, we can still keep things to a minimum by using only what is absolutely necessary. Feeding a balanced, fresh, whole-food diet limits toxin exposure and helps the body's ability to manage what it is exposed to. When autoimmune conditions do occur, integrative care and redoubling the effort toward healthy living are the most effective means to recapture a balanced immune system.

The level to which Western therapy comes into play in the treatment of autoimmune disease is directly related to the severity of the condition. Systemic disease such as IMHA, ITP, or Evans syndrome clearly requires immediate Western medical intervention and sometimes hospitalization. Skin- and eye-related conditions do not frequently require emergency care, but some degree of Western therapy is still indicated. Regardless of the type of autoimmune disease, changing to a fresh, whole-food diet and cleanup of drugs and toxins are always recommended.

Autoimmune Conditions of the Blood

After emergency, life-saving therapy is completed, pets will need to be on some degree of immunosuppressive therapy such as prednisone or azathioprine. The ultimate goal of therapy is to slowly wean them off of the medication in the future. Complementary therapy including diet, whole-food supplementation, liver support, probiotics, antioxidants, and omega fatty acids provides good patient support. Whenever possible, hyperbaric oxygen therapy should be utilized.

Autoimmune Conditions of the Skin and Eye

While these conditions are not life-threatening, they can be very uncomfortable. Western medical therapy to mitigate inflammation and discomfort is highly recommended for skin conditions. When it comes to the eyes, both KCS and pannus can cause blindness if untreated. Supportive care with complementary and alternative medicine is excellent adjunctive treatment.

AFTERWORD

Happiness is the highest form of health.

— DALAI LAMA

If the Dalai Lama is right, most pets are healthier than people. Even when they are physically sick, dogs and cats have a great ability to live in the moment. That said, physical health contributes to spiritual health. Just as the black and white halves of the symbol for yin and yang combine to form a perfect circle, spiritual and physical health integrates as two halves of a whole. The spiritual aspect of a pet's circle usually takes care of itself. Pets are naturally Zen. But maintaining a complete circle relies on lifestyle and health care that support a lifetime of excellent physical health.

As humans, our natural inclination is toward short-term thinking. If our pet's (or our own) health seems fine right now, the tendency is to keep everything the same. It's a good coping mechanism that prevents us from obsessively worrying when things are okay. However, a little long-term planning pays off in spades—particularly when it comes to health care.

There can be no better course of action regarding health care than having a comprehensive, integrative health and wellness plan. Regardless of whether planning begins when a pet is young and healthy or after an illness has occurred, a good plan provides direction when our human brain becomes distracted and strays off course.

Integrative, proactive health care involves not only regular visits to your veterinarian but also an understanding of what you can do on a day-to-day basis to maintain and improve your pet's health. You have a great ability to affect positive change in the health and lifestyle of your pet, and there are nutritional and medical answers out there for the health challenges they may face. Combining Western medical care with herbs, nutritional supplementation, and nonconventional treatments such as acupuncture, chiropractic, and physical rehabilitation is an excellent means to support and restore good health.

Even though complementary and alternative care often focuses on traditional forms of medicine, our technological age has brought us new tools with which we can positively affect quality of life. Modalities such as stem cells, electromagnetic field therapy, and hyperbaric oxygen therapy are routinely saving and extending the lives of pets. The rediscovery of herbs like cannabis holds enormous promise for the treatment of many medical conditions. While these modalities may not be part of mainstream medicine (yet), their efficacy is undeniable for those who make the effort to seek out and avail themselves of what is out there.

Too often in life we accept premises and statements as fact without evaluating the details. An advertisement may claim a product is "ideal" or a label may boast of "high quality" with little or no information to back it up. Similar shortcomings are found in the medical field as well.

Western veterinarians, with the best of intentions, may recommend treatment options without knowing there are better, less invasive alternatives. Conversely, false and unsubstantiated claims made by proponents of alternative medicine may give pet owners unrealistic expectations and cause them to turn away from effective Western medical care.

These realities present a challenge to making informed decisions regarding how to best care for your pet. The best advice is to seek out medical providers who share your philosophy toward health care and allow them to guide you along the way. As a pet owner, you are not supposed to have all the answers, but the information you've gained here will help you know the right questions to ask when issues arise.

As time goes on, medicine will continue to integrate organically. The scientifically documented effects of complementary and alternative care continue to attract the attention of open-minded health-care providers. Until the "singularity" of medicine occurs, however, it is up to pet owners and integrative health-care providers to combine the best that both worlds have to offer.

We create a wonderful symbiotic relationship with the animals in our lives. We support each other emotionally and, in many cases, physically. Throughout this book, you have read stories documenting the bonds between people and their pets. Make no mistake: The lengths that people will go to in order to restore and maintain a pet's health benefits both human and animal. It's no secret that people who have pets frequently live longer than those who do not.

The decisions we make regarding medical care, nutrition, and lifestyle affect the quality and quantity of life of our four-legged family members and their two-legged guardians. In the final analysis, nothing matters more than the relationships we forge in life. The depths of these bonds know no bounds, and they are worth preserving for as long as possible.

APPENDIX A

If the secret to a long and healthy life is good living, then the secret to good living is preventive care, health, and wellness. Whether it is the result of lifestyle, nutrition, medical care, or anything else, optimal results usually don't happen by chance. The most successful pet owners are the ones who take time to consider how they are best able to provide for their pet.

The following appendix examines caring for a healthy pet at all stages, from choosing the right pet to geriatric care. Taking a proactive approach helps prevent illness and, if illness does occur, provide for early diagnosis and more successful treatment.

What Pet to Get and When

Choosing a pet may be the only time in our lives we get to pick a relative. Caring for a pet should begin even before you bring him or her home. Possibly the single most impactful decision you will make during the entire time you have a pet is choosing the right one. Variables to navigate include choosing dog or cat, young or adult, and purebred or mixed.

Making these kinds of decisions really is about lifestyle. The best pet to get is one that will be comfortable living in the environment and at the pace of life that is comfortable to you. The following are some important lifestyle considerations to keep in mind as you decide on your pet:

- How much time are you at home versus working?
- Are you an "outdoorsy" person, or do you spend more time at home?
- How large is your living space?
- Do you have an enclosed yard?

- If you have children, what are their ages and levels of maturity?

- If you have other pets, how do they get along with other animals?

- How much time, energy. and money are you willing to commit to your pet's grooming needs? (Even short-haired pets can have high-maintenance fur!)

Failing to consider these kinds of factors can lead to a very stressful experience. Look for a pet that naturally agrees with your pace of life. Make your decisions based on personality, not aesthetics. Forcing a square peg into a round hole is asking for trouble. For example, a person who is at work for 12 hours a day might not want to get a high-energy dog that needs lots of exercise. A bored dog cooped up by himself leads to a pretty good chance the couch is going be eaten when you come home. If you do choose a dog that needs a lot of attention and exercise, you may want to consider the use of a dog walker or "day care" to keep your dog occupied.

Look before you leap. If you've decided to adopt from a shelter or rescue, spend some time with the animal before you make a decision. If you choose a pet from a breeder, check references and make sure the dog or cat was bred responsibly and has excellent genetics.

The Decision of Pet Insurance

The health-care options available to pets are more effective now than they have ever been. Top-notch care, however, can get pricey; the term "holistic" is not synonymous with "inexpensive." Many of the drugs and supplies used are exactly the same as those used in human medicine, and pharmaceutical companies don't discount a drug just because it is used on animals.

The solution to the rising costs associated with better health care is pet insurance. Like any insurance, what suits you best has to do with what kind of coverage you want, deductibles, etc. Given that integrative care is the gold standard, look for a policy that covers holistic treatment. The last thing you ever want to do is make a treatment decision based on finances.

Insurance plans change all the time, so there is no point in recommending anything specific here. Consult with trusted friends and colleagues, and do an Internet search for "Pet Insurance Comparisons." Ask your veterinarian which policies their clients seem most happy with.

Introducing New Pets to Old

Bringing a new pet into a household with existing pets has the potential to be a stressful experience, depending on the personalities of the new and existing pets. (In many cases, introductions of pets of the opposite sex seem to go more smoothly than having two of the same gender.) There are, however, ways to smooth out rough spots in the transition. The name of the game with introductions is take it slow and be patient. There are excellent resources out there to help guide new pet introductions. Books, articles, and videos by the renowned veterinary behaviorist Dr. Sophia Yin are a great place to start.

Dog Introductions: The best way to introduce dogs is on neutral ground. To prevent territory aggression, have the dogs meet at the park or some other place where neither of them are on their "home turf." Have the dogs meet several times over several days before bringing the new dog home. (If this isn't possible, even a single meeting in neutral territory can be helpful.) Once home, be sure to supervise interactions until you feel comfortable a workable relationship has developed.

Cat Introductions: Cats are tricky when it comes to introductions because they don't like change of any kind. When bringing home an additional cat, keep it in a room with the door closed and allow the cats to sniff each other under the door. Allow the new cat to explore the house while the "old" cat is in the room. Do this for several days, and then reverse the arrangement.

It may take as long as a couple of weeks before the cats can be allowed full contact with one another. Even then, there may be some hissing and spitting. However, most cats will find a way to get along or, at least, peacefully coexist.

Dog–Cat Introductions: When introducing dogs to cats, take it slow. Unless the animals are particularly tolerant of the other species, it's going to take time. Cats typically feel threatened and scared, while dogs may either feel scared or want to chase the cat.

Allow the dog and cat to sniff one another under a closed door as in cat introductions. Consider keeping the dog on a leash even in the house whenever the animals are in the same room until you feel comfortable a relationship has been established. Sometimes it takes a few good swats from the cat for a dog to realize it's in their best interest to keep some distance.

Puppy and Kitten Socialization

The first weeks and months a puppy or kitten is at home lay the foundations of behavior for their entire life. Your veterinarian can direct you to good local trainers if you need one. Books and videos from veterinary behaviorist Dr. Sophia Yin are excellent resources in this field as well.

Puppy Socialization: Socialization of young dogs is critical, especially for dogs with a tendency toward nervousness or anxiety. The optimal "window" for socialization is before the dog is 14 weeks old, so get started early. Be sure to introduce your puppy to new experiences at a young age in order to expand their horizons and create a well-adjusted dog. However, this must be done under controlled conditions to prevent disease transmission and inadvertently traumatizing your dog.

Early puppy socialization classes with a trainer and taking your pup to meet friends' dogs are good ways to encourage social behavior. Any dog the puppy comes in contact with should be healthy and current on his vaccines. To prevent serious illness, never take an unvaccinated puppy to dog parks, sidewalks, or anywhere there is dog traffic you are not in control of. The risks of disease are too great.

Kitten Socialization: Kittens kind of socialize themselves. Since they are not out and about like dogs, there is not the same concern for disease transmission. Kittens can get a little aggressive with their play tactics, though. Even though it may be cute when they bite you when they are small, it's not so great when they weigh 15 pounds. Discourage this behavior by disengaging play when they get too rough. Then, once they calm down, you can play with them again.

Choosing a Veterinarian

Given that you are reading a book about integrative medicine, you are likely looking for a veterinarian who is at least open to integrative care. Whatever you're looking for, it's important to find a veterinarian who shares your health care philosophy. You should feel confident that their treatment recommendations fit with how you want your pet's care managed. If you are unsure what your best choice is, see what the "word on the street" is. Ask for recommendations at holistic pet stores in your area, dog parks, and trusted friends and colleagues. Also, the American Holistic Veterinary Association has a listing of holistic practitioners on their website: www.ahvma.org. Just click on "Find a Vet."

When all is said and done, keeping pets healthy is a group effort. Integrative care often provides more hands-on time with a veterinary professional. These frequent interactions provide a greater opportunity for you to communicate questions or concerns and for early diagnosis of new conditions. If you feel your pet is acting differently or his pattern has changed for no apparent reason, get in touch with your veterinarian. Maybe it's nothing, but as you know, the earlier a problem is diagnosed, the greater the chance of a positive outcome.

Schedule Regular Physical Examinations and Diagnostic Testing

Beyond everything you do at home, regular veterinary visits are among the most important ways to make sure your pet stays healthy. As your pet gets older, you'll want to move from annual examinations to semiannual (twice yearly) examinations.

- Cats (1–10 years old): annual examinations
- Cats (10+ years old): semiannual examinations
- Small to medium breeds of dog (1–10 years old): annual examinations
- Small to medium breeds of dog (10+ years old): semiannual examinations
- Large to giant breeds of dog (1–7 years old): annual examinations
- Large to giant breeds of dog (7+ years old): semiannual examinations

During the physical exam, your veterinarian will want to run routine lab work on your pet to make sure they have not been exposed to parasites and everything is okay systemically. In many cases, the early onset of disease can be detected in blood or urine before symptoms arise. Just as with physical examinations, you'll want to move to more frequent screenings as your pet gets older, from biennial (every two years) to annual testing.

- All pets, all ages: annual fecal screening for parasites
- Cats and small to medium breeds of dog (1–10 years old): biennial blood and urine testing
- Cats and small to medium breeds of dog (10+ years old): annual blood and urine testing
- Large to giant breeds of dog (1–7 years old): biennial blood and urine testing
- Large to giant breeds of dog (7+ years old): annual blood and urine testing

APPENDIX B

Choosing the Right Procedures for Your Pet:
Vaccines and Routine Surgical Procedures

Being a pet owner requires taking preventive steps to make sure your pet (and the pet population at large) stays healthy. While certain procedures involve short-term discomfort, the long-term benefits they provide are substantial—just like having your child vaccinated. Since pets don't plan for the future, pet owners and veterinarians must make the decisions that will provide them with a lifetime of good health.

Declawing Cats

Let's get this procedure out of the way right now. In short, there is absolutely no legitimate reason to declaw a cat. Please don't do it.

The process of declawing cats is equivalent to a person having their fingertips amputated at the last knuckle. The procedure itself is painful, and it may lead to lifelong chronic pain. Alternatives to declawing are scratching posts, nail trimming, and placing soft rubber caps on the nails.

Microchipping

Implanting a microchip in pets is commonplace in most veterinary practices. It's a tiny device about the size of a grain of rice that is implanted with a syringe. After the microchip is placed, you register the chip number with your address and contact information. Should a lost pet be brought in to a veterinary hospital, shelter, etc., the chip can be scanned and the owner contacted.

There are a couple of common misconceptions regarding microchips that I'd like to dispel here. First, microchips cannot be used to "track" a pet; the scanners work only when they are a few inches away from the animal. Claims of cancer and other severe complications from microchips are vastly exaggerated. Some isolated incidences may have occurred, but the benefits far outweigh any perceived risk.

Should a fire or natural disaster occur, owners and pets may become separated, and there is little chance for animal control to reconnect them without some kind of positive identification like a microchip. In fact, according to the Humane Society of the United States, of the 15,000 animals that were rescued after Hurricane Katrina, only 3,000 were reunited with their owners.

In short, microchips are recommended for all pets.

Routine Parasite Preventives

Fleas and Ticks

The relative necessity for flea and tick products depends on geographic location, season, and the pet's lifestyle. In hot and humid areas, the presence of these parasites can present major health problems, so good medical care necessitates regular treatment to prevent infestation. In more temperate areas, however, fleas and ticks are more of a nuisance.

There are many flea and tick products on the market, and more are coming and going all the time. Which product to choose for your pet and how often to use it depend on the pet's sensitivity to fleas and how bad the fleas are in your area. For more information, refer to the discussion in Chapter 11.

Gastrointestinal Worms and Deworming

Deworming generally refers to gastrointestinal worms such as hookworms and roundworms. Like all parasites, prevalence is a function of climate, with warmer, more humid areas having more severe issues. There are several ways to address GI parasitism in pets.

Regardless of where you live, an annual fecal examination is recommended to screen for parasites. If a pet is on a heartworm preventive, they are likely getting dewormed regularly as part of that product. Otherwise, deworming can be accomplished on an as-needed basis.

When GI parasites are confirmed via fecal testing, the best bet is to deworm your dog or cat through conventional medical means and be done with it. Although there are natural dewormers such as diatomaceous earth, they are often unreliable in the treatment of worms.

(These products may be helpful as preventives.) Pharmaceutical dewormers generally take one to three days to be effective.

It is commonplace and relatively safe to use dewormers on puppies and kittens, but it may not be necessary. During the course of the puppy or kitten vaccines, your veterinarian should ask for a stool sample to check for parasites. If the test is positive, deworming is appropriate and safe. If the test is negative, however, it may be just as well to hold off. Since parasites cannot always be found in every sample, it is best to have two fecal screenings done during the course of the puppy or kitten vaccines. If both are negative, there should be no need to deworm.

Heartworm

Heartworm is a parasitic disease where worms literally live in the heart of an infested dog. (Although cats can also contract heartworm, it is rare.) Mosquitoes transmit heartworm, so disease prevalence is dependent on weather. Warm, humid climates have more heartworm cases.

Depending on where you live, you may or may not have options regarding heartworm for your dog. Temperate climates, like where I live in Oakland, don't have much heartworm. Since incidences here are relatively rare, the options are to put a dog on heartworm preventive and/or test annually. Even though infection is unlikely, if a dog comes up positive, we will have caught the infestation very early, which makes treatment easier.

In high-rate heartworm areas, such as the southeastern U.S., heartworm prevention for dogs is a necessity. The odds are just too great to try and go without protection. These pets should be on heartworm preventive year-round *and* receive an annual heartworm test.

There are many brands of heartworm preventives on the market. They all use some version of drugs like ivermectin or milbemycin. These drugs kill the larval forms of heartworm before they become adults and set up shop in the heart. While high doses of these drugs can be dangerous to dogs, the doses used for heartworm prevention are very safe. Any risk is far outweighed by the risk of contracting heartworm.

One final note regarding heartworm prevention: There is no such thing as an effective natural or holistic heartworm preventive. Please don't attempt this. If a dog gets heartworm due to ineffectual prevention, the results can literally be fatal.

Spay and Neuter

The decision of if and when to spay or neuter a pet weighs heavily on some pet owners. If you or someone in your family is hesitant to spay or neuter your pet, you are not alone. Many people are a little hesitant. There are, however, plenty of great reasons to spay or neuter and very few reasons not to. It can benefitsyour dog or cat from a physical, behavioral, and safety standpoint. It also benefits you financially and socially. Let me explain.

Spaying or neutering pets eliminates the chances of unwanted reproduction and cancer of the testicles, ovaries, and uterus. Spaying decreases the chances of mammary (breast) cancer. In addition, neutering dogs prevents enlargement of the prostate in male dogs as they age. All of these factors improve the quality and quantity of life of dogs and cats.

Behaviorally, the reduction in testosterone and estrogen after spaying often makes pets better pets. Behaviors like aggression between animals, urine marking or spraying, and a tendency to "roam" looking for mates are all minimized. Pets are safer, since they get into fewer fights and are less likely to be hit by cars. There is also far less of a chance they will be surrendered by their owners because of behavioral issues.

In addition to benefits to your pet, having them spayed or neutered benefits you as well. The decrease in fighting and elimination of medical issues as described below make their health care easier and less expensive. It's also cheaper to license a spayed or neutered pet. Last, there is a social stigma to having an intact pet. If your pet is trying to mate or your female cat in heat is keeping the neighborhood awake with her howling all night, you are not winning any popularity contests.

Perceived Drawbacks of Spay and Neuter

There are purebred dogs and cats that are left intact in order to continue their breed. Even within this narrow field, however, breeding of pets should be done very judiciously and only as often as is necessary. These pets can and should be spayed or neutered after they are successfully bred.

Other common reasons I hear for not wanting to spay or neuter are "I want my pet to experience having a litter" and "I want my children to experience the miracle of our pet having babies." Yet there is absolutely no evidence to suggest that dogs or cats are longing for the joys of parenthood. Under most circumstances, their offspring are separated from them eight weeks after birth anyway. It's not like they have the "joy" of watching their kids grow up!

Parents who want to breed their pets for the benefit of their children's experience would be better served to think it through a little more. A more educational alternative is for the family to volunteer at the SPCA or a local rescue group. This allows children to enjoy puppies and kittens and also realize the reality of pet overpopulation. The ASPCA estimates 2,700,000 dogs and cats are euthanized in shelters every year. There is no reason to breed more.

What to Do and When

Classically, veterinarians recommend spaying and neutering before pets are 6 months old. The goal here is to perform the surgery before they hit puberty. This eliminates most hormonally associated behavioral issues and, in females, eliminates the chances of mammary (breast) cancer later in life. Although this has been "written in stone" in the veterinary community for many years, new research is about to shake things up.

Recent studies indicate certain breeds of dogs have lower incidences of specific cancers, orthopedic disease, urinary incontinence, and age-related cognitive decline if they are spayed or neutered later. In other words, waiting longer leads to better health in the long term. While there are definitely differences between the breeds, there does appear to be a trend toward better health in pets that were spayed or neutered later. To date, the published studies have only evaluated golden retrievers, labrador retrievers, and German shepherds, and it is unknown if these trends will hold true with all breeds of dogs.

There have been no similar studies done in cats, and the behavioral issues associated with intact male and female cats is so significant, it would be unrealistic to expect the majority of pet owners to "stick it out" and wait to spay and neuter.

In the final analysis, the question is really not *if* you should spay or neuter your pet, but *when*. Based on what we know as of 2016, recommendations for spay and neuter are as follows:

- Small to medium dogs: Spay or neuter at 12 to 18 months of age
- Large or giant breeds: Spay or neuter at 18 to 24 months of age
- Cats: Spay or neuter at or around 6 months of age

Last, if an intact male dog does not have behavioral issues, there is no absolute necessity to neuter him. Careful veterinary monitoring for the development of testicular cancer or prostate enlargement as he gets older may necessitate neutering down the road. Outside of these concerns, leaving males intact poses no major health risks. The same cannot be said for females, who run the risk of ovarian, uterine, or mammary cancer as well as uterine infections, which can be life-threatening. They should be spayed as described above.

Your Pet's Vaccine Guide

Dog and cat owners are often unclear about what to vaccinate their pets for and how often. In truth, the veterinary community is not in complete agreement on the topic. There are several reasons for the disparity amongst veterinarians that range from disagreement between researchers to simple unwillingness to change.

It is true that vaccines are not benign drugs. Under normal circumstances, vaccines stimulate the immune system, leading to antibody production and effective immunity against disease. However, the body might respond to a vaccine with excessive or aberrant immune stimulation, and this may lead to medical issues in your pet. Although the research is ongoing and not conclusive, vaccines in pets have been implicated in the onset of autoimmune diseases (see Chapter 23) and cancerous processes. Cats are susceptible to a cancer called feline injection-site sarcoma, which results in aggressive tumors that require extensive treatment. However, the risk to your cat is as low as 1 in 10,000.

Despite any controversy, appropriately administered vaccines are absolutely necessary. The fact is, without protection from diseases like canine distemper and parvo, many dogs would die before reaching adulthood. The same is true for cats with panleukopenia, and both species are susceptible to rabies.

Vaccines are effective and have saved countless pets. Like every other drug, however, vaccines should be used judiciously.

Vaccine Dos and Don'ts

The big "don't" when it comes to vaccines is: Don't overvaccinate. To that end, in the following sections, I discuss the difference between core and non-core canine and feline vaccinations as well as vaccine titers.

Core vaccines are the ones that should be given to all pets to protect them from life-threatening diseases. The only exceptions are pets with an underlying medical condition that precludes the ability to safely vaccinate; such decisions should be made with your veterinarian based on what is safest for your pet.

Non-core vaccinations are available for pets whose lifestyle may put them in contact with specific diseases. These non-core vaccines are recommended for certain animals based largely on lifestyle and geographic location.

Vaccine titers are a means by which your pet's level of immunity can be measured through a blood sample. It measures the level of antibodies that the animal's immune system has produced in response to a vaccine against a specific disease. Through this method, we can determine whether your pet is protected.

The bottom line is, vaccinate for what is absolutely necessary based on core vaccination protocols, legal necessities, and your pet's lifestyle. Don't vaccinate for diseases your pet will never come in contact with.

To prevent adverse reactions, it is best if pets receive no more than two vaccines at any one time, and wait at least one month before giving the next vaccinations.

As they get older, dogs and cats may need fewer vaccines. Older pets tend to be outside less and have less direct contact with other animals. Talk with your veterinarian about what is necessary for your pet at the stage of life he or she is currently in.

Core Canine Vaccines

The vaccine schedules discussed below are guidelines for safe and effective vaccination. Timing and protocol variation based on the needs of an individual pet are commonplace. Consult with your veterinarian about what is best for your dog.

Canine distemper and parvo vaccination: Canine distemper and parvo (short for canine parvovirus type 2) are deadly viruses that commonly affect younger, unvaccinated dogs. Distemper often causes severe respiratory infection and sometimes neurologic disease; it is most commonly transmitted through coughing dogs. Parvo causes severe gastrointestinal disease, including vomiting and profound bloody diarrhea that is infectious to other dogs.

Because parvo is so contagious, it is critical that puppies not be allowed to go anywhere with a lot of dog traffic and/or stray dogs. Until they are fully vaccinated, keep their interactions restricted to controlled environments like puppy class or friends' houses.

There are many vaccines available that protect against distemper and parvo. However, Nobivac, made by Intervet, is the only one that contains only distemper and parvo. All others are combined with vaccinations against diseases such as leptospirosis, canine adenovirus, and parainfluenza. I believe that vaccines combining three, four, or even five different diseases are unnecessary and should be avoided because they may increase the chances of adverse reactions.

Canine distemper and parvo titers can be used to determine the necessity of further vaccinations after the initial core vaccine series. Dogs who show adequate antibody levels to distemper and parvo are presumed to be immune and need no further vaccinations; however, they will need to be retested every three years.

- Puppies need three doses at 3- to 4-week intervals starting at 8 to 10 weeks of age—for example, at 8, 12, and 16 weeks of age.

- One-year-old dogs should have a distemper–parvo titer (see below) or a single vaccine. The Nobivac vaccine will have a three-year duration.

- Starting at one or four years old, distemper–parvo titers are recommended every three years.

Rabies vaccination: Most people are at least passingly familiar with rabies. This virus, which is transmitted through the saliva of an infected animal, is 100 percent fatal to pets. Only a handful of humans have ever survived a rabies infection, and because of its transmissibility to humans, rabies vaccinations in dogs are legally required. However, medical exemptions can be granted based on approval of the local animal services or public health departments.

The legal specifics of when rabies vaccines need to be given vary by geographic location. Your veterinarian will let you know what the requirements are.

Rabies vaccine titers are available and often required for the transportation of dogs overseas. Although a rabies titer does indicate protection from the rabies virus, it is not acceptable as an alternative to vaccination in the eyes of the law.

There are two different kinds of rabies titers. If you are traveling overseas, the Fluorescent Antibody Virus Neutralization (FAVN) test may be required. If the titer is being used to demonstrate immunity for reasons other than travel, the Rapid Fluorescent Foci Inhibition Test (RFFIT) is recommended. It can take weeks to get rabies titer results back, so be sure to plan ahead with regard to travel.

- Puppies should have a rabies vaccine between 16 and 20 weeks of age, as per local ordinance. Some people prefer to wait until their puppies are six months old; however, remember that unvaccinated animals are at risk.

- A one-year booster is required in most areas, and then the vaccine is required every three years.

- Rabies vaccine titers are often required for overseas transport of your pet. They are not a legal substitute for vaccination.

Non-Core Canine Vaccines

Leptospirosis: Leptospirosis is a bacterial disease transmitted through the urine of infected animals. It is contracted when a dog drinks from a contaminated water source such as a puddle. Leptospirosis infections can be quite serious and lead to liver or kidney failure (see Chapters 18 and 19). It is also transmissible to humans.

Dogs spending a lot of time outdoors may be at greater risk for leptospirosis. Your veterinarian can discuss with you the relative incidence in your area.

It is possible for vaccinated dogs to get leptospirosis.

- Initially, dogs are given two vaccines, approximately one month apart.

- A booster vaccine is required annually to maintain immunity.

Bordetella: *Bordetella bronchiseptica* is a bacterium that causes the disease colloquially known as "kennel cough." However, saying a dog has "kennel cough" is like saying a person has "a cold." Kennel cough is simply a description of symptoms that can be caused by many different organisms. The Bordetella vaccine protects against only the one bacterial organism.

Kennel cough is transmitted through the air when infected dogs cough, which is why transmission is most common in enclosed areas such as boarding facilities. To help prevent outbreaks, the vaccine is frequently required by boarding, daycare, and grooming facilities.

The vast majority of dogs who get kennel cough recover with no treatment or with a short course of antibiotics and cough suppressants. Severe disease from kennel cough caused by secondary pneumonia is rare, and the vaccine does not prevent all dogs from getting sick.

Bordetella vaccines can be oral, intranasal, or injectable. The oral and intranasal forms are best.

- Vaccination is needed every 6 to 12 months, depending on risk assessment and the requirements of any facilities that you frequent.

Lyme: Lyme is a bacterial disease transmitted by ticks, so along with vaccination, tick control is a major part of Lyme prevention. The disease affects both dogs and humans, although humans tend to get the worst of it. The prevalence of Lyme disease varies greatly by geographic region. Depending on where you live, a Lyme vaccination may be considered a core vaccine.

- Initial vaccination is a series of two vaccines given one month apart, and then a third given six months later.

- Annual boosters are recommended to maintain immunity.

Rattlesnake toxoid: Obviously, there is no vaccine that is going to prevent a snake from biting a nosy dog. The rattlesnake toxoid was developed to help minimize the severity of rattlesnake bites in dogs. "Vaccinated" dogs tend to have less severe reactions to rattlesnake venom and may need less antivenin. However, any dog bitten by a rattlesnake needs immediate medical attention, regardless of vaccination status.

Dogs living in rattlesnake endemic areas, or those who travel to the backcountry, may benefit from vaccination.

- The rattlesnake vaccine is initially given as a series of two vaccines, one month apart. Boosters are recommended every 6 to 12 months depending on the level of risk.

- If the booster is given annually, it is best to give it in the spring, when snakes have the most venom and bites are potentially the most dangerous.

Core Feline Vaccines

The vaccine schedules discussed below are guidelines for safe and effective vaccination. Timing and protocol variation based on the needs of an individual pet are commonplace. Consult with your veterinarian about what is best for your kitty.

FVRCP: FVRCP is a combination vaccine that protects against feline viral rhinotracheitis (FVR), feline calicivirus (C), and panleukopenia (P). Rhinotracheitis and calicivirus cause upper respiratory symptoms rather like bad head colds and are rarely life-threatening. Panleukopenia, however, is similar to parvo in dogs, a potentially fatal disease that causes severe GI distress.

Feline panleukopenia titers can be used to determine the necessity of further vaccinations after the initial core vaccine series. Cats who show adequate antibody levels to panleukopenia are presumed to be immune. There is no titer for rhinotracheitis or calicivirus.

- Kittens are usually given three doses at 3- to 4-week intervals, usually at 8, 12, and 16 weeks. Alternatively, two vaccines can be given when they are 8 or 9 weeks old, and then at 12 or 13 weeks old, as long as they stay strictly indoors so their disease exposure prior to completing their vaccine series is minimal.

- A booster vaccine at one year of age is effective for three years. You may use a panleukopenia titer afterward to determine whether further vaccinations are needed.

- Adult cats who are allowed outdoors may benefit from an FVRCP booster every three years, as protection against upper respiratory viruses.

Rabies: Most people are at least passingly familiar with rabies. This virus, which is transmitted through the saliva of an infected animal, is 100 percent fatal to pets. Only a handful of humans have ever survived a rabies infection, and because of its transmissibility to humans, rabies vaccinations in cats are legally required. However, medical exemptions can be granted based on approval of the local animal services or public health departments. The legal specifics of when rabies vaccines need to be given vary by geographic location. Your veterinarian will let you know what the requirements are.

There are several rabies vaccines available. Purevax, made by Merial, seems to cause the fewest reactions. Purevax vaccines are available as both one-year and three-year protection durations.

Rabies vaccine titers are available and often required for the transportation of cats overseas. Although a rabies titer does indicate protection from the rabies virus, it is not acceptable as an alternative to vaccination in the eyes of the law.

There are two different kinds of rabies titers. If you are traveling overseas, the Fluorescent Antibody Virus Neutralization (FAVN) test may be required. If the titer is being used to demonstrate immunity for reasons other than travel, the Rapid Fluorescent Foci Inhibition

Test (RFFIT) is recommended. It can take weeks to get rabies titer results back, so be sure to plan ahead with regard to travel.

- All kittens should be given a rabies vaccination between 16 and 20 weeks of age. Some people prefer to wait until their kittens are six months old; however, remember that unvaccinated animals are at risk.

- Strictly indoor cats do not need a rabies booster. (The single vaccine as a kitten may help provide some immunity in case the cat gets outside.)

- Cats allowed outdoors should have a booster at one year, and then every one or three years, depending on the vaccine used.

- Rabies vaccine titers are often required for overseas transport of your pet. They are not a legal substitute for vaccination.

Non-Core Feline Vaccines

Feline leukemia: Feline leukemia virus (FeLV) is a retrovirus much like human immunodeficiency virus (HIV) in humans. Despite the name, the virus rarely causes leukemia, but it can lead to immune dysfunction and secondary illness in much the same way HIV progresses to acquired immune deficiency syndrome (AIDS). Also similar to HIV, it can take years for cats infected with FeLV to show any symptoms of disease.

FeLV is contracted through the bite or scratch of an infected cat. "Casual" contact is not generally considered a major risk for contracting the disease, and cats living in the same household for years may not transmit the virus from one to the other. Regardless, infected cats should be kept strictly indoors to prevent transmission. Outdoor cats and cats living with an FeLV-infected cat should be vaccinated.

- Kittens should initially be given two vaccines, approximately one month apart.

- A booster vaccine is needed at one year of age and every three years afterward.

Feline immunodeficiency virus: Feline immunodeficiency virus (FIV) is a retrovirus like FeLV. Over time, the virus suppresses the immune system, leading other conditions like infections and organ disease. Just like FeLV, FIV infection can take years to show symptoms. FIV is usually contracted through the bite or scratch of an infected cat, and "casual" contact is not generally considered a risk for contracting the disease.

There are two problems with the FIV vaccine: (1) It is not particularly effective, and (2) FIV-vaccinated cats will test positive for FIV. Unfortunately, this can lead to FIV-vaccinated cats that turn up at shelters being euthanized under suspicion of being FIV positive. For these reasons, vaccinating for FIV is not rcommended.

APPENDIX C

Home-Prepared Diets for Dogs and Cats

It's easy to get bogged down in little details and make things more difficult than they need to be. At the end of the day, however, feeding your pet is simple. In fact, the entire process can be summed up in three steps:

- Determine how many calories your cat or dog needs per day based on the RER table in Chapter 5.

- Choose the recipe you are going to make and buy the ingredients and supplements required.

- Follow the recipe instructions.

Read through all the information provided below once, and then use this section as a reference.

How the Recipes Are Nutritionally Balanced

Dr. Susan Lauten has painstakingly crafted each of the recipes so they are perfectly balanced for optimal nutrition for long-term feeding. Dr. Lauten holds a master's degree in Animal Nutrition and a doctorate in Biomedical Sciences from Auburn University. She also completed a postdoctoral fellowship at the University of Tennessee (UT) College of Veterinary Medicine. At UT, she was one of the founders of the clinical nutrition service at the teaching hospital. She continues her work through her pet service, PetNutritionConsulting.com.

It is crucial to add all of the supplements as instructed in each recipe in order for the food to be nutritionally balanced. Multiple supplements are used in the diets because no single supplement provides vitamins and minerals in the appropriate amounts for dogs and cats.

Although it is possible to make pet food at home with fewer supplements, it would require a much higher number of food ingredients, creating more complex recipes with dozens of ingredients that even the most highly motivated pet owners are loath to do. For those who are truly motivated to make balanced, home-prepared foods with minimal supplementation, I strongly recommend a consultation with a nutritionist like Dr. Lauten. The goal of this book, however, is to provide your pet with optimal nutrition while keeping your life relatively easy.

Every recipe in this book is compatible for any healthy adult dog or cat (whichever type of animal is indicated by the recipe). For example, if you have two pets and one has kidney disease, you can feed the healthy one the kidney diet as well. While certain recipes are designed to maximize health for pets with a specific condition, their nutrient profile is excellent for all adult pets.

Caution: Puppy and kitten diets should not be fed to seniors, because the levels of calcium and phosphorus are too high.

How to Transition Your Pet to a Home-Prepared Diet

Any diet change should be done gradually, particularly when changing food formats such as going from kibble to fresh food. Many animals, cats in particular, are creatures of habit and routine, so a gradual change will help them get used to it. Furthermore, it allows your pet's digestive tract time to adjust. An abrupt diet change can lead to vomiting and/or diarrhea.

Begin the transition by feeding one-third of the new diet with two-thirds of the existing diet. Over the course of one to two weeks, slowly increase the amount of the new and decrease the amount of the old. For animals with sensitive tummies, feel free to take more time for the transition. Most pets do great with the change as long as we give their GI tract a little time.

How to Source Ingredients and Supplements

Buying the highest-quality ingredients leads to a higher-quality product. Although there is an ongoing and heated debate about the nutritional benefits of organic products, if you can afford to buy organic, I recommend it. While the nutritional value may or may not be different from conventional, the lack of traditional pesticides and herbicides is a bonus.

It is best not to make substitutions when it comes to ingredients in these recipes. Even different cuts of chicken (thighs versus breasts, for example) have different nutrient profiles, so they are not interchangeable. Exchanging one ingredient for another can lead to a poorly balanced diet and cause medical problems over time. Although feeding a variety of foods is recommended, home-prepared diets must be rebalanced with every change. Always consult with a veterinarian or nutritionist to discuss how to rotate through foods safely.

Dr. Lauten and I feel that the following ingredients in the recipes warrant extra caution:

- **Canola oil:** Conventionally produced canola oil is genetically modified (GMO), so please use organic.

- **Rice:** Basmati rice is preferred, as it tends to have fewer issues with chemical contamination. Do not substitute white rice for brown (or brown for white), as they have different nutrient profiles.

- **Meat:** Try to source domestic (and organic) whenever possible. This will cut down on the possibility of contaminants.

Sourcing high-quality ingredients for supplements is crucial. (Low-quality fish oil, for example, can contain contaminants such as lead and other heavy metals.) The easiest way to source high-quality supplements is to use reputable brands. If you are unsure, ask for help at your local health food store or naturopathic pharmacy.

Ultimately, you want supplements produced by reputable companies that can show independent laboratory testing of their products to confirm accuracy of the ingredient label and the absence of contaminants. When in doubt, research companies online to find out what are the best supplements available in your area. If a company is testing for contaminants, they will talk about it in their literature and on their website. A few minutes of research will really pay off.

Because of the challenges in finding ideal supplements, we have provided brand name recommendations for every supplement required in the recipes. The goal is to eliminate any stress or guesswork required to help you make an ideal diet for your pet. In some cases, vitamin E for example, the supplement is so ubiquitous, a brand recommendation is not necessary.

All of the supplements can be purchased through online retailers such as iherb.com or amazon.com. I've listed all the supplements that will be needed, along with the recommended brands and guidelines for substitutions, in Appendix D.

How to Prepare the Food

Convenience is always a consideration when preparing a homemade diet. Feel free to double or triple any recipe, then divide the food into meal-sized portions and freeze. (This is safe to do for both cooked and raw preparations.) When ready to feed your pet, transfer frozen meals to the refrigerator to thaw the day before you need them. Do not thaw meat at room temperature because this can lead to bacterial contamination.

At feeding time, warm the food to body temperature to increase palatability and make it easier to digest. The best method is to warm the bag or container of food in hot water. Warming food in a microwave or in a pan on the stovetop can lead to overheating and destroy the vitamins.

If feeding your pet raw, make sure the vegetables are chopped into small pieces. You can also use a blender to make vegetables small enough for efficient digestion. Certain ingredients always require cooking: potatoes, butternut squash, noodles, rice, and other grains.

When a particular cooking method is specified for a recipe, it is often done to control the fat content or another aspect of nutrition. It is best not to substitute specific cooking methods, if possible.

When it comes to seasoning, less is more. Our pets do not have the same craving for "seasoned" food as we do. However, you may use small amounts of garlic in the recipes, which is both a flavoring agent *and* an herb with antibacterial and antiviral properties.

Caution: Never use onions or products containing onions—they are toxic to dogs and cats.

Raw vs. Cooked Diets

Most pets do great on fresh foods, whether raw or cooked. All of the recipes in this book can be prepared using cooked or raw ingredients, as you desire. The nutritional analysis stays the same either way.

If you decide to experiment with cooked versus raw food, monitor for differences in your pet's appetite, stool quality, and activity level. Pets with inflammatory bowel disease (IBD), dietary sensitivities, or allergies may find more relief with one method over the other. I recommend feeding a cooked diet to puppies under six months of age to prevent the possibility of food-borne bacterial illness.

If your pet has never eaten raw food, start by feeding him cooked fresh foods. First, cook a recipe as normal so they get accustomed to it. Feed the cooked food for two or three days. Then, feed your pet a lightly cooked batch of food for two or three days. The next time you make a batch of the recipe, leave it raw. By doing this, you are allowing their digestive system to become accustomed to digesting raw food.

Caution: Raw feeding contains the potential for foodborne illness. Raw meat, even that purchased for human consumption, often has a certain amount of bacterial contamination. Be sure to use hot soapy water or an appropriate cleaner to wash plates, utensils, and countertops that have come in contact with raw meat. For pets or people with compromised immune systems, or households with small children, cooking the food is the safest way to go.

A Special Note for Large-Breed Puppies

The following section has been contributed by Dr. Susan Lauten, who is, among other things, an expert on the topic of large-breed puppy nutrition. (She wrote her Ph.D. dissertation on the topic.) There are very few resources for pet owners to find appropriate recipes for home-prepared diets for large- and giant-breed dogs, and early nutrition is critical for long-term health in these puppies.

In the mammalian kingdom, it is impossible to find newborns that grow to full height within the first year of life. This, however, is exactly the case in giant-breed dogs. Newborn puppies that weigh about a pound at birth frequently weigh 130 pounds by their first birthday. This exceptional growth rate makes these puppies more sensitive to dietary changes during their growth period, particularly between three and five months of age.

The nutritional components that play an important role in this remarkable growth rate include energy, vitamin D, calcium, phosphorus, and associated hormones. High-protein foods do not contribute to dietary imbalances causing growth deformities and skeletal disease.[1] However, excess energy or calories is one contributing factor of degenerative orthopedic disease (DOD) and other developmental diseases that large-and giant-breed puppies frequently encounter.

Dietary Energy (Calories)

Despite the incredible growth rate of large-breed puppies, lack of nutrition will not affect the adult size of the animal. It will, however, slow their growth rate. Although DOD can also be seen in puppies with an insufficient calcium intake, veterinarians more frequently see it as a consequence of excess food.

Those roly-poly, cute, overfed puppies you often see are, unfortunately, the *most* in danger of developing DOD. Young puppies fed an excess amount of calories will not result in fat, normal-sized puppies, but instead faster-growing puppies. The problem is that the undeveloped skeletal system of these puppies is not able to adequately support quick growth, and this leads to bone and joint problems. Commonly encountered problems related to overfeeding are hip and elbow dysplasia, cartilage abnormalities (osteochondrosis dessicans), painful bone inflammation (panosteitis), and elbow damage (fragmentation and fissures of the coronoid process).[2] Inflamed joints (arthritis) are also associated with excess energy intake during the rapid growth phase. Arthritis decreases the life expectancy of dogs by 1.8 years compared with dogs provided restricted energy intake.[3]

In a large study of Labrador puppies, one group was fed as much as they wanted while another group was fed 75 percent of the food eaten by the first group. The expected growth rate differences appeared, but gradually disappeared beginning at six months of age.[4] Developmental orthopedic disease, however, occurred in the puppies that ate as much as they wanted.

The take-home message is that regardless of how you feed them, the puppies will achieve the same adult size. The puppies whose food intake was restricted, however, had a much lower rate of orthopedic problems.

Calcium and Phosphorus

Levels of calcium and phosphorus in the diet are crucial for large, fast-growing puppies. Prior to six months of age, puppies' bodies cannot regulate how much calcium they absorb, and excesses of calcium in the diet can affect bone development, leading to DOD. In older puppies (five to six months and older) and adults, the body absorbs calcium from the diet through an active process involving hormones and Vitamin D.

Once the process switches from passive to active, the amount of dietary calcium is less critical because the body will only absorb what it needs. For those who have had too much calcium at an early age, however, the damage may have already been done.

How Much to Feed

Anyone who has a large-breed puppy knows how incredibly fast they grow. Owners should regularly recalculate their puppy's energy requirement as it can change from week to week. In order to determine how much food to feed, we need to determine the dog's resting energy requirement (RER) and, from that, its daily energy requirement (DER). (See Chapter 5 for more details on RER and DER.)

The daily energy requirement for puppies is determined as follows:

Weaning to 4 months of age:	DER = 3 × RER
4 months to 1 year of age:	DER = 2 × RER
Over 1 year of age (spayed/neutered):	DER = 1.6 × RER
Over 1 year of age (intact):	DER = 1.8 × RER

Utilizing a body condition score (BCS) chart is an excellent point of reference to determine if the puppy is of an appropriate weight. (See Chapter 5 for more information and charts.) On the 5-point scale, 2.5 is considered ideal weight. On the 9-point scale, 5 is average. When it comes to large-breed puppies, it is best to err slightly on the light side. In other words, keeping the puppy at a "2" on the 5-point scale or a "4.5" on the 9-point scale is best.

What Kind of Food

To prevent skeletal growth disturbances in large-breed dogs, it is critical to offer a diet specifically formulated for large-breed puppies. These diets restrict energy (calorie) intake and provide defined levels of calcium and phosphorus and ratios different from those found in regular puppy foods. Avoid dietary supplements, because they can cause an imbalance in the diet and contribute to developmental orthopedic disease.

Owners of large-breed puppies should look for foods with the following nutrient profiles:

Protein 24–29%

Fat 11–16%

Fiber 2.4–5.6%

Calcium 0.8–1.4%

Phosphorus 0.7–1.2%

Calcium Phosphorus Ratio (Ca:P) 1.1:1–1.2:1

Energy Density . . . . 3.4–4.1 kcal on a dry-matter basis

Puppies need specific quantities of food, and you and your veterinarian will need to assess the puppy's body condition weekly to make adjustments to the feeding regimen. If you make home-prepared meals, you'll need a recipe that has been formulated by a qualified nutritionist to prevent developmental orthopedic disease. The effects of skeletal disturbances and obesity resulting from improper diets can result in deformities in bones and joints that are irreversible. These effects often lead to chronic pain and poor quality of life as the dog ages, which in turn may lead to early death or euthanasia.

The potential pitfalls of improper nutrition in large-breed puppies can be catastrophic. While not all nutritional considerations are as dramatic, these pups are an example of how important it is to feed a balanced diet to our pets. As you can see, it is about so much more than quality ingredients.

Recipes for Dogs

Canine Growth (Puppy): Medium-Sized Breeds and Smaller

Caution: Puppy diets should not be fed to seniors, because the levels of calcium and phosphorus are too high.

CHICKEN, OATS, AND VEGGIES

Yield: 1,972.41 grams
Calories: 2,343.35 (per recipe): 1.2 kcal/g, 254 kcal/cup, 1,188 kcal/kg
As fed: Protein 13.9%, Fat 4.3%, Fiber 1%, Carbohydrates 6.1%, Moisture 74%
All ingredients can be served raw, except for: quick oats

 2½ pounds chicken breast, skinless
 3 ounces chicken livers
 1½ cups unenriched quick oats (to yield 3 cups cooked)
 1½ cups green beans
 1½ cups cauliflower
 1½ cups kale
 3 tablespoons organic canola oil
 1,000 mg omega-3 fish oil
 ½ teaspoon iodized salt
 1½ teaspoons calcium carbonate powder
 4½ teaspoons dicalcium phosphate
 3 tablets Kirkland Signature Daily Multi, crushed

Place the chicken in a pot with just enough water to barely cover the meat. Bring to a boil, cook for 15 minutes, then add liver and cook for 5 minutes or until meat reaches an internal temperature of 165°F. Drain, retaining broth to pour over the finished recipe before serving. When chicken is cool enough to handle, chop meat and liver into bite-size pieces.

Follow package instructions to yield 3 cups of cooked quick oats.

Chop green beans and cauliflower into bite-size pieces, then boil in water for 10 minutes, or until tender.

Slice the kale into ½-inch strips, and put into the hot chicken broth to wilt. Remove the wilted kale and place it with the other cooked vegetables, keeping the broth separate. Refrigerate the broth, and pour some over each portion of food before serving.

Allow all hot ingredients to rest and come to room temperature, either on the counter or in the refrigerator. Then combine the chicken meat, liver, oats, and vegetables with the canola oil and the omega-3 fish oil.

Combine the salt and rest of the supplements in a small bowl. Sprinkle this mixture over the food as evenly as possible, and combine well. Pour some of the broth over the food just before serving.

BEEF, SWEET POTATO, AND LENTILS

Yield: 3,233.68 grams
Calories: 4,320.03 (per recipe): 1.3 kcal/g, 303 kcal/cup, 1,336 kcal/kg
As fed: Protein 10.2%, Fat 6.4%, Fiber 1.9%, Carbohydrates 8.5%, Moisture 72.5%
All ingredients can be served raw, except for: sweet potatoes, lentils

  3 cups sweet potatoes

  3 pounds 85% lean ground beef

  1½ cups lentils (to yield 3 cups cooked; canned is okay)

  1 cup cauliflower

  1 cup broccoli

  2 cups green beans

  100 IU vitamin E (from capsules)

  ¾ teaspoon iodized salt

  2 tablespoons bone meal powder

  1½ tablets Kirkland Signature Daily Multi, crushed

  30 mg zinc citrate

  200 mcg selenium

  700 mg choline

  500 mg L-tryptophan

Preheat the oven to 400°F. Peel the sweet potatoes, and chop into bite-size cubes. Bake in the oven for 20 to 30 minutes, or until fork-tender. Potatoes may also be mashed, if desired.

While the potatoes are cooking, break the ground beef into 2-inch chunks and place in a pot with just enough water to cover. Bring water to a boil, then allow the meat to cook for 10 minutes or until browned, occasionally breaking the meat up into chunks with a fork to ensure all the beef is cooked. Use a strainer to drain the meat, but reserve the broth. Chill this broth in the refrigerator, and remove the fat that comes to the top. A bit of this reserved broth can be poured over each portion of food before serving.

Prepare dry lentils according to the package instructions to yield 3 cups of cooked lentils. If using canned lentils, simply drain the lentils before using.

Bring a pot of water to a boil. Chop cauliflower, broccoli, and green beans into bite-size pieces. Add all vegetables to the pot, and cook for 10 minutes or until tender. Drain.

Allow all hot ingredients to rest and come to room temperature, either on the counter or in the refrigerator, then mix everything together with the contents of the vitamin E capsules.

Combine the salt and rest of the supplements in a small bowl. Sprinkle this mixture over the food as evenly as possible, and combine well. Pour some of the reserved broth over the food just before serving.

Canine Growth (Puppy): Large and Giant Breeds

Caution: Puppy diets should not be fed to seniors, because the levels of calcium and phosphorus are too high.

BEEF AND QUINOA

Yield: 3,992.68 grams
Calories: 6,228.33 (per recipe): 1.6kcal/g, 354 kcal/cup, 1,559 kcal/kg
As fed: Protein 11.3%, Fat 7.2%, Fiber 1%, Carbohydrates 11.3%, Moisture 67.6%
All ingredients can be served raw, except for: quinoa, butternut squash

   4 pounds 85% lean ground beef

   3 cups quinoa (to yield 9 cups cooked)

   2 cups kale

   2 cups butternut squash

   1 tablespoon organic canola oil

   400 IU vitamin D3 (from capsules)

   2,000 mg omega-3 fish oil (from capsules)

   1 teaspoon iodized salt

   ⅝ teaspoon potassium chloride powder

   1¼ teaspoons calcium carbonate powder

   5½ teaspoons bone meal powder

   4 tablets Kirkland Signature Daily Multi, crushed

   45 mg zinc citrate

   36 mg iron bisglycinate

   1,000 mg L-tryptophan

15 mg chelated copper

650 mcg iodine (from kelp tablets)

Crumble the ground beef, and broil or panfry over medium-high heat for 15 minutes or until browned. Reserve the rendered fat with the meat.

Prepare the quinoa according to the package to yield 9 cups of cooked quinoa. Slice kale into 1-inch strips and mix into the hot quinoa to wilt.

Chop the butternut squash into 1-inch cubes and boil in water for 15 minutes or until tender. Drain, and then lightly mash the squash so that it will be easy for a puppy to eat. (The smaller the puppy, the smaller the pieces.)

Allow all hot ingredients to rest and come to room temperature, either on the counter or in the refrigerator, then mix with the canola oil and the contents of the vitamin D and omega-3 fish oil capsules.

Combine the salt and rest of the supplements in a small bowl. Sprinkle this mixture over the food as evenly as possible, and combine well.

TURKEY AND DRESSING

Yield: 1,841.58 grams
Calories: 2,692.77 (per recipe): 1.5 kcal/g, 332 kcal/cup, 1,462 kcal/kg
As fed: Protein 13.7%, Fat 5.9%, Fiber 1%, Carbohydrates 10%, Moisture 68.6%
All ingredients can be served raw, except for: potatoes

1 cup potatoes

1½ pounds ground turkey

1 teaspoon dried sage

1 cup carrots

1 cup green peas

5 slices whole-wheat bread

½ cup dried cranberries

1 tablespoon organic canola oil

3,000 mg omega-3 fish oil (from capsules)

100 IU vitamin E (from capsules)

1 teaspoon iodized salt

½ teaspoon potassium chloride powder

2⅜ teaspoons calcium carbonate powder

1 tablet Kirkland Signature Daily Multi, crushed

27 mg iron bisglycinate

30 mg zinc citrate

700 mg choline

Preheat the oven to 400°F. Peel potatoes and bake 30 minutes or until tender, then mash with a fork.

While the potatoes are baking, place the turkey and sage in a pot with just enough water to cover. Bring water to a boil, then allow the meat to cook for 10 minutes, or until meat turns from pink to white. Occasionally break the meat up into chunks with a fork to ensure all the meat is cooked. Drain, keeping the sage with the turkey, and reserve the broth to soften the bread and pour over finished recipe.

Bring a pot of water to a boil. Chop carrots into bite-size cubes, then add to the pot and cook for 5 minutes. Add the peas and cook until both carrots and peas are tender, approximately 3 to 4 minutes. Drain.

Allow all hot ingredients to rest and come to room temperature, then combine with the bread, cranberries, canola oil, and the contents of the fish oil and vitamin E capsules.

Combine the salt and the supplements in a small bowl. Sprinkle this mixture over the food as evenly as possible, and combine well.

Canine Adult Maintenance

RABBIT AND MILLET

Yield: 861.1 grams

Calories: 1,363.20 (per recipe): 1.6 kcal/g, 360 kcal/cup, 1,583 kcal/kg

As fed: Protein 10.2%, Fat 6%, Fiber 1%, Carbohydrates 15%, Moisture 66.9%

All ingredients can be served raw, except for: millet

8 ounces rabbit meat, deboned

1 cup millet (to yield 3 cups cooked)

½ cup carrots

2 tablespoons organic canola oil

100 IU vitamin E (from capsules)

⅛ teaspoon iodized salt

⅛ teaspoon potassium chloride powder

1 tablet Kirkland Signature Daily Multi, crushed

1 teaspoon calcium carbonate powder

350 mg choline

250 mg pantothenic acid

Bring a pot of water to a boil. Add the rabbit to the pot and cook for about 20 minutes or until meat reaches an internal temperature of 160°F. Set aside.

Cook millet according to the package instructions to yield 3 cups of cooked millet.

Chop the carrots into bite-size pieces. Cook the carrots in boiling water for about 10 minutes or until tender, and drain.

Allow all hot ingredients to rest and come to room temperature, either on the counter or in the refrigerator, then mix with the canola oil and the contents of the vitamin E capsule.

Combine the salt and the rest of the supplements in a small bowl. Sprinkle this mixture over the food as evenly as possible, and combine well.

SALMON AND OATS

Yield: 2,615.12 grams
Calories: 2,803.08 (per recipe): 1.1 kcal/g, 243 kcal/cup, 1,072 kcal/kg
As fed: Protein 10.1%, Fat 4.3%, Fiber 1%, Carbohydrates 6.9%, Moisture 77%
All ingredients can be served raw, except for: quick oats

2 pounds salmon fillets

3 cups unenriched quick oats (to yield 6 cups cooked)

½ cup carrots

½ cup broccoli

½ cup kale

4 ounces sardines with bones, canned in oil

1 tablespoon organic canola oil

3½ teaspoons calcium carbonate powder

1 tablet Kirkland Signature Daily Multi, crushed

30 mg zinc citrate

1,050 mg choline

Broil salmon fillets on high for 3 to 6 minutes, or until fish is opaque and flakes easily with a fork.

Cook oats according to the package to yield 6 cups of cooked oatmeal.

Bring a pot of water to a boil. Chop the carrots and broccoli into bite-size pieces, and slice the kale into ½-inch strips. Add the carrots to the pot and cook for 5 minutes. Add the broccoli and cook until both carrots and broccoli are tender, approximately 3 to 4 minutes. Drain, then add the sliced kale to the hot cooked vegetables to wilt.

Allow all hot ingredients to rest and come to room temperature, either on the counter or in the refrigerator, then combine the vegetables, salmon, sardines, and canola oil.

Combine the supplements in a small bowl. Sprinkle this mixture over the food as evenly as possible, and combine well.

Canine Senior Maintenance Diet

TURKEY AND PORK

Yield: 4,806.08 grams
Calories: 7,320.38 (per recipe): 1.5 kcal/g, 345 kcal/cup, 1,523 kcal/kg
As fed: Protein 14.3%, Fat 8.2%, Fiber 1%, Carbohydrates 5.3%, Moisture 76%
All ingredients can be served raw, except for: sweet potatoes

    1½ pounds sweet potatoes

    4 pounds ground turkey

    2 pounds ground pork

    ½ cup kale

    8 large eggs

    1 pound green beans

    ¾ pint blueberries

    100 IU vitamin E (from capsules)

    ½ teaspoon iodized salt

    ¾ cup ground flaxseed

    2 tablets Kirkland Signature Daily Multi, crushed

    2 tablespoons calcium carbonate powder

    325 mcg iodine (from kelp tablets)

Preheat the oven to 400°F. Peel the sweet potatoes, chop into bite-size cubes, and bake in the oven for 20 to 30 minutes, or until fork-tender. Mash up the sweet potatoes lightly.

While the potatoes are cooking, place the turkey and pork in a pot with just enough water to cover. Bring to a boil, then cook for 10 minutes or until meat is done. Drain and reserve the leftover broth.

Slice the kale into ½-inch strips and add to the hot broth to wilt. Remove the wilted kale and place it with the other cooked vegetables, keeping the broth separate. Refrigerate the broth, and remove the solid fat that rises to the top of the broth and discard. A bit of this reserved broth can be poured over each portion of food before serving.

Bring a large pot of water to a boil. Add the eggs, and cook for 16 minutes or until hard-boiled. Chop the green beans into bite-size pieces. Remove the eggs from the pot and boil the green beans for 3 to 5 minutes or until tender. Drain. Peel and chop or mash the eggs.

Allow all hot ingredients to rest and come to room temperature, either on the counter or in the refrigerator, then mix with the blueberries and the contents of the vitamin E capsule.

Combine the salt, flaxseed, and rest of the supplements in a small bowl. Sprinkle this mixture over the food as evenly as possible, and combine well. Pour reserved broth over portions before serving.

WHITEFISH AND QUINOA

Yield: 2,586.21 grams
Calories: 3,432.64 (per recipe): 1.3 kcal/g, 301 kcal/cup, 1,327 kcal/kg
As fed: Protein 10.4%, Fat 4.2%, Fiber 1.3%, Carbohydrates 12.9%, Moisture 69.4%
All ingredients can be served raw, except for: quinoa

    2.5 pounds whitefish fillet

    1⅔ cups quinoa (to yield 5 cups cooked)

    2 cups carrots

    2 cups green beans

    1 cup kale

    1 cup dried cranberries

    1½ tablespoons organic canola oil

    2,000 mg omega-3 fish oil (from capsules)

    100 IU vitamin E (from capsules)

    1½ tablets Kirkland Signature Daily Multi, crushed

    4 teaspoons calcium carbonate powder

30 mg zinc citrate

200 mcg selenium

500 mg pantothenic acid

700 mg choline

100 mcg vitamin B12

Broil whitefish on high for 3 to 6 minutes, or until fish is opaque and flakes easily with a fork.

Cook the quinoa according to the package directions to yield 5 cups of cooked quinoa.

Bring a pot of water to a boil. Chop the carrots and green beans into bite-size pieces. Add the carrots to the pot and cook for 5 minutes, then add the green beans and cook until both carrots and green beans are tender, approximately 3 to 4 minutes. Drain. Slice the kale into ½-inch strips and mix into hot vegetables to wilt.

Allow all hot ingredients to rest and come to room temperature, either on the counter or in the refrigerator, then combine with the cranberries, canola oil, and the contents of the fish oil and vitamin E capsules.

Combine the rest of the supplements in a small bowl. Sprinkle this mixture over the food as evenly as possible, and combine well.

Canine Skin Allergies

Note: Skin allergy diets can also be useful for other allergic conditions and GI sensitivities. This recipe is meant for a dog with severe skin allergies and should be used for a limited time before new ingredients are added and replaced one at a time.

BLACK BEANS AND QUINOA

Yield: 1,140.26 grams
Calories: 1,827.12 (per recipe): 1.6 kcal/g, 365 kcal/cup, 1,609 kcal/kg
As fed: Protein 6.1%, Fat 6.1%, Fiber 1.7%, Carbohydrates 21%, Moisture 64%
All ingredients can be served raw, except for: quinoa

1 cup quinoa (to yield 3 cups cooked)

3 cups canned black beans, drained and rinsed

¼ cup hemp oil, organic

¼ teaspoon sea salt

1½ teaspoons calcium carbonate powder

250 mcg iodine (from kelp tablets)

200 mcg selenium

1 teaspoon taurine powder

5,000 IU dry vitamin A

30 mg zinc citrate

350 mg choline

500 mg methionine

Cook the quinoa according to the package directions to yield 3 cups of cooked quinoa. Allow to come to room temperature on counter or in refrigerator. Add the beans and oil, and mix well.

Combine the salt and the supplements in a small bowl. Sprinkle this mixture over the food as evenly as possible, and combine well.

Canine Degenerative Joint Disease

PORK

Yield: 1,846.38 grams
Calories: 2,498.53 (per recipe): 1.4 kcal/g, 307 kcal/cup, 1,353 kcal/kg
As fed: Protein 9.3%, Fat 5.4%, Fiber 2%, Carbohydrates 12.6%, Moisture 71%
All ingredients can be served raw, except for: sweet potatoes

1½ pounds sweet potatoes

1½ pounds pork loin

1 cup broccoli, chopped

1 cup carrots

½ cup blueberries

1½ cups canned garbanzo beans, drained and rinsed

3 tablespoons organic canola oil

2,000 mg omega-3 fish oil (from capsules)

350 mg choline

1½ teaspoons calcium carbonate powder

325 mcg iodine (from kelp tablets)

45 mg zinc citrate

2 tablets Kirkland Signature Daily Multi, crushed

2.5 mg chelated copper

18 mg iron bisglycinate

Preheat the oven to 400°F. Peel the sweet potatoes, then chop the potatoes and bake along with the pork loin. Bake the potatoes for 20 to 30 minutes, or until fork-tender, and bake the roast until it comes to an internal temperature of 160°F. Allow to cool, then mash the potato and finely chop the pork.

While the meat and potatoes are cooking, bring a pot of water to a boil. Chop the broccoli and the carrots into bite-size pieces. Add the carrots to the pot, and cook for 5 minutes. Then add the broccoli and cook until both carrots and broccoli are tender, approximately 3 to 4 minutes. Drain.

Allow all hot ingredients to rest and come to room temperature on the counter or in the refrigerator, then mix together with the blueberries, beans, canola oil, and the contents of the fish oil capsules.

Combine the rest of the supplements in a small bowl. Sprinkle this mixture over the food as evenly as possible, and combine well.

Canine Struvite Crystals/ Stone Diet

TURKEY AND PASTA

Yield: 3,348.64 grams
Calories: 3,427.08 (per recipe): 1.0 kcal/g, 232 kcal/cup, 1,023 kcal/kg
As fed: Protein 11.4%, Fat 4.6%, Fiber 1%, Carbohydrates 4.1%, Moisture 78%
All ingredients can be served raw, except for: macaroni

8 ounces whole-wheat macaroni

4 pounds ground turkey

1 pound cauliflower

1 pound zucchini

3 tablespoons carrots

12 ounces apple (without core and seeds)

1 tablespoon organic canola oil

3½ teaspoons calcium carbonate powder

1,300 mcg iodine (from kelp tablets)

4 tablets Kirkland Signature Daily Multi, crushed

350 mg choline

Prepare pasta according to the package directions to yield about 4 cups of cooked pasta.

Panfry the turkey over medium-high heat until opaque. (You can also choose another cooking method that doesn't add fat.)

Bring a pot of water to a boil. Chop the cauliflower, zucchini, carrots, and apple into bite-size pieces. Add fruits and vegetables to the pot, and boil for 10 minutes or until tender.

Allow all hot ingredients to rest and come to room temperature, either on the counter or in the refrigerator, then mix with the canola oil.

Combine the supplements in a small bowl. Sprinkle this mixture over the food as evenly as possible, and combine well.

Canine Oxalate Crystals

Note: Calcium oxalate stones generally cannot be dissolved through diet. Dogs with discrete stones need them removed (see Chapter 13). This diet is beneficial for reducing the formation of calcium oxalate crystals, thus preventing the formation and recurrence of oxalate stones.

BISON AND EGG NOODLES

Yield: 802.32 grams
Calories: 1,559.62 (per recipe): 1.9 kcal/g, 441 kcal/cup, 1,944 kcal/kg
As fed: Protein 6.7%, Fat 10.6%, Fiber 1%, Carbohydrates 17.7%, Moisture 63.3%
All ingredients can be served raw, except for: egg noodles

  3 ounces ground bison

  1 ¾ cups enriched egg noodles (to yield 3½ cups cooked)

  2 large eggs

  3½ tablespoons organic canola oil

  1,000 mg omega-3 fish oil (from capsules)

  ⅛ teaspoon iodized salt

  1½ tablets Kirkland Signature Daily Multi, crushed

  125 mg pantothenic acid

  ½ teaspoon potassium chloride powder

  ¾ teaspoon calcium carbonate powder

  350 mg choline

Crumble the ground bison, and panfry over medium-high heat for 15 minutes or until browned. To add a bit of moisture to the meal, you may pour 2 tablespoons of water over the meat while cooking to deglaze the pan.

Boil pasta according to the package instructions to yield 3½ cups of cooked pasta.

Bring a pot of water to a boil. Add the eggs, and cook for 16 minutes or until hard-boiled. Peel and chop or mash the eggs.

Allow all hot ingredients to rest and come to room temperature, either on the counter or in the refrigerator, then mix with the canola oil and the contents of the fish oil capsules.

Combine the salt and the rest of the supplements in a small bowl. Sprinkle this mixture over the food as evenly as possible, and combine well.

Canine Elimination Diet (Limited-Ingredient Diet): GI Disease

Note: While this diet is best when the goal is a limited-ingredient diet (see Appendix E), the diets for skin allergies can also be useful for GI sensitivities.

TURKEY AND QUINOA

Yield: 1,974.64 grams
Calories: 2,649.05 (per recipe): 1.3 kcal/g, 304 kcal/cup, 1,342 kcal/kg
As fed: Protein 10.2%, Fat 3%, Fiber 1.5%, Carbohydrates 15.9%, Moisture 69%
All ingredients can be served raw, except for: quinoa

    1 pound light meat turkey, ground
    2⅔ cups quinoa (to yield 8 cups cooked)
    5 teaspoons organic canola oil
    ¼ teaspoon iodized salt
    1 teaspoon potassium chloride powder
    1 tablet Kirkland Signature Daily Multi, crushed
    15 mg zinc citrate
    1 tablespoon calcium carbonate powder
    350 mg choline
    250 mg pantothenic acid

Place the turkey in a pot with just enough water to cover. Bring to a boil and cook for 10 minutes or until cooked through. Drain and reserve the leftover broth. Chill the broth in the refrigerator, and remove the fat that comes to the top. Pour the broth over each portion of food before serving.

Cook the quinoa according to the package directions to produce 8 cups of quinoa.

Allow all hot ingredients to rest and come to room temperature, either on the counter or in the refrigerator, then mix with the canola oil.

Combine the salt and the supplements in a small bowl. Sprinkle this mixture over the food as evenly as possible, and combine well.

TURKEY AND MILLET

Yield: 3,227.88 grams
Calories: 4,377.75 (per recipe): 1.4 kcal/g, 307 kcal/cup, 1,356 kcal/kg
As fed: Protein 12.5%, Fat 4.8%, Fiber 1%, Carbohydrates 10.2%, Moisture 71.4%
All ingredients can be served raw, except for: millet

> 4 pounds ground turkey
>
> 2½ cups millet (to yield 8 cups cooked)
>
> 4,000 mg omega-3 fish oil (from capsules)
>
> 100 IU vitamin E (from capsules)
>
> 4 ¾ teaspoons calcium carbonate powder
>
> 1,050 mg choline
>
> 1 tablet Kirkland Signature Daily Multi, crushed
>
> 2,500 IU dry vitamin A

Place the turkey in a pot with just enough water to cover. Bring to a boil, and cook for 10 minutes or until meat turns from pink to white. Drain and reserve the leftover broth. Chill the broth in the refrigerator, and remove the fat that comes to the top. Pour the broth over each portion of food before serving.

Cook the millet according to the package directions to produce 8 cups of millet.

Allow all hot ingredients to rest and come to room temperature on the counter or in the refrigerator, then mix with the contents of the fish oil and vitamin E capsules.

Combine the supplements in a small bowl. Sprinkle this mixture over the food as evenly as possible, and combine well.

Canine Pancreatitis

PORK AND BARLEY

Yield: 1,459 grams
Calories: 1,760 (per recipe): 1.2 kcal/g, 273 kcal/cup, 1,206 kcal/kg
As fed: Protein 8%, Fat 1.8%, Fiber 2.4%, Carbohydrates 18%, Moisture 69.5%
All ingredients can be served raw, except for: sweet potato, barley

  1 pound lean pork tenderloin
  1⅔ cups pearl barley (to yield 5 cups cooked)
  1 cup sweet potato
  1 tablespoon Flora pumpkin seed oil
  2 tablets Kirkland Signature Daily Multi, crushed
  1½ teaspoons calcium carbonate powder
  350 mg choline

Place the pork in a crockpot with enough water to cover half the pork, and cook on low for 8 hours. Shred the pork right in the crockpot, then allow to come to room temperature on the counter or in the refrigerator.

Cook the barley according to the package directions to yield 5 cups of cooked barley.

Preheat the oven to 400°F. Peel the sweet potato, and chop into bite-size cubes. Bake in the oven for 20 to 30 minutes, or until fork-tender. Potato may be mashed, if desired.

Combine the shredded meat with reserved broth, barley, potato, and pumpkin seed oil.

Combine the supplements in a small bowl. Sprinkle this mixture over the food as evenly as possible, and combine well.

Canine Low Fat (Weight Management)

BISON AND QUINOA

Yield: 1,712.22 grams
Calories: 1,727.70 (per recipe): 1.0 kcal/g, 229 kcal/cup, 1,009 kcal/kg
As fed: Protein 7.3%, Fat 2%, Fiber 2.1%, Carbohydrates 13.1%, Moisture 76%
All ingredients can be served raw, except for: quinoa, summer squash

1⅔ cups quinoa (to yield 5 cups cooked)

12 ounces lean bison steak

1½ cups broccoli, chopped

1 cup summer squash, any variety

1 cup carrots

1 cup kale

1½ teaspoons organic canola oil

1,000 mg omega-3 fish oil (from capsules)

⅛ teaspoon sea salt

1 tablet Kirkland Signature Daily Multi, crushed

2¼ teaspoons calcium carbonate powder

100 mcg vitamin B12

30 mg zinc citrate

500 mg pantothenic acid

1,050 mg choline

Cook the quinoa according to the package directions to yield 5 cups of cooked quinoa.

Bring a pot of water to a boil. Chop the bison, broccoli, squash, and carrots into bite-size pieces. Slice the kale into strips about ½-inch wide. Add bison to the boiling water and cook until it reaches an internal temperature of 160°F, then remove from the pot and add the squash and carrots. After 5 minutes, add the broccoli and kale to the pot and cook for another 3 minutes or until all vegetables are tender. Drain.

Allow all hot ingredients to rest and come to room temperature either on the counter or in the refrigerator, then mix with the canola oil and the contents of the fish oil capsules.

Combine the salt and rest of the supplements in a small bowl. Sprinkle this mixture over the food as evenly as possible, and combine well.

Canine Low Fat, Low Fiber (Weight Management)

CHICKEN AND RICE

Yield: 2,211.33 grams
Calories: 2,649.74 (per recipe): 1.2 kcal/g, 271 kcal/cup, 1,194 kcal/kg
As fed: Protein 14.6%, Fat 2.8%, Fiber 1%, Carbohydrates 1%, Moisture 73%
All ingredients can be served raw, except for: rice

3 pounds chicken breast, skinless

1 cup white basmati rice (to yield 3 cups cooked)

2 cups carrots

2 cups green beans

½ cup red bell pepper, diced

2 tablespoons organic canola oil

100 IU vitamin E (from capsules)

⅝ teaspoon potassium chloride powder

2 tablets Kirkland Signature Daily Multi, crushed

1 ¾ teaspoons calcium carbonate powder

325 mcg iodine (from kelp tablets)

30 mg zinc citrate

Place the chicken in a pot and add just enough water to barely cover the meat. Bring to a boil, then cook for 15 minutes or until meat reaches an internal temperature of 165°F. When chicken is cool enough to handle, drain and shred the meat.

Cook the rice according to the package directions to yield 3 cups of cooked rice.

Bring a pot of water to a boil. Chop the carrots, green beans, and pepper into pieces small enough for the animal that is going to be fed. Add carrots to boiling water and cook for 5 minutes. Then add the green beans and pepper, and cook for 3 to 4 minutes or until all vegetables are tender.

Allow all hot ingredients to rest and come to room temperature on the counter or in the refrigerator, then mix with the canola oil and the contents of the vitamin E capsules.

Combine the rest of the supplements in a small bowl. Sprinkle this mixture over the food as evenly as possible, and combine well.

Canine Heart Disease Diet

CHICKEN AND PASTA

Yield: 842.68 grams
Calories: 1,399.11 (per recipe): 1.7 kcal/g, 377 kcal/cup, 1,660 kcal/kg
As fed: Protein 6.5%, Fat 10.9%, Fiber 1.1%, Carbohydrates 11.4%, Moisture 69.5%
All ingredients can be served raw, except for: macaroni

5 ounces chicken breast, skinless

8 ounces enriched macaroni

3 cups green beans

6 tablespoons organic canola oil

2,000 mg omega-3 fish oil (from capsules)

⅛ teaspoon iodized salt

¼ teaspoon potassium chloride powder

1 tablet Kirkland Signature Daily Multi, crushed

500 mg methionine

2 grams L-carnitine powder

1 teaspoon taurine powder

⅞ teaspoon bone meal powder

250 mg pantothenic acid

30 mg zinc citrate

350 mg choline

Place the chicken in a pot and add just enough water to barely cover the meat. Bring to a boil, then cook for 15 minutes or until meat reaches an internal temperature of 165°F. When chicken is cool enough to handle, shred the meat and remove from the pot. Retain the broth to pour over the finished recipe before serving.

Cook the macaroni according to the package directions. This will yield about 4 cups of cooked pasta. Drain.

Bring a pot of water to a boil. Chop the green beans into bite-size pieces. Place the green beans in the pot and cook for 3 to 5 minutes, or until tender. Drain.

Allow all hot ingredients to rest and come to room temperature, either on the counter or in the refrigerator, then mix with the canola oil and the contents of the fish oil capsules.

Combine the salt and the rest of the supplements in a small bowl. Sprinkle this mixture over the food as evenly as possible, and combine well.

Canine Diabetes Diet

CHICKEN AND WHOLE-WHEAT PASTA

Yield: 1,236.97 grams
Calories: 1,001.33 (per recipe): 1.1 kcal/g, 257 kcal/cup, 1,135 kcal/kg
As fed: Protein 11.5%, Fat 3%, Fiber 1.5%, Carbohydrates 10.6%, Moisture 74.4%
All ingredients can be served raw, except for: sweet potato, macaroni

2 tablespoons sweet potato

1½ pounds chicken thighs, skinless, bone-in

½ pound chicken breast, skinless, bone-in

1½ cups whole-wheat enriched macaroni (to yield 3 cups cooked)

1 cup cauliflower

1 cup green beans

1 tablespoon organic canola oil

2,000 mg omega-3 fish oil (from capsules)

1 tablet Kirkland Signature Daily Multi, crushed

2 teaspoons calcium carbonate powder

350 mg choline

30 mg zinc citrate

Preheat the oven to 400°F. Peel and chop the sweet potato into bite-size pieces, then bake for 15 minutes or until fork-tender. You can mash it, if you wish.

While the potato is cooking, place the chicken in a pot and add just enough water to barely cover the meat. Bring to a boil, then cook for 15 minutes or until meat reaches an internal temperature of 165°F. When chicken is cool enough to handle, drain, remove the bones, and chop into bite-size pieces. Retain the broth to pour over the finished recipe before serving.

Cook the pasta according to the package directions to yield 3 cups of cooked macaroni.

Bring a pot of water to a boil. Chop the cauliflower and green beans into bite-size pieces. Add the vegetables to the pot and cook for 10 minutes or until tender. Drain.

Allow all hot ingredients to rest and come to room temperature, either on the counter or in the refrigerator, then mix with the canola oil and the contents of the fish oil capsules.

Combine the rest of the supplements in a small bowl. Sprinkle this mixture over the food as evenly as possible, and combine well. Pour reserved broth over each portion of food before serving.

Canine Liver Diet

WHITEFISH AND BROWN RICE

Yield: 2,246.46 grams
Calories: 2,619.66 (per recipe): 1.2 kcal/g, 264 kcal/cup, 1,166 kcal/kg
As fed: Protein 5.4%, Fat 3%, Fiber 1.3%, Carbohydrates 16.8%, Moisture 73.3%
All ingredients can be served raw, except for: rice

    14 ounces whitefish fillet
    2 cups brown basmati rice (to yield 8 cups cooked)
    ½ cup green beans
    ½ cup zucchini, sliced
    ½ cup carrots
    2 tablespoons organic canola oil
    1,000 mg omega-3 fish oil (from capsules)
    400 IU vitamin D3 (from capsules)
    1,200 IU vitamin E (from capsules)
    ¼ teaspoon iodized salt
    ½ teaspoon potassium chloride powder
    2⅛ teaspoons calcium carbonate powder
    30 mg zinc citrate
    9 mg iron bisglycinate
    50 mg vitamin B complex
    700 mg choline
    1 tablet Kirkland Signature Daily Multi, crushed

Place the whitefish in a pot and add just enough water to barely cover the fillet. Bring to a simmer, then cook for 7 to 10 minutes, or until fish is opaque and flakes easily with a fork. Drain, and reserve the broth to pour over the finished recipe before serving.

Cook the rice according to the package directions to yield 8 cups of cooked brown rice.

Bring a pot of water to a boil. Chop the green beans, zucchini, and carrots into bite-size pieces. Add the vegetables to the pot, and cook for 10 minutes or until tender. Drain.

Allow all hot ingredients to rest and come to room temperature, either on the counter or in the refrigerator, then mix with the canola oil and the contents of the fish oil, vitamin D, and vitamin E capsules.

Combine the salt and the rest of the supplements in a small bowl. Sprinkle this mixture over the food as evenly as possible, and combine well.

COTTAGE CHEESE AND EGGS

Yield: 945.9 grams
Calories: 1,399.03 (per recipe): 1.3 kcal/g, 307 kcal/cup, 1,356 kcal/kg
As fed: Protein 12.5%, Fat 4.8%, Fiber 1%, Carbohydrates 10.2%, Moisture 71.4%
All ingredients can be served raw, except for: rice

> 3 large eggs
>
> 1 cup 2% cottage cheese
>
> 1 cup white basmati rice (to yield 3 cups cooked)
>
> 2 slices white bread, crumbled
>
> 5 teaspoons organic canola oil
>
> 2,000 mg omega-3 fish oil (from capsules)
>
> 1,200 IU vitamin E (from capsules)
>
> ⅓ teaspoon psyllium powder
>
> 1 tablet Kirkland Signature Daily Multi, crushed
>
> ¼ teaspoon calcium carbonate powder
>
> 315 mg zinc citrate
>
> 700 mg choline
>
> 60 mg L-carnitine
>
> 1 teaspoon taurine powder
>
> ¾ teaspoon potassium chloride powder
>
> 1 teaspoon bone meal powder

Scramble the eggs in a small amount of canola oil, then mix in the cottage cheese.

Cook the rice according to the package directions to yield 3 cups of cooked rice.

Allow all hot ingredients to rest and come to room temperature, either on the counter or in the refrigerator, then mix with the bread, canola oil, and the contents of the fish oil and vitamin E capsules. (If you desire the bread to be softer, you can add a bit of water or low-sodium chicken broth.)

Combine the rest of the supplements in a small bowl. Sprinkle this mixture over the food as evenly as possible, and combine well.

Canine Renal Diet

PORK AND WHITE RICE

Yield: 2,425.52 grams
Calories: 3,869.92 (per recipe): 1.2 kcal/g, 264 kcal/cup, 1,166 kcal/kg
As fed: Protein 5.4%, Fat 3%, Fiber 1.3%, Carbohydrates 16.8%, Moisture 73.3%
All ingredients can be served raw, except for: rice

   1 pound lean pork loin

   3⅓ cups white basmati rice (to yield 10 cups cooked)

   1 cup green beans

   1 cup carrots

   6 tablespoons organic canola oil

   400 IU vitamin D3 (from capsules)

   3,000 mg omega-3 fish oil (from capsules)

   ½ teaspoon iodized salt

   ¼ teaspoon potassium chloride powder

   1 tablet Kirkland Signature Daily Multi, crushed

   2¼ teaspoons calcium carbonate powder

   5 mg chelated copper

   2 teaspoons taurine powder

   90 mg zinc citrate

   500 mg pantothenic acid

   30 to 50 mg riboflavin 5' phosphate

   100 mcg vitamin B12

   1,050 mg choline

Bring a pot of water to a boil. Slice the pork into bite-size pieces, then boil for 15 minutes or until meat reaches an internal temperature of 160°F. Drain, reserving the broth to pour over the finished recipe before serving.

Cook the rice according to the package directions to yield 10 cups of cooked rice.

Bring a pot of water to a boil. Chop the green beans and carrots into bite-size pieces, then add to the pot and cook for 8 minutes or until tender. Drain.

Allow all hot ingredients to rest and come to room temperature, either on the counter or in the refrigerator, then mix with the canola oil and the contents of the vitamin D and fish oil capsules.

Combine the salt and the rest of the supplements in a small bowl. Sprinkle this mixture over the food as evenly as possible, and combine well.

CHICKEN, LIVER, AND RICE

Yield: 3,112.2 grams
Calories: 4,923.5 (per recipe): 1.6 kcal/g, 360 kcal/cup, 1,582 kcal/kg
As fed: Protein 6%, Fat 4.3%, Fiber 1%, Carbohydrates 22.8%, Moisture 65.1%
All ingredients can be served raw, except for: rice

14 ounces chicken thighs, skinless

2 ounces chicken liver

5⅓ cups white basmati rice (to yield 16 cups cooked)

6 tablespoons organic canola oil

3,000 mg omega-3 fish oil (from capsules)

400 IU vitamin D3 (from capsules)

½ teaspoon iodized salt

2 teaspoons taurine powder

1,500 mg methionine

1 tablespoon potassium chloride powder

1 tablespoon calcium carbonate powder

1 tablet Kirkland Signature Daily Multi, crushed

120 mg zinc citrate

1,500 mg choline

1 teaspoon magnesium citrate

100 mcg vitamin B12

Place the chicken thighs and livers in a pot and add just enough water to barely cover the meat. Bring to a boil, cook for 15 minutes, then add liver and cook for 5 minutes or until meat reaches an internal temperature of 165°F. When the chicken is cool enough to handle, drain and chop into bite-size pieces. Retain the broth to pour over the finished recipe before serving.

Cook the rice according to the package directions to yield 16 cups of rice.

Allow all hot ingredients to rest and come to room temperature, either on the counter or in the refrigerator, then mix with the canola oil and the contents of the fish oil and vitamin D capsules.

Combine the salt and the rest of the supplements in a small bowl. Sprinkle this mixture over the food as evenly as possible, and combine well.

Canine Cancer Diet

CHICKEN AND BEEF

Yield: 703.07 grams
Calories: 1,279.07 (per recipe): 1.8 kcal/g, 413 kcal/cup, 1,819 kcal/kg
As fed: Protein 21.9%, Fat 9.4%, Fiber 1%, Carbohydrates 1%, Moisture 66%
All ingredients can be served raw.

13 ounces chicken breast, skinless
6 ounces 80% ground beef
2 tablespoons chicken livers, chopped
¼ cup spinach
¼ cup kale, chopped
1 tablespoon organic canola oil
100 IU vitamin E (from capsules)
3,000 mg omega-3 fish oil (from capsules)
¼ teaspoon potassium chloride powder
1 tablet Kirkland Signature Daily Multi, crushed
1 teaspoon calcium carbonate powder
30 mg zinc citrate

Place the chicken in a pot and add just enough water to barely cover the meat. Bring to a boil, then cook for 15 minutes or until meat reaches an internal temperature of 165°F. Drain, reserving broth to pour over the finished recipe before serving. When chicken is cool enough to handle, chop into bite-size pieces.

Crumble the ground beef and panfry with the chicken liver over medium-high heat for 15 minutes or until browned. Remove the beef and liver from pan, then add the spinach and kale back to the same pan with the canola oil. Cook for 3 to 5 minutes, stirring regularly, until the greens wilt.

Allow all hot ingredients to rest and come to room temperature, either on the counter or in the refrigerator, then add the contents of the vitamin E and fish oil capsules.

Combine the rest of the supplements in a small bowl. Sprinkle this mixture over the food as evenly as possible, and combine well.

CHICKEN AND SWEET POTATO

Yield: 667.01 grams
Calories: 840.01 (per recipe): 1.3 kcal/g, 286 kcal/cup, 1,259 kcal/kg
As fed: Protein 18.2%, Fat 3%, Fiber 1%, Carbohydrates 5.4%, Moisture 71.4%
All ingredients can be served raw, except for: sweet potato, summer squash

¼ cup sweet potato

13 ounces chicken breast, skinless

¼ cup summer squash, any variety

¼ cup spinach

¼ cup green peas

1 teaspoon organic canola oil

2,000 mg omega-3 fish oil (from capsules)

100 IU vitamin E (from capsules)

¼ teaspoon iodized salt

½ teaspoon potassium chloride powder

¾ teaspoon calcium carbonate powder

1 tablet Kirkland Signature Daily Multi, crushed

500 mg vitamin C, buffered

Preheat the oven to 400°F. Peel and chop the sweet potato into bite-size pieces, then bake for 15 minutes or until fork-tender. You can mash it, if you wish.

While the potato is cooking, place the chicken in a pot and add just enough water to barely cover the meat. Bring to a boil, then cook for 15 minutes or until meat reaches an internal temperature of 165°F. When chicken is cool enough to handle, drain and shred. Retain the broth to pour over the finished recipe before serving.

Bring a pot of water to a boil. Chop the summer squash into bite-size pieces, add to the pot and cook for 5 minutes, then add the spinach and peas and cook 5 more minutes, or until tender. Drain.

Allow all hot ingredients to rest and come to room temperature, either on the counter or in the refrigerator, then add canola oil and the contents of the fish oil and vitamin E capsules.

Combine the salt and the rest of the supplements in a small bowl. Sprinkle this mixture over the food as evenly as possible, and combine well.

Recipes for Cats

Kitten Diet

Caution: Kitten diets should not be fed to seniors, because the levels of calcium and phosphorus are too high.

CHICKEN

Yield: 366.25 grams
Calories: 412.86 (per recipe): 1.1 kcal/g, 256 kcal/cup, 1,100 kcal/kg
As fed: Protein 19%, Fat 2.61%, Fiber 1%, Carbohydrates 2.4%, Moisture 74%
All ingredients can be served raw.

  10 ounces chicken breast, skinless
  1½ ounces chicken livers
  1 cup green beans
  ⅛ teaspoon sea salt
  ½ teaspoon taurine powder
  ¼ teaspoon bone meal powder
  ⅜ teaspoon calcium carbonate powder
  1 tablet Kirkland Signature Daily Multi, crushed
  15 mg zinc citrate

Place the chicken breasts in a pot and add just enough water to barely cover the meat. Bring to a boil, cook for 15 minutes, then add liver and cook for 5 minutes or until meat reaches an internal temperature of 165°F. When the chicken is cool enough to handle, drain and chop into bite-size pieces. Retain the broth to pour over the finished recipe before serving.

Bring a pot of water to a boil. Chop the green beans into bite-size pieces, then add to the pot and cook for 3 to 5 minutes or until tender. Drain.

Allow all hot ingredients to rest and come to room temperature, either on the counter or in the refrigerator, then mix well.

Place 2 tablespoons of the reserved broth in a small bowl, and dissolve the salt and supplements in it. Pour this over the chicken mixture and stir well. Before serving each portion to your pet, add a bit of the reserved broth.

CHICKEN AND LIVER

Yield: 274.08 grams
Calories: 432.24 (per recipe): 1.6 kcal/g, 358 kcal/cup, 1,577 kcal/kg
As fed: Protein 17.8%, Fat 7.4%, Fiber 1%, Carbohydrates 4%, Moisture 68.6%
All ingredients can be served raw, except for: quick oats

> 7 ounces chicken breast, skinless
> 1 tablespoon chicken livers
> 2½ tablespoons unenriched quick oats (to yield 5 tablespoons cooked)
> 1 tablespoon carrots
> 1 tablespoon green peas
> 1 tablespoon organic canola oil
> ⅛ teaspoon iodized salt
> ½ teaspoon taurine powder
> ⅓ tablet Kirkland Signature Daily Multi, crushed
> ⅝ teaspoon bone meal powder
> 1/16 teaspoon potassium chloride powder
> 80 mcg iodine (from kelp tablets)
> 15 mg zinc citrate
> 175 mg choline
> 300 mcg biotin

Place the chicken breast in a pot and add just enough water to barely cover the meat. Bring to a boil, cook for 15 minutes, then add liver and cook for 5 minutes or until meat reaches an internal temperature of 165°F. When the chicken is cool enough to handle, drain and chop into bite-size pieces. Reserve the broth for later use.

Cook oats according to the package directions to yield 5 tablespoons of oatmeal.

Bring a pot of water to a boil. Chop carrots into bite-size cubes, then add to the pot and cook for 5 minutes. Add the peas and cook until both carrots and peas are tender, approximately 3 to 4 minutes. Drain.

Allow all hot ingredients to rest and come to room temperature, either on the counter or in the refrigerator, then mix with the canola oil.

Place 2 tablespoons of the reserved broth in a small bowl, and dissolve the salt and supplements in it. Pour this over the chicken mixture and stir well. Before serving each portion to your pet, add a bit of the reserved broth.

Feline Adult Maintenance

VENISON AND BARLEY

Yield: 434.85 grams
Calories: 945.98 (per recipe): 2.2 kcal/g, 493 kcal/cup, 2,175 kcal/kg
As fed: Protein 13.7%, Fat 13.4%, Fiber 1%, Carbohydrates 10.5%, Moisture 60%
All ingredients can be served raw, except for: barley

> 8 ounces ground bison
>
> ⅓ cup pearl barley (to yield 1 cup cooked)
>
> 2 tablespoons carrots
>
> 5 teaspoons organic canola oil
>
> ¼ teaspoon potassium chloride powder
>
> ½ teaspoon bone meal powder
>
> 1 tablet Kirkland Signature Daily Multi, crushed
>
> ½ teaspoon taurine powder
>
> 700 mg choline
>
> 300 mcg biotin

Crumble the ground bison, and broil or panfry over medium-high heat for 15 minutes or until browned. Reserve the rendered fat with the meat.

Cook the barley according to the package directions to yield 1 cup of cooked barley.

Bring a pot of water to a boil. Chop the carrots into bite-size pieces, and boil for 10 minutes or until tender. Drain.

Allow all hot ingredients to rest and come to room temperature, either on the counter or in the refrigerator, then mix with the canola oil.

Combine the supplements in a small bowl. Sprinkle this mixture over the food as evenly as possible, and combine well.

BEEF AND SWEET POTATO

Yield: 694.27 grams
Calories: 1,422.96 (per recipe): 2.2 kcal/g, 498 kcal/cup, 2,195 kcal/kg
As fed: Protein 19.2%, Fat 12.2%, Fiber <1%, Carbohydrates 7.2%, Moisture 59.8%
All ingredients can be served raw, except for: sweet potato, rice

2 tablespoons sweet potato

1 pound 85% lean ground beef

¼ cup brown basmati rice (to yield 1 cup cooked)

1 tablespoon organic canola oil

1 teaspoon calcium carbonate powder

1 tablet Kirkland Signature Daily Multi, crushed

½ teaspoon taurine powder

400 mcg folic acid

525 mg choline

18 mg iron bisglycinate

25 mg vitamin B1 (thiamine)

300 mcg biotin

Preheat the oven to 400°F. Peel the sweet potato, chop into bite-size cubes, and bake in the oven for 20 minutes, or until fork-tender. Mash up the sweet potato, if desired.

While the potato is cooking, crumble the ground beef, and panfry over medium-high heat for 15 minutes or until browned. Reserve the rendered fat with the meat.

Cook the rice according to the package directions to yield 1 cup of cooked rice.

Allow all hot ingredients to rest and come to room temperature, either on the counter or in the refrigerator, then mix with the organic canola oil.

Combine the supplements in a small bowl. Sprinkle this mixture over the food as evenly as possible, and combine well.

Feline Senior Diet

BEEF AND SQUASH

Yield: 262.91 grams

Calories: 423.97 (per recipe): 1.6 kcal/g, 366 kcal/cup, 1,613 kcal/kg

As fed: Protein 12.7%, Fat 11.6%, Fiber 1%, Carbohydrates 1%, Moisture 72.2%

All ingredients can be served raw, except for: summer squash

6 ounces 85% lean ground beef

3 ounces summer squash, any variety

1 teaspoon organic canola oil

½ teaspoon calcium carbonate powder

1 tablet Kirkland Signature Daily Multi, crushed

350 mg choline
½ teaspoon taurine powder
200 mcg folic acid
300 mcg biotin

Crumble the ground beef, and panfry over medium-high heat for 15 minutes or until browned. Reserve the rendered fat with the meat.

Bring a pot of water to a boil. Add the squash, and cook for 10 minutes or until tender. Mash well.

Allow all hot ingredients to rest and come to room temperature, either on the counter or in the refrigerator, then combine with the canola oil.

Combine the supplements in a small bowl. Sprinkle this mixture over the food as evenly as possible, and combine well.

TURKEY, EGG, AND RICE

Yield: 358.32 grams
Calories: 723.30 (per recipe): 2.0 kcal/g, 458 kcal/cup, 2,019 kcal/kg
As fed: Protein 19.5%, Fat 11.9%, Fiber 1%, Carbohydrates 4%, Moisture 62.3%
All ingredients can be served raw, except for: rice

8 ounces ground turkey
1 tablespoon organic canola oil
1 large egg
1½ tablespoons brown basmati rice (to yield 5 tablespoons cooked)
¼ teaspoon iodized salt
¼ teaspoon potassium chloride powder
1 tablet Kirkland Signature Daily Multi, crushed
½ teaspoon taurine powder
¼ teaspoon bone meal powder
⅜ teaspoon calcium carbonate powder
300 mcg biotin

Panfry the turkey over medium-high heat for 4 minutes or until meat turns from pink to white. Remove the turkey from the pan. Add the canola oil to the pan and scramble the egg.

Prepare the rice according to the package instructions to yield 5 tablespoons of cooked rice.

Allow all hot ingredients to rest and come to room temperature, either on the counter or in the refrigerator, then mix well.

Combine the salt and the supplements in a small bowl. Sprinkle this mixture over the food as evenly as possible, and combine well.

Feline Skin Allergies

Note: Skin allergy diets can also be useful for other allergic conditions and GI sensitivities.

FLOUNDER AND POTATO

Yield: 165.36 grams
Calories: 195.82 (per recipe): 1.6 kcal/g, 365 kcal/cup, 1,609/kg
As fed: Protein 6.1%, Fat 6.1%, Fiber 1.7%, Carbohydrates 21%, Moisture 64%
All ingredients can be served raw, except for: potato

> ¼ cup potato
> 4 ounces flounder fillet
> 2 teaspoons organic canola oil
> ¼ tablet Kirkland Signature Daily Multi, crushed
> ¼ teaspoon calcium carbonate powder
> 250 mg pantothenic acid
> ½ teaspoon taurine powder
> 300 mcg biotin

Preheat the oven to 400°F. Peel the potato, chop into bite-size cubes, and bake in the oven for 20 minutes, or until fork-tender. Mash with a fork.

While the potato is cooking, place the flounder in a pot and add just enough water to barely cover the fillet. Bring to a simmer, then cook for 7 to 10 minutes, or until fish is opaque and flakes easily with a fork. Drain.

Allow all hot ingredients to rest and come to room temperature, either on the counter or in the refrigerator, then mix with the canola oil.

Combine the supplements in a small bowl. Sprinkle this mixture over the food as evenly as possible, and combine well.

Feline Degenerative Joint Disease

TURKEY AND SWEET POTATO

Yield: 429.21 grams
Calories: 549.72 (per recipe): 1.3 kcal/g, 290 kcal/cup, 1,281 kcal/kg
As fed: Protein 6.5%, Fat 5.5%, Fiber 1%, Carbohydrates 2.8%, Moisture 73%
All ingredients can be served raw, except for: sweet potato

¼ cup sweet potato

8 ounces dark meat turkey, skinless

10 grams turkey or chicken liver

2 teaspoons organic canola oil

1,000 mg omega-3 fish oil (from capsules)

½ teaspoon calcium carbonate powder

1 teaspoon taurine powder

⅜ teaspoon calcium phosphate powder

350 mg choline

1 tablet Kirkland Signature Daily Multi, crushed

175 mcg iodine (from kelp tablets)

9 mg iron bisglycinate

300 mcg biotin

Preheat the oven to 400°F. Peel the sweet potato, chop into bite-size cubes, and bake in the oven for 20 minutes, or until fork-tender. Mash with a fork.

While the sweet potato is baking, place the turkey in a pot and add just enough water to barely cover the meat. Bring to a boil, cook for 10 minutes, then add liver and cook for 5 minutes or until meat reaches an internal temperature of 165°F. When the meat is cool enough to handle, drain and chop into bite-size pieces. Retain the broth for later use.

Allow all hot ingredients to rest and come to room temperature, either on the counter or in the refrigerator, then mix with the canola oil and the contents of the omega-3 fish oil capsule.

Place ¼ cup of the reserved broth in a small bowl, and dissolve the rest of the supplements in it. Pour this over the turkey mixture and stir well. Before serving each portion to your pet, add a bit of the reserved broth.

Feline Struvite Crystals/Stones

CHICKEN AND RICE

Yield: 239.52 grams
Calories: 493.14 (per recipe): 2.1 kcal/g, 467 kcal/cup, 2,059 kcal/kg
As fed: Protein 21.3%, Fat 10.1%, Fiber 1%, Carbohydrates 6%, Moisture 61%
All ingredients can be served raw, except for: rice, sweet potato

2 tablespoons sweet potato

5⅓ ounces chicken breast, skinless

3 tablespoons long grain white rice

½ ounce clams, canned

4 teaspoons organic canola oil

1/16 teaspoon potassium chloride powder

⅜ teaspoon calcium carbonate powder

½ tablet Kirkland Signature Daily Multi, crushed

½ teaspoon taurine powder

45 mg zinc citrate

350 mg choline

300 mcg biotin

Preheat the oven to 400°F. Peel the sweet potato, chop into bite-size cubes, and bake in the oven for 20 minutes, or until fork-tender. Mash with a fork.

While the sweet potato is baking, place the chicken in a pot and add just enough water to barely cover the meat. Bring to a boil, and cook for 15 minutes or until meat reaches an internal temperature of 165°F. When the meat is cool enough to handle, drain and shred or chop into bite-size pieces. Retain the broth to pour over the finished recipe before serving.

Cook the rice according to the package directions to produce 3 tablespoons of cooked rice.

Allow all hot ingredients to rest and come to room temperature, either on the counter or in the refrigerator, then mix with the drained clams, a few drops of the tinned clam juice, and the canola oil.

Combine the supplements in a small bowl. Sprinkle this mixture over the food as evenly as possible, and combine well.

BEEF AND COUSCOUS

Note: The ingredients in this diet will help maintain a more acid pH in the body.

Yield: 179.64 grams
Calories: 347.07 (per recipe): 0.9 kcal/g, 438 kcal/cup, 1,932 kcal/kg
As fed: Protein 18.9%, Fat 9.6%, Fiber 1%, Carbohydrates 6.9%, Moisture 63%
All ingredients can be served raw, except for: couscous

6 ounces 85% lean ground beef

5 tablespoons couscous

2 tablespoons green beans

⅓ tablet Kirkland Signature Daily Multi, crushed

¼ teaspoon calcium carbonate powder

350 mg choline

½ teaspoon taurine powder

300 mcg biotin

Break the ground beef into 2-inch chunks and place in a pot with just enough water to cover. Bring water to a boil, then allow the meat to cook for 10 minutes or until browned, occasionally breaking the meat up into chunks with a fork to ensure all the beef is cooked. Use a strainer to drain the meat, but reserve the broth for later use.

Cook the couscous according to the package directions to yield 5 tablespoons of cooked couscous.

Bring a pot of water to a boil. Chop the green beans into bite-size pieces, then add to pot and cook for 3 to 5 minutes or until tender. Drain.

Allow all hot ingredients to rest and come to room temperature, either on the counter or in the refrigerator, then mix well.

Place 2 tablespoons of the reserved broth in a small bowl, and dissolve the supplements in it. Pour this over the beef mixture and stir well. Before serving each portion to your pet, add a bit of the reserved broth.

Feline Oxalate Crystal Diet

Note: Calcium oxalate stones generally cannot be dissolved through diet. Cats with discrete stones need them removed (see Chapter 13). This diet is beneficial for reducing the formation of calcium oxalate crystals, thus preventing the formation and recurrence of oxalate stones.

COD AND PEAS

Yield: 377.08 grams
Calories: 530.09 (per recipe): 1.9 kcal/g, 441 kcal/cup, 1,944 kcal/kg
As fed: Protein 6.7%, Fat 10.6%, Fiber 1%, Carbohydrates 17.7%, Moisture 63.3%
All ingredients can be served raw.

5⅓ ounces Atlantic cod fillet

1 cup green peas

2 tablespoons organic canola oil

2 tablespoons clam juice

¼ teaspoon calcium carbonate powder

⅔ teaspoon psyllium powder

¼ tablet Kirkland Signature Daily Multi, crushed

½ teaspoon taurine powder

½ tsp kelp powder

15 mg zinc citrate

175 mg choline

300 mcg biotin

Preheat the oven to 350°F, and bake cod for 15 to 20 minutes or until fish is opaque and flakes easily with a fork.

Bring a pot of water to a boil. Add the peas to the pot and cook for 3 to 4 minutes or until tender. Drain and mash with a fork.

Allow all hot ingredients to rest and come to room temperature, either on the counter or in the refrigerator, then combine with the canola oil.

Place the clam juice in a small bowl, and dissolve the supplements in it. Pour this over the fish mixture and stir well.

Feline Elimination Diet (Limited-Ingredient Diet): GI Disease

Note: While these diets are best when the goal is a limited-ingredient diet, the diets for skin allergies can also be useful for GI sensitivities.

PORK AND SWEET POTATO

Yield: 616.54 grams
Calories: 691.30 (per recipe): 1.1 kcal/g, 254 kcal/cup, 1,121 kcal/kg
As fed: Protein 16.2%, Fat 2.7%, Fiber 1%, Carbohydrates 5%, Moisture 74%
All ingredients can be served raw, except for: sweet potato

¾ cup sweet potato

1 pound lean pork tenderloin

1½ teaspoons organic canola oil

1 tablet Kirkland Signature Daily Multi, crushed

¾ teaspoon calcium carbonate powder

700 mg choline

½ teaspoon taurine powder

300 mcg biotin

Preheat the oven to 400°F. Peel the sweet potato, chop into bite-size pieces, then bake for 20 to 30 minutes, or until fork-tender. Mash with a fork.

Place the pork in a pot, and add just enough water to cover the meat. Bring the water to a boil, then cook for 20 minutes or until meat reaches an internal temperature of 160°F. Drain, then shred the meat.

Allow all hot ingredients to rest and come to room temperature, either on the counter or in the refrigerator, then mix with the canola oil.

Combine the supplements in a small bowl. Sprinkle this mixture over the food as evenly as possible, and combine well.

BISON AND BARLEY

Yield: 676.62 grams
Calories: 1,289.35 (per recipe): 1.9 kcal/g, 432 kcal/cup, 1,906 kcal/kg
As fed: Protein 13.3%, Fat 9.1%, Fiber 1%, Carbohydrates 13%, Moisture 62.6%
All ingredients can be served raw, except for: barley

> 1 pound ground bison
> ⅔ cup pearl barley (to yield 2 cups cooked)
> 1½ teaspoons organic canola oil
> ¼ teaspoon potassium chloride powder
> ¾ teaspoon calcium carbonate powder
> 1 tablet Kirkland Signature Daily Multi, crushed
> 700 mg choline
> ½ teaspoon taurine powder
> 300 mcg biotin

Break the ground bison into 2-inch chunks and place in a pot with just enough water to cover. Bring water to a boil, then allow the meat to cook for 10 minutes or until browned, occasionally breaking the meat up into chunks with a fork to ensure all the beef is cooked. Use a strainer to drain the meat, but reserve the broth for later use.

Cook the barley according to the package directions to yield 2 cups of cooked barley.

Allow all hot ingredients to rest and come to room temperature, either on the counter or in the refrigerator, then mix with the canola oil.

Place 2 tablespoons of the reserved broth in a small bowl, and dissolve the supplements in it. Pour this over the food and stir well. Before serving each portion to your pet, add a bit of the reserved broth.

Feline Pancreatitis

TURKEY AND RICE

Yield: 1,280.24 grams
Calories: 1,678.03 (per recipe): 13 kcal/g, 297 kcal/cup, 1,310 kcal/kg
As fed: Protein 7.5%, Fat 1.8%, Fiber 1%, Carbohydrates 20.4%, Moisture 69%
All ingredients can be served raw, except for: sweet potato, rice

½ cup sweet potato

½ cup white basmati rice (to yield 1½ cups cooked)

11 ounces 99% fat-free ground turkey

1 tablespoon flaxseed oil

2,000 mg omega-3 fish oil (from capsules)

½ teaspoon iodized salt

½ teaspoon taurine powder

1 teaspoon calcium carbonate powder

2 tablets Kirkland Signature Daily Multi, crushed

30 mg zinc citrate

700 mg choline

18 mg iron bisglycinate

300 mcg biotin

Preheat the oven to 400°F. Peel the sweet potato and chop into bite-size cubes. Bake in the oven for 20 minutes, or until fork-tender, then mash.

While the potato is baking, prepare the rice according to the package directions to yield 1½ cups of cooked rice.

Place the turkey in a pot with just enough water to cover. Bring to a boil, and cook for 10 minutes or until meat turns from pink to white. Drain and reserve the leftover broth to pour over portions of food before serving.

Allow all hot ingredients to rest and come to room temperature, either on the counter or in the refrigerator, then mix with the flaxseed oil and the contents of the fish oil capsules.

Combine the salt and the supplements in a small bowl. Sprinkle this mixture over the food as evenly as possible, and combine well.

Feline Low Fat, Low Fiber (Weight Management)

TILAPIA AND CHICKEN

Note: To enable easier measurements of the supplements in this recipe, we recommend that at least four recipes' worth are made at a time.

Yield: 270.86 grams

Calories: 308.77 (per recipe): 1.1 kcal/g, 257 kcal/cup, 1,135 kcal/kg

As fed: Protein 20.6%, Fat 2.9%, Fiber <1%, Carbohydrates 1.9%, Moisture 73.6%

All ingredients can be served raw, except for: sweet potato

  2 tablespoons sweet potato

  6 ounces tilapia

  One (3.25-oz.) jar of stage 1 infant food: chicken with broth, any brand

  ½ teaspoon organic canola oil

  ⅜ teaspoon calcium carbonate powder

  ½ teaspoon taurine powder

  5 mg iron bisglycinate

  1 mg chelated copper

  1.25 mg manganese

  15 mg zinc citrate

  80 mcg iodine (from kelp tablets)

  ⅛ tablet vitamin B50 complex

  350 mg choline

  300 mcg biotin

Preheat the oven to 350°F. Peel the sweet potato and bake along with the tilapia for 15 to 20 minutes. When potatoes are tender, remove and mash with a fork. Fish is done when it is opaque and flakes easily with a fork.

Allow all hot ingredients to rest and come to room temperature, either on the counter or in the refrigerator, then mix with the baby food and canola oil. (Stage 1 infant foods are plain purées meant for babies who are 4 to 8 months old.)

Combine the supplements in a small bowl. Sprinkle this mixture over the food as evenly as possible, and combine well.

Feline Low Fat (Weight Management)

TILAPIA AND SQUASH

Yield: 1,223.76 grams
Calories: 1,049.55 (per recipe): 1.0 kcal/g, 195 kcal/cup, 861 kcal/kg
As fed: Protein 8.4%, Fat 1.9%, Fiber 1.6%, Carbohydrates 1%, Moisture 79%
All ingredients can be served raw, except for: rice, butternut squash

  1 pound tilapia

  ½ cup white basmati rice (to yield 1½ cups cooked)

  1 cup butternut squash

  1 cup carrots

  1 cup green beans

  1 tablespoon organic canola oil

  1 tablet Kirkland Signature Daily Multi, crushed

  ⅓ teaspoon psyllium

  ⅞ teaspoon calcium carbonate powder

  15 mg zinc citrate

  525 mg choline

  ½ teaspoon taurine powder

  300 mcg biotin

Preheat the oven to 350°F, and bake tilapia for 15 to 20 minutes or until fish is opaque and flakes easily with a fork.

Prepare the rice according to the package directions to yield 1½ cups of cooked rice.

Bring a pot of water to a boil. Chop the squash, carrots, and green beans into bite-size pieces. Add to pot and cook for 10 minutes or until tender. Drain.

Allow all hot ingredients to rest and come to room temperature, either on the counter or in the refrigerator, then mix with the canola oil.

Combine the supplements in a small bowl. Sprinkle this mixture over the food as evenly as possible, and combine well.

Feline Heart Disease

TURKEY AND SWEET POTATO

Yield: 433.6 grams
Calories: 588.61 (per recipe): 1.7 kcal/g, 377 kcal/cup, 1,660 kcal/kg
As fed: Protein 6.5%, Fat 10.9%, Fiber 1.1%, Carbohydrates 11.4%, Moisture 69.5%
All ingredients can be served raw, except for: sweet potato

¼ cup sweet potato

8 ounces dark meat turkey, skinless

1 tablespoon turkey or chicken liver, chopped

1 tablespoon organic canola oil

2,000 mg omega-3 fish oil (from capsules)

½ tablet Kirkland Signature Daily Multi, crushed

⅜ teaspoon bone meal powder

⅝ teaspoon calcium carbonate powder

1 teaspoon taurine powder

350 mg choline

300 mcg biotin

Preheat the oven to 400°F. Peel the sweet potato, and chop into bite-size cubes. Bake in the oven for 20 minutes, or until tender, then mash with a fork.

Place the turkey in a pot and add just enough water to barely cover the meat. Bring to a boil, cook for 10 minutes, then add liver and cook for 5 minutes or until meat reaches an internal temperature of 165°F. When the meat is cool enough to handle, drain and chop into bite-size pieces. Retain the broth for later use.

Allow all hot ingredients to rest and come to room temperature, either on the counter or in the refrigerator, then mix with the canola oil and the contents of the fish oil capsules.

Place 2 tablespoons of the reserved broth in a small bowl, and dissolve the supplements in it. Pour this over the food and stir well. Before serving each portion to your pet, add a bit of the reserved broth.

Feline Diabetes

TURKEY AND LENTILS

Yield: 286.33 grams
Calories: 443.33 (per recipe): 1.5 kcal/g, 351 kcal/cup, 1,548 kcal/kg
As fed: Protein 17.8%, Fat 8.1%, Fiber 1%, Carbohydrates 3.4%, Moisture 69%
All ingredients can be served raw, except for: lentils

    8 ounces ground turkey
    2 tablespoons lentils (to yield ¼ cup cooked; canned is okay)
    1 teaspoon organic canola oil
    1,000 mg omega-3 fish oil (from capsules)
    ½ teaspoon calcium carbonate powder
    ½ tablet Kirkland Signature Daily Multi, crushed
    ½ teaspoon taurine powder
    350 mg choline
    300 mcg biotin

Place the turkey in a pot and add just enough water to barely cover the meat. Bring to a boil, then cook for 10 minutes or until meat turns from pink to white. Drain and reserve the broth for later use.

Cook the lentils according to the package directions to yield ¼ cup of cooked lentils.

Allow all hot ingredients to rest and come to room temperature, either on the counter or in the refrigerator, then mix with the canola oil and the contents of the fish oil capsules.

Place 2 tablespoons of the reserved broth in a small bowl, and dissolve the rest of the supplements in it. Pour this over the turkey mixture and stir well. Before serving each portion to your pet, add a bit of the reserved broth.

SARDINES AND RICE

Yield: 288.93 grams
Calories: 512.76 (per recipe): 1.8 kcal/g, 404 kcal/cup, 1,783 kcal/kg
As fed: Protein 17.3%, Fat 9.1%, Fiber 1%, Carbohydrates 5.3%, Moisture 65.1%
All ingredients can be served raw, except for: rice

1½ tablespoons brown basmati rice (to yield ⅓ cup cooked)

1 large egg

6 ounces sardines in water, without skin and bone

⅓ tablet Kirkland Signature Daily Multi, crushed

½ teaspoon taurine powder

½ teaspoon calcium carbonate powder

300 mcg biotin

Cook the rice according to the package directions to yield ⅓ cup of rice.

Bring a pot of water to a boil. Add the egg, and cook for 16 minutes or until hard-boiled. Peel and chop or mash the eggs.

Allow all hot ingredients to rest and come to room temperature, either on the counter or in the refrigerator, then combine with the drained sardines.

Combine the supplements in a small bowl. Sprinkle this mixture over the food as evenly as possible, and combine well. Use a small amount of the leftover sardine water in the tin to moisten the food if necessary.

Feline Liver Diet

COD AND POTATO

Yield: 336.03 grams
Calories: 486.72 (per recipe): 1.5 kcal/g, 329 kcal/cup, 1,448 kcal/kg
As fed: Protein 11.1%, Fat 5.4%, Fiber 1.3%, Carbohydrates 13.7%, Moisture 67.3%
All ingredients can be served raw, except for: potato

1 cup potato

4 ounces Atlantic cod fillet

¼ egg

1 tablespoon organic canola oil

1 teaspoon canola oil

1,000 mg omega-3 fish oil (from capsules)

⅛ teaspoon calcium carbonate powder

1 tablet Kirkland Signature Daily Multi, crushed

1 level teaspoon L-carnitine

¾ teaspoon taurine powder

250 mg L-arginine

⅓ teaspoon psyllium powder

350 mg choline

300 mcg biotin

Preheat the oven to 400°F. Peel the potato, and chop into bite-size cubes. Bake in the oven for 20 minutes, or until tender, then mash with a fork.

Place the cod in a pot and add just enough water to barely cover the fillet. Bring to a simmer, then cook for 7 to 10 minutes, or until fish is opaque and flakes easily with a fork.

Bring a pot of water to a boil. Add one egg to the pot, and cook for 16 minutes or until hard-boiled. Peel and slice the egg into 4 even pieces, reserving ¾ for a later use.

Add the ¼ egg to the fish and potato, and allow to come to room temperature on the counter or in the refrigerator. Mix together with the canola oil and the contents of the fish oil capsules.

Combine the rest of the supplements in a small bowl. Sprinkle this mixture over the food as evenly as possible, and combine well.

CHICKEN AND PASTA

Yield: 169.51 grams
Calories: 367.46 (per recipe): 2.2 kcal/g, 492 kcal/cup, 2,167 kcal/kg
As fed: Protein 16.1%, Fat 10.8%, Fiber 1%, Carbohydrates 12.7%, Moisture 57.2%
All ingredients can be served raw, except for: macaroni

   3 ounces dark meat chicken, skinless

   ¼ cup enriched macaroni (to yield ½ cup cooked)

   2 teaspoons organic canola oil

   ¼ tablet Kirkland Signature Daily Multi, crushed

   ⅛ teaspoon potassium chloride powder

   ⅛ teaspoon calcium carbonate powder

   ⅛ teaspoon bone meal powder

   ½ teaspoon taurine powder

   5 mg iron bisglycinate

   15 mg zinc citrate

   ¼ teaspoon L-carnitine powder

   ⅙ teaspoon (approximately) psyllium powder

   300 mcg biotin

Place the chicken in a pot and add just enough water to barely cover the meat. Bring to a boil, then cook for 15 minutes or until meat reaches an internal temperature of 165°F. When chicken is cool enough to handle, drain and shred the meat, reserving the broth to pour over the finished recipe before serving.

Cook the pasta according to the package directions to yield ½ cup pasta, then cut it up into smaller, bite-size pieces.

Allow all hot ingredients to rest and come to room temperature, either on the counter or in the refrigerator, then combine with the canola oil.

Combine the supplements in a small bowl. Sprinkle this mixture over the food as evenly as possible, and combine well.

Feline Renal Diet

BISON AND COUSCOUS

Yield: 300.48 grams
Calories: 674.77 (per recipe): 1.2 kcal/g, 264 kcal/cup, 1,166 kcal/kg
As fed: Protein 5.4%, Fat 3%, Fiber 1.3%, Carbohydrates 16.8%, Moisture 73.3%
All ingredients can be served raw, except for: couscous

  6 ounces ground bison
  ½ cup couscous
  2 tablespoons carrots, sliced
  1 ounce clams, canned
  1 tablespoon organic canola oil
  2,000 mg omega-3 fish oil (from capsules)
  2 teaspoon clam juice
  ⅜ teaspoon calcium carbonate powder
  ½ teaspoon taurine powder
  400 mcg folic acid
  18 mg iron bisglycinate
  2 mg chelated copper
  60 mg zinc citrate
  160 mcg iodine (from kelp tablets)
  ½ teaspoon potassium chloride powder
  350 mg choline
  1 tablet Kirkland Signature Daily Multi, crushed
  300 mcg biotin

Break the ground bison into 2-inch chunks and place in a pot with just enough water to cover. Bring water to a boil, then allow the meat to cook for 10 minutes or until browned, occasionally breaking the meat up into chunks with a fork to ensure all the beef is cooked. Use a strainer to drain the meat, but reserve the broth for later use.

Prepare the couscous according to the package directions to yield ½ cup of cooked couscous.

Bring a pot of water to a boil. Chop the carrots into bite-size pieces, then add to pot and cook for 10 minutes or until tender. Drain.

Allow all hot ingredients to rest and come to room temperature, either on the counter or in the refrigerator, then mix with the clams, canola oil, and the contents of the fish oil capsules.

Place the clam juice in a small bowl, and dissolve the rest of the supplements in it. Pour this over the food and stir well. Before serving each portion to your pet, add a bit of the reserved broth.

PORK AND RICE CEREAL

Yield: 187.16 grams
Calories: 279.25 (per recipe): 1.5 kcal/g, 338 kcal/cup, 1,491 kcal/kg
As fed: Protein 10.9%, Fat 6.3%, Fiber 1%, Carbohydrates 11.6%, Moisture 69.6%
All ingredients can be served raw, except for: brown rice cereal

    3 ounces pork tenderloin
    ½ (3.25-oz.) jar of stage 1 infant food: butternut squash
    2 teaspoons organic canola oil
    ⅓ cup instant infant brown rice cereal
    ¼ tablet Kirkland Signature Daily Multi, crushed
    ¼ teaspoon calcium carbonate
    350 mg choline
    ½ teaspoon taurine powder
    300 mcg biotin

Place the pork in a pot, and add just enough water to cover the meat. Bring the water to a boil, then cook for 20 minutes or until meat reaches an internal temperature of 160°F. Drain, then shred the meat. Reserve the broth to make the cereal and pour over the finished recipe before serving.

Allow the pork to rest and come to room temperature, either on the counter or in the refrigerator, then combine with the baby food and canola oil. (Stage 1 infant foods are plain purées meant for babies who are 4 to 8 months old.)

Prepare the baby cereal according to the package directions, using the reserved pork broth in place of water. Add the supplements to the cereal, then combine well with the pork mixture.

Feline Cancer Diet

SALMON AND MILLET

Yield: 462.77 grams
Calories: 719.74 (per recipe): 1.6 kcal/g, 353 kcal/cup, 1,555 kcal/kg
As fed: Protein 21.2%, Fat 6.1%, Fiber 1%, Carbohydrates 2.6%, Moisture 69%
All ingredients can be served raw, except for: millet

1 pound pink salmon fillet

4 teaspoons millet (to yield ¼ cup cooked)

2 tablespoons carrots

1 teaspoon organic canola oil

3,000 mg omega-3 fish oil (from capsules)

100 IU vitamin E (from capsules)

1¼ teaspoons calcium carbonate

½ teaspoon taurine powder

1 capsule Thorne Research Citramins

30 to 50 mg riboflavin 5' phosphate

800 mcg folic acid

300 mcg biotin

Broil salmon fillets on high for 3 to 6 minutes, or until fish is opaque and flakes easily with a fork.

Cook the millet according to the package directions to yield ¼ cup of cooked millet.

Bring a pot of water to a boil. Chop the carrots into bite-size pieces, add to the pot, and cook for 10 minutes or until tender.

Allow all hot ingredients to rest and come to room temperature, either on the counter or in the refrigerator, then mix with the canola oil and the contents of the fish oil and vitamin E capsules.

Combine the rest of the supplements in a small bowl. Sprinkle this mixture over the food as evenly as possible, and combine well.

STEAK AND SWEET POTATO

Yield: 519.53 grams
Calories: 1,190.77 (per recipe): 2.3 kcal/g, 520 kcal/cup, 2,292 kcal/kg
As fed: Protein 25%, Fat 12.7%, Fiber 1%, Carbohydrates 2%, Moisture 58.4%
All ingredients can be served raw, except for: sweet potato

¼ cup sweet potato

1 pound 90% lean ground beef

2 teaspoons organic canola oil

2,000 mg omega-3 fish oil (from capsules)

1 tablet Kirkland Signature Daily Multi, crushed

1 teaspoon calcium carbonate powder

350 mg choline

160 mcg iodine (from kelp tablets)

½ teaspoon taurine powder

300 mcg biotin

Preheat the oven to 400°F. Peel the sweet potato, and chop into bite-size cubes. Bake in the oven for 20 to 30 minutes, or until tender. Potato may be mashed, if desired.

Break the ground beef into 2-inch chunks and place in a pot with just enough water to cover. Bring water to a boil, then allow the meat to cook for 10 minutes or until browned, occasionally breaking the meat up into chunks with a fork to ensure all the beef is cooked. Use a strainer to drain the meat, but reserve the broth for later use.

Allow all hot ingredients to rest and come to room temperature, either on the counter or in the refrigerator, then mix with the canola oil and the contents of the fish oil capsules.

Place 2 tablespoons of the reserved broth in a small bowl, and dissolve the rest of the supplements in it. Pour this over the food and stir well. Before serving each portion to your pet, add a bit of the reserved broth.

APPENDIX D

Vitamin and Mineral
Supplement Recommendations

All of the supplements recommended in this book's recipes can be purchased online at sites such as iherb.com or Amazon.com. In addition, many local vitamin stores will have these supplements. The Kirkland multivitamin can be purchased at Costco's online or physical stores.

To achieve the best results, consult with an experienced veterinarian regarding what supplements are best for your pet. If your veterinarian is unfamiliar with natural medicine, please review your pet's supplements with them anyway. Medicine is a collaborative effort and there is no benefit in keeping secrets.

A Note on Doses

When sourcing your own supplements, there will be occasions when the dose recommended in the recipe does not exactly match what you are able to purchase. Not to worry. The supplement dosing in the recipes has some wiggle room. For example, if a recipe calls for 250 mg choline and you purchased 300 mg capsules, it is fine. Try to get as close to the recommended doses as possible. Ultimately, however, even alterations of 20% above (or 10% below) the recommended amount will be fine.

Be cautious—do not make dosing mistakes by factors of 10! For example, if the recipe calls for 400 IU of Vitamin D, do not use 4000 IU instead.

Supplements and Recommended Brands

In an effort to make your life easier, the best brands of supplements to use in these recipes have been listed below. However, there may be instances where the specific brands are not available. When sourcing supplements on your own, do your research to choose the highest-quality products from the most reputable manufacturer. Remember, small differences in the quantity or chemical makeup of a supplement can have a large impact on nutrition and safety.

When using human supplements or raw herbs, be sure to seek veterinary advice on dosing and preparation. Supplements that are specifically formulated for pets are generally regarded as safe. Products containing the seal of the National Animal Supplement Council (NASC) can be relied upon to be of high quality. The NASC is a private organization that monitors supplements for animals. Supplement manufacturers voluntarily submit their products to the NASC for evaluation of both ingredient quality and accuracy of labeling.

The following is an alphabetical listing of every supplement indicated for the recipes.

- Biotin: Solgar biotin 300 mcg tablet
- Bone meal powder: KAL bone meal powder
- Calcium carbonate: NOW vegetarian calcium carbonate powder, or an equal amount of ground eggshells
- Calcium phosphate: Freeda calcium phosphate powder
- Choline: Solgar 350 mg capsule, Nature's Way 500 mg tablets
- Citramins: This is a proprietary product made by Thorne Research. You may substitute any mineral supplement that contains 15 mg iron and 900 mcg copper.
- Copper: TwinLab copper 2 mg capsule, Carlson chelated copper 5 mg capsule
- Dicalcium phosphate: UPCO or Freeda dicalcium phosphate
- Folic acid: NOW Foods 800 mcg tablets
- Iron bisglycinate: NOW Foods 18 mg capsule
- Kelp tablets: NOW Foods kelp (325 mcg iodine per dose), Nature's Way kelp caps (300 mcg iodine per dose), Country Life Norwegian kelp (225 mcg iodine per dose), Solgar North Atlantic kelp tablets (225 mcg iodine per dose)
- L-arginine: NOW Foods L-arginine 1,000 mg tablet
- L-carnitine: NOW Foods L-carnitine powder
- L-tryptophan: NOW Foods L-tryptophan 500 mg capsule
- Magnesium citrate: NOW Foods magnesium citrate powder
- Manganese: TwinLab manganese 10 mg tablet

- Methionine: Solgar methionine 500 mg capsule, Solaray 500 mg capsule

- Multivitamin: Kirkland Signature Multi Vitamins & Minerals. If you choose to source an alternative multivitamin, check the label for the "% daily value" for each vitamin and mineral. Choose one that offers no more than 100 percent of the requirement for vitamin D (400 IU) and iron (18 mg). Avoid brands with very high doses of any vitamin or mineral; most values should be close to 100 percent.

- Omega-3 fish oil: Be sure to source a highly reputable brand due to concerns for contaminants in fish oil. Generally, 1,000 mg is equivalent to one capsule or ¼ teaspoon of liquid fish oil.

- Pantothenic acid: NOW Foods pantothenic acid 500 mg capsule

- Potassium chloride: NOW Foods calcium chloride powder

- Psyllium powder: Metamucil capsules are equivalent to 1 teaspoon of psyllium husks

- Riboflavin 5' phosphate: Thorne riboflafin 5' phosphate 36.5 mg capsule

- Salt, iodized: Any brand of iodized salt is acceptable.

- Selenium: NOW Foods selenium 200 mcg capsule

- Taurine: NOW Foods taurine powder

- Vitamin A: Dry vitamin A 10,000 IU capsule ("Dry" refers to the vitamin in powdered rather than in an oil base. In this case, dry vitamin A has been chosen for its better absorption.)

- Vitamin B1 (thiamine): NOW Foods 100 mg tablets

- Vitamin B12: Solgar 1,000 mcg capsule

- Vitamin B50 complex: NOW Foods B50 Complex (If you choose to source your own brand, match the NOW Foods B50 Complex blend of 50 mg B1, 50 mg B2, 50 mg B3, 50 mg B6, 400 mcg folate, 50 mcg B12, 50 mcg biotin, 50 mg pantothenic acid, 25 mg PABA, 25 mg choine, 25 mg inositol.)

- Vitamin C, buffered: Nature's Way buffered vitamin C 500 mg capsules

- Vitamin D3 (cholecalciferol): Jarrow Formulas vitamin D3 1,000 IU softgels

- Vitamin E: Any reputable brand for vitamin E is acceptable.

- Zinc citrate: TwinLab (30 mg) capsules

APPENDIX E

Special Diets: Limited-Ingredient Diet Trial, Bland Diet, and Rice Water Fast

Limited-Ingredient Diet Trials

A limited-ingredient diet (LID) trial, also known as a feeding trial or elimination diet, is a period of time during which a pet will only be fed a very restricted list of foods. Most commonly, diet trials are conducted with pets who have severe allergies or chronic gastrointestinal (GI) issues, such as inflammatory bowel disease. The goal is to see if some or all of the pet's symptoms resolve on the LID.

Diet trials are held for three to eight weeks, as it takes this long for the body to cleanse itself of food antigens that are absorbed into the blood and tissues. During that period, it is imperative that your pet eat only the foods of the trial—no snacks or treats allowed. The diet often consists of a single protein and carbohydrate source so as to rule out as many variables as possible. Any stray bites of other foods during the trial period can cause symptoms and cloud the results of the test.

What to Feed on an LID

When it comes to a diet trial, the biggest concern is what food to use. The goal is to use a protein source that is the least likely to cause a reaction. Ideally, you'd use a single protein and carbohydrate source that your pet has never had before. It is unlikely for a pet to have a severe inflammatory reaction to a new food. Usually allergies and sensitivities are built up over time due to repeated exposure of a substance to the immune system.

Western medicine veterinarians most frequently recommend "prescription" diets to use for food trials. These veterinary exclusive diets are specifically designed for sensitive animals, and often contain a single protein and carbohydrate source. They also tend to have ingredients infrequently found in pet foods such as venison, rabbit, etc. Alternatively, these diets may contain "hydrolyzed" proteins, in which a more common protein such as chicken is broken down into much smaller protein molecules. The intent is that the immune system does not recognize the smaller protein bits as chicken, and therefore doesn't respond with an inflammatory response.

The potential shortcoming of prescription diets is much the same as with any highly processed food. The processing methods can lead to the production of proinflammatory compounds that might affect an already inflamed pet, making for an unsuccessful food trial. While prescription diets can be effective, a better option is homemade foods. Preparing your own foods for an LID allows you to feed your pet fresh food and minimize chance contamination by molds, toxins, or other trace proteins found in processed diets.

How to Conduct the Diet Trial

Home-prepared diets for the purposes of a food trial can be put together in several ways. Balanced recipes for skin allergies and/or GI problems in dogs and cats are listed in Appendix C. When it comes to a relatively short-term diet trial however, even these recipes are not necessary. Any reasonably healthy dog or cat will do fine for three to eight weeks on an unbalanced diet. After the diet trial is over, however, switching to a long-term balanced diet is essential.

All you need to do is choose a protein and carbohydrate source that your pet has not had before, and feed your pet a proportion of two-thirds protein and one-third carbohydrates. Raw food is acceptable for diet trials; simply remember to take the appropriate precautions regarding raw feeding (see Appendix C).

Diet trials are a trial-and-error process. After three to eight weeks, if there are no changes in symptoms in your pet, it may be because your pet has no food sensitivity. On the other hand, your pet may be continuing to have a reaction to something in the ingredients you are feeding. Consider picking other ingredients and running the trial again.

Transitioning to Food after the Trial

If you see a marked improvement or resolution of allergy symptoms in your pet, your next goal is to find a balanced long-term diet that keeps your pet's allergies at bay. Options for this include a home-prepared recipe such as those included in Appendix C or a commercially prepared diet with an appropriate source of proteins and carbohydrates.

After finishing the diet trial, be sure to transition your pet to a new diet slowly (see Appendix C for tips). When choosing a diet, the closer to a fresh, whole-food diet you are feeding, the better. Raw versus cooked is less important, and is simply a matter of the individual pet's and your personal preferences.

Diets for Acute GI Upset

Vomiting and diarrhea due to dietary indiscretion is very common in dogs and cats. As long as there is no suspicion of an ingested foreign body, these pets generally require minimal medical care, although dehydration can become an issue if the vomiting is severe. Most frequently, veterinarians recommend a "bland diet" for a few days, which is easily digestible and allows the GI tract to recover. When the diarrhea is severe, a rice water fast may be necessary, as even a bland diet will go right through them.

If your pet is vomiting frequently, a veterinary consultation is a good idea. Your veterinarian may be able to give your pet medication to help stop the vomiting or recommend fluids to ward off dehydration. Once the vomiting is under control, begin either the bland diet or the rice water fast for a few days.

The Standard Bland Diet

Combining an easily digestible protein and carbohydrate source is the best nutritional method to help your pet overcome their short-term GI upset. Boiled chicken and white rice are the standard ingredients, although substitutions can be made for pets that have sensitivities to chicken or rice.

RECIPE

Boil 1 cup of white rice in 4 cups of water. Continue to boil until the rice grains to break up into mush, about 20 minutes. Drain and allow to cool. This will yield about 3 cups of cooked rice.

While the rice is cooking, boil 3 cups of white meat chicken in a separate pot for about 15 minutes, or until it reaches an internal temperature of 165°F. Allow to cool, then cut or shred the meat.

Combine the rice and chicken in a 50:50 proportion.

Feed your pet rice and chicken rather than their regular diet for several days, until the diarrhea resolves. Then slowly mix in their regular food while decreasing the bland diet over two to four days to allow them to adjust back to their normal diet.

The Rice Water Fast

For more severe GI upset, sometimes a rice water is better than the standard bland diet. Rice water has been used in developing countries to sustain people with severe GI problems such as dysentery. Proteins released by the rice grains soothe the inflamed GI tract and aid in recovery while the water provides hydration and electrolytes. Although I most often give this treatment to dogs, it can be offered to cats as well.

RECIPE

Boil 1 cup of white rice in 4 cups of water. Continue to boil until the rice grains to break up into mush, about 20 minutes. Drain the rice, retaining the milky water, and allow the rice to cool.

Once the milky rice water cools, feed it directly to your pet. To aid with palatability, you may add small amounts of baby food to the water.

As your pet is feeling better, mix the mushy rice with baby food and form it into small balls to feed to your pet.

As your pet improves, add boiled chicken to the rice balls in a 50:50 proportion.

Feed your pet this rice water fast rather than their regular diet for several days, until the diarrhea resolves. Then slowly mix in their regular food while decreasing the bland diet over two to four days to allow them to adjust back to their normal diet.

ENDNOTES

Introduction

1. Bennett, Simeon. "Life expectancy increased by 5 years since 2000, but health inequalities persist." http://www.who.int/mediacentre/news/releases/2016/health-inequalities-persist/en.

2. Abbott, R. B. et al. "Medical student attitudes toward complementary, alternative and integrative medicine." *Evidence-Based Complementary and Alternative Medicine.* 2011.

3. Patwardhan, B. "Drug discovery and development: Traditional medicine and ethnopharmacology perspectives." *SciTopics.* 2009.

4. Ramesh, V. et al. "Novel Bioactive Wild Medicinal Mushroom—Xylaria sp. R006 (Ascomycetes) against Multidrug Resistant Human Bacterial Pathogens and Human Cancer Cell Lines." *International Journal of Medicinal Mushrooms.* 2015;17(10):1005-17.

5. Chowdhury, M., Kubra, K., and Ahmed, S. "Screening of antimicrobial, antioxidant properties and bioactive compounds of some edible mushrooms cultivated in Bangladesh." *Annals of Clinical Microbiology and Antimicrobials.* 2015;14(8). doi: 10.1186/s12941-015-0067-3.

6. Ghalib, H. "The hunt for the next Artemisinin: African researchers screen herbal remedies for drug discovery leads." *TDRnews.* 2007;(79):8–13. See more at: http://www.scidev.net/global/indigenous/feature/integrating-modern-and-traditional-medicine-facts-and-figures.html#sthash.WAwuwud8.dpuf

7. Sanchez-Ramos, J. "The entourage effect of the phytocannabinoids." *Annals of Neurology.* 2015;77(6):1083. doi: 10.1002/ana.24402. Epub April 9, 2015.

Chapter 1

1. Freedman, A.H. et al. "Genome Sequencing Highlights Genes Under Selection and the Dynamic Early History of Dogs." *PLOS Genetics.* Jan. 16, 2014. http://journals.plos.org/plosgenetics/article?id=10.1371/journal.pgen.1004016

2. Ogden, C. L. et al. "Prevalence of childhood and adult obesity in the United States, 2011–2012." *Journal of the American Medical Association.* 2014;311(8):806–814. http://www.petobesityprevention.org/pet-obesity-fact-risks/

3. Lund, E. M. et al. "Prevalence and Risk Factors for Obesity in Adult Dogs from Private US Veterinary Practices." *International Journal of Applied Research and Veterinary Medicine.* 2006;4(2):177–186. http://jarvm.com/articles/Vol4Iss2/Lund.pdf

4. Nijland, M. L., Stam, F., and Seidell, J.C. "Overweight in dogs, but not in cats, is related to overweight in their owners." *Public Health Nutrition.* Epub June 23, 2009. doi: 10.1017/S136898000999022X.

5. Hand, M. S. et al., eds. *Small Animal Clinical Nutrition,* 5th ed. Topeka, KS: Mark Morris Institute; 2002:157–250.

6. Cowell, C. S. et al. "History of Pet Food Manufacture in the United States." Hand, M.S. et al., eds. *Small Animal Clinical Nutrition*, 4th ed. Walsworth Publishing Company; 2000:129.

7. Hand, M. S. et al., eds. *Small Animal Clinical Nutrition*, 5th ed. Topeka, KS: Mark Morris Institute; 2002:157–250.

8. Laflamme, D. and Gunn-Moore, D. "Nutrition of aging cats." *Veterinary Clinics of North America, Small Animal Practice*. 2014;44(4):761–774. doi: 10.1016/j.cvsm.2014.03.001.

9. Kahn, S. E., Hull, R. L., and Utzschneider, K. M. "Mechanisms linking obesity to insulin resistance and type 2 diabetes." *Nature*. Dec. 14, 2006:840–846.Endnote 1

Chapter 2

1. Bradshaw, J. W. "The evolutionary basis for the feeding behavior of domestic dogs (*Canis familiaris*) and cats (*Felis catus*)." *Journal of Nutrition*. July 2006;136(7). http://www.ncbi.nlm.nih.gov/pubmed/16772461

2. Hand, M. S. et al., eds. *Small Animal Clinical Nutrition*, 5th ed. Topeka, KS: Mark Morris Institute; 2002:49–105.

3. Seefeldt, S. L. and Chapman, T. E. "Body water content and turnover in cats fed dry and canned rations." *American Journal of Veterinary Research*. 1979;40(2):183–185.

4. Fram, M. S. and Belitz, K. "Occurrence and Concentrations of Pharmaceutical Compounds in Groundwater Used for Public Drinking-water Supply in California." *Science of the Total Environment*. 2011;409(18):3409–3417.

5. Gonda, I. et al. "Branched-chain and Aromatic Amino Acid Catabolism into Aroma Volatiles in Cucumis Melo L. Fruit." *Journal of Experimental Botany*. March 2010;61(4):1111–1123.

6. Lignou, S. et al. "Sensory and Instrumental Analysis of Medium and Long Shelf-life Charentais Cantaloupe Melons (*Cucumis melo* L.) Harvested at Different Maturities." *Food Chemistry*. April 1, 2014;148:218–229.

7. Axelsson, E. et al. "The genomic signature of dog domestication reveals adaptation to a starch-rich diet." *Nature*. 2013;495(7441):360–364. doi: 10.1038/nature11837.

8. Daley, C. A. et al. "A review of fatty acid profiles and antioxidant content in grass-fed and grain-fed beef." *Nutrition Journal*. 2010. doi: 10.1186/1475-2891-9-10

9. Scott, D. W., Miller, W. H., and Griffin, C. E., eds. "Skin Immune System and Allergic Diseases." *Muller & Kirk's Small Animal Dermatology*. Philadelphia: W.B. Saunders; 2001.

10. Wenstrom, K. D. "The FDA's New Advice on Fish: It's Complicated." *American Journal of Obstetrics & Gynecology*. Nov. 2014;211(5):475–478. http://www.ncbi.nlm.nih.gov/pubmed/25072735

11. "Best Fish Oil?" ConsumerLab.com. July 4, 2015. https://www.consumerlab.com/reviews/fish_oil_supplements_review/omega3/

12. Hand, M. S. et al., eds. *Small Animal Clinical Nutrition*, 5th ed. Topeka, KS: Mark Morris Institute; 2002:49–105.

13. Guyton, K. Z. et al. "Carcinogenicity of tetrachlorvinphos, parathion, malathion, diazinon, and glyphosate." *The Lancet. Oncology* 2015;16(5): 490–1. doi: 10.1016/S1470-2045(15)70134-8. PMID 25801782.

14. Giesy, J. P., Dobson, S., and Solomon, K. R. "Ecotoxicological Risk Assessment for Roundup Herbicide." *Reviews of Environmental Contamination and Toxicology*. 2000;167:35–120. doi: 10.1007/978-1-4612-1156-3_2. ISBN 978-0-387-95102-7.

15. "Greener Pastures: How grass-fed beef and milk contribute to healthy eating." Union of Concerned Scientists. March 2006:58. http://www.ucsusa.org/sites/default/files/legacy/assets/documents/food_and_agriculture/greener-pastures.pdf

16. Aursand, M. et al. "Description of the processes in the value chain and risk assessment of decomposition substances and oxidation products in fish oils" Norwegian Scientific Committee for Food Safety. 2011. http://www.vkm.no/dav/4be9bee090.pdf ISBN 978-82-8259-035-8. Accessed Oct. 19, 2012.

17. Lenox, C. E. and Bauer, J. E. "Potential adverse effects of omega-3 fatty acids in dogs and cats." *Journal of Veterinary Internal Medicine*. 2013;27(2):217–226.

18. Hand, M. S. et al., eds. *Small Animal Clinical Nutrition*, 5th ed. Topeka, KS: Mark Morris Institute; 2002:49–105.

19. *Nutrient Requirements of Dogs and Cats*. National Research Council of the National Academy of Sciences. Washington, DC: National Academies Press; 2006:317.

20. Hand, M. S. et al., eds. *Small Animal Clinical Nutrition*, 5th ed. Topeka, KS: Mark Morris Institute; 2002:1143–1153.

21. Plantinga, E. A., Bosch, G., and Hendriks, W. H. "Estimation of the dietary nutrient profile of free-roaming feral cats: possible implications for nutrition of domestic cats." *British Journal of Nutrition*. Oct. 2011:S35–48. doi: 10.1017/S0007114511002285.

22. Brown, S. *Unlocking the Canine Ancestral Diet*. Wenatchee, WA: Dogwise Publishing; 2009.

23. Axelsson, E. et al. "The genomic signature of dog domestication reveals adaptation to a starch-rich diet." *Nature*. 2013;495(7441):360–364. doi: 10.1038/nature11837.

24. Patrick, J. S. "Deconstructing the Regulatory Façade: Why Confused Consumers Feed their Pets Ring Dings and Krispy Kremes." Harvard Law School. April 2006. http://dash.harvard.edu/bitstream/handle/1/10018997/Patrick06.html

25. Cowell, C. S. et al. "History of Pet Food Manufacture in the United States." Hand, M.S. et al., eds. *Small Animal Clinical Nutrition*, 4th ed. Walsworth Publishing Company; 2000:129.

26. Plantinga, E. A., Bosch, G., and Hendriks, W. H. "Estimation of the dietary nutrient profile of free-roaming feral cats: possible implications for nutrition of domestic cats." *British Journal of Nutrition*. Oct. 2011:S35–48. doi: 10.1017/S0007114511002285.

27. Hand, M. S. et al., eds. *Small Animal Clinical Nutrition*, 5th ed. Topeka, KS: Mark Morris Institute; 2002:49–105.

Chapter 3

1. Cowell, C. S. et al. "History of Pet Food Manufacture in the United States." Hand, M.S. et al., eds. *Small Animal Clinical Nutrition*, 4th ed. Walsworth Publishing Company; 2000:129.

2. Hand, M. S. et al., eds. *Small Animal Clinical Nutrition*, 5th ed. Topeka, KS: Mark Morris Institute; 2002:157–190.

3. Fox, M. W., Hodgkins, E., and Smart, M. E. *Not Fit for a Dog!: The Truth about Manufactured Dog and Cat Food*.

4. Riaz, M. N. "Stability of Vitamins during Extrusion." *Critical Reviews in Food Science and Nutrition*. 2009;49(4):361–368.

5. "How Dry Pet Food Is Made." Pet Food Institute. 2013. http://www.petfoodinstitute.org/?page=DryPetFood

6. "U.S. Pet Industry Spending Figures & Future Outlook." American Pet Products Association. 2015. http://www.americanpetproducts.org/press_industrytrends.asp

7. Patrick, J. S. "Deconstructing the Regulatory Façade: Why Confused Consumers Feed their Pets Ring Dings and Krispy Kremes." Harvard Law School. April 2006. http://dash.harvard.edu/bitstream/handle/1/10018997/Patrick06.html

8. "Fair Packaging and Labeling Act." FTC. https://www.ftc.gov/enforcement/rules/rulemaking-regulatory-reform-proceedings/fair-packaging-labeling-act

9. "Fair Packaging and Labeling Act." U.S. Food and Drug Administration. http://www.fda.gov/RegulatoryInformation/Legislation/ucm148722.htm

10. "FDA's Regulation of Pet Food." U.S. Food and Drug Administration. http://www.fda.gov/AnimalVeterinary/ResourcesforYou/ucm047111.htm

11. Dzanis, D. A. "Which pet food nutrient values should you follow?" PetfoodIndustry.com. March 7, 2013. http://www.petfoodindustry.com/articles/3518-which-petfood-nutrient-values-should-you-follow.

12. "U.S. Pet Industry Spending Figures & Future Outlook." American Pet Products Association. 2015. http://www.americanpetproducts.org/press_industrytrends.asp

Chapter 4

1. Nestle, M. *Pet Food Politics: The Chihuahua in the Coal Mine*. Berkeley, CA: University of California Press; 2010.

2. Dozier, W. A., Dale, N. M., and Dove, C. R. "Nutrient Composition of Feed Grade and Pet Food Grade Poultry By-Product Meal." *Journal of Applied Poultry Research*. 2003;12:526–530.

3. Hand, M. S. et al., eds. *Small Animal Clinical Nutrition*, 5th ed. Topeka, KS: Mark Morris Institute; 2002:11b.

4. van Rooijen, C. et al. "Quantitation of Maillard reaction products in commercially available pet foods." *Journal of Agricultural and Food Chemistry*. Sept. 3, 2014;62(35):8883–8891. doi: 10.1021/jf502064h.

5. van Rooijen, C. et al. "The Maillard reaction and pet food processing: effects on nutritive value and pet health." *Nutrition Research Reviews*. December 2013;26(2):130–148. doi: 10.1017/S0954422413000103.

6. Vistoli, G. et al. "Advanced glycoxidation and lipoxidation end products (AGEs and ALEs): an overview of their mechanisms of formation." *Free Radical Research*. August 2013:3–27. doi: 10.3109/10715762.2013.815348.

7. Finley, R. et al. "The risk of salmonellae shedding by dogs fed Salmonella-contaminated commercial raw food diets." *Canadian Veterinary Journal*. 2007;48(1):69–75.

8. Stogdale, l. and Diehl, G. "Just how pathogenic to pets and humans are the bacteria in the concentrations found in raw pet foods." *Canadian Veterinary Journal*. 2005;46(11):967.

9. Kang, J. H. and Kondo, F. "Determination of bisphenol A in canned pet foods." *Research in Veterinary Science*. October 2002;73(2):177–82.

10. Lorber, M. et al. "Exposure assessment of adult intake of bisphenol A (BPA) with emphasis on canned food dietary exposures." Environ Int. April 2015;77:55–62. doi: 10.1016/j.envint.2015.01.008. Epub Jan. 30, 2015.

Chapter 5

1. "2009 Summary Report on Antimicrobials Sold or Distributed for Use in Food-Producing Animals." U.S. Food and Drug Administration. September 2014. http://www.fda.gov/downloads/ForIndustry/UserFees/AnimalDrugUserFeeActADUFA/UCM231851.pdf

2. Davis, D. R., Epp, M. D., and Riordan, H. D. "Changes in USDA food composition data for 43 garden crops, 1950 to 1999." *Journal of the American College of Nutrition*. December 2004;23(6):669–682.

3. Eastbrook, B. *Tomatoland: How Modern Industrial Agriculture Destroyed Our Most Alluring Fruit*. Kansas City: Andrews McMeel Publishing; 2011.

4. Brooks, D. et al. "2014 AAHA Weight Management Guidelines for Dogs and Cats." AAHA.org. 2014. https://www.aaha.org/public_documents/professional/guidelines/weight_management_guidelines.pdf

5. Hand, M. S. et al., eds. *Small Animal Clinical Nutrition*, 5th ed. Topeka, KS: Mark Morris Institute; 2002.

Chapter 6

1. Larsen, L. L. and Berry, J. A. "The regulation of dietary supplements." Journal of the American Academy of Nurse Practitioners. 2003;15(9):410–4.

2. https://www.blumenthal.senate.gov/newsroom/press/release/fda-issues-warnings-on-mislabeled-supplements-following-blumenthal-and-durbins-call-to-action

3. https://ods.od.nih.gov/factsheets/MVMS-HealthProfessional/

4. Guarner, F. and Malagelada, J. "Gut flora in health and disease." *The Lancet.* Feb. 8, 2003; 361(9356):512–519. doi: 10.1016/S0140-6736(03)12489-0.

5. Sears, C. L. "A dynamic partnership: Celebrating our gut flora." *Anaerobe.* October 2005;11(5):247–251. doi: 10.1016/j.anaerobe.2005.05.001.

6. Vighi, G. et al. "Allergy and the gastrointestinal system." *Clinical and Experimental Immunology.* September 2008:153. doi: 10.1111/j.1365-2249.2008.03713.x

7. Gershwin, M. E., Nestel, P., and Keen, C. L., eds. *Handbook of Nutrition and Immunity.* Berlin: Springer Science & Business Media; 2004.

8. http://www.mayoclinic.org/diseases-conditions/crohns-disease/basics/definition/con-20032061

9. http://www.ccfa.org/what-are-crohns-and-colitis/what-is-crohns-disease/

10. Chandler, M. "Probiotics – not all created equally." *Journal of Small Animal Practice.* 2014;55(9):439–441. doi: 10.1111/jsap.12263

11. S. Falk-Petersen et al., "Lipids and fatty acids in ice algae and phytoplankton from the Marginal Ice Zone in the Barents Sea." *Polar Biology.* 1998;20(1):41–47. "Product Review: Omega-3 Fatty Acids (EPA and DHA) from Fish/Marine Oils." ConsumerLab.com. March 15, 2003. Accessed Aug. 14, 2007.

12. "Conversion Efficiency of ALA to DHA in Humans." DHA-EPA Omega-3 Institute. 2013. http://www.dhaomega3.org/Overview/Conversion-Efficiency-of-ALA-to-DHA-in-Humans Retrieved Accessed 21 Oct. 21,ober 2007.

13. Hand, M. S. et al., eds. *Small Animal Clinical Nutrition,* 5th ed. Topeka, KS: Mark Morris Institute; 2002:96–97.

14. Bauer, J. E. "Therapeutic use of fish oils in companion animals." *Journal of the American Veterinary Medical Association.* December 2011;239(11):1441–1451.

15. Pan, Y. et al. "Dietary supplementation with medium-chain TAG has long-lasting cognition-enhancing effects in aged dogs." *British Journal of Nutrition.* June 2010;103(12):1746–54. doi: 10.1017/S0007114510000097. Epub Feb. 9, 2010.

16. Henderson, S.T. et al. "Study of the ketogenic agent AC-1202 in mild to moderate Alzheimer's disease: a randomized, double-blind, placebo-controlled, multicenter trial." *Nutrition & Metabolism.* Aug. 10, 2009;6:31. doi: 10.1186/1743-7075-6-31.

17. Takeuchi, H. et al. "The application of medium-chain fatty acids: edible oil with a suppressing effect on body fat accumulation." *Asia Pacific Journal of Clinical Nutrition.* 2008;17(Suppl 1):320–3.

18. Azzam, R. and Azar, N. J. "Marked Seizure Reduction after MCT Supplementation." *Case Reports in Neurological Medicine.* 2013. doi: 10.1155/2013/809151. Epub Dec. 8, 2013.

19. Kono, H. et al. "Medium-chain triglycerides enhance secretory IgA expression in rat intestine after administration of endotoxin." *American Journal of Physiology. Gastrointestinal Liver Physiology.* June 2004;286(6):G1081–9.

20. Omura, Y. et al. "Caprylic acid in the effective treatment of intractable medical problems of frequent urination, incontinence, chronic upper respiratory infection, root canalled tooth infection, ALS, etc., caused by asbestos & mixed infections of Candida albicans, Helicobacter pylori & cytomegalovirus with or without other microorganisms & mercury." *Acupuncture & Electro-Therapeutics Research.* 2011;36(1–2):19–64.

21. Nebeling, L. C. and Lerner, E. "Implementing a ketogenic diet based on medium-chain triglyceride oil in pediatric patients with cancer." *Journal of the American Dietetic Association.* 1995;95(6):693–7.

Chapter 7

1. Cameron, T. "Glandular Therapy." *IVC Journal.* Summer 2012;2(3):12–14.

2. Murphy, K. Chapter 15. *Janeway's Immunobiology,* 8th ed. New York, NY: Garland Science; 2012:611–668. ISBN 0815342438.

3.   Choi, J., Kim, S. T,, and Craft, J. "The pathogenesis of systemic lupus erythematosus-an update." *Current Opinion in Immunology*. December 2012;24(6):651–657. doi: 10.1016/j.coi.2012.10.004

4.   Soyer, O. U. et al. "Mechanisms of peripheral tolerance to allergens." *Allergy* 2012;68(2):161–170. doi: 10.1111/all.12085.

5.   Round, J. L., O'Connell, R. M., and Mazmanian, S. K. "Coordination of tolerogenic immune responses by the commensal microbiota." *Journal of Autoimmunity*. May 2010;34(3): J220–J225. doi: 10.1016/j.jaut.2009.11.007

6.   Weiner, H. L. "Oral tolerance, an active immunologic process mediated by multiple mechanisms." *Journal of Clinical Investigation*. Oct, 15, 2000;106(8):935–937.

7.   Faria, A. M. and Weiner, H. L. "Oral Tolerance." *Immunological Reviews*. July 2005;206:232–259. http://doi.org/10.1111/j.0105-2896.2005.00280.x

8.   Ishikawa, Y. et al. "Inhibitory effect of honeybee-collected pollen on mast cell degranulation in vivo and in vitro." *Journal of Medicinal Food*. March 2008;11(1):14–20. doi: 10.1089/jmf.2006.163.

9.   Sonestedt, E. et al. "Fat and carbohydrate intake modify the association between genetic variation in the FTO genotype and obesity." *American Journal of Clinical Nutrition*. November 2009;90(5)1418–25.

10. Yoshida, K. et al. "Broccoli sprout extract induces detoxification-related gene expression and attenuates acute liver injury." *World Journal of Gastroenterology*. Sept. 21, 2015;21(35):10091–103. doi: 10.3748/wjg.v21.i35.10091.

11. Schmutz, J. et al. "Quality assessment of the human genome sequence." *Nature*. 2004;429(6990):365–368. doi: 10.1038/nature02390

12. https://www.genome.gov/11006943/human-genome-project-completion-frequently-asked-questions/

13. Mardis, E. R. "Anticipating the 1,000 dollar genome." *Genome Biology*. 2006;7(7):112. doi: 10.1186/gb-2006-7-7-112. PMC 1779559. PMID 17224040.

14. Davies, K. *The $1,000 Genome: The Revolution in DNA Sequencing and the New Era of Personalized Medicine*. New York: Free Press; 2010. ISBN 1-4165-6959-6

Chapter 8

1.   http://umm.edu/health/medical/altmed/treatment/herbal-medicine

2.   Elvin-Lewis, M. "Should we be concerned about herbal remedies." *Journal of Ethnopharmacology*. May 2001;75(2–3):141–164. doi: 10.1016/S0378-8741(00)00394-9. PMID 11297844.

3.   Ernst, E. "Harmless herbs? A review of the recent literature." *American Journal of Medicine*. 1998;104(2):170–178. doi: 10.1016/S0002-9343(97)00397-5. PMID 9528737.

4.   Vanschoonbeek, K. et al. "Thrombosis: Variable Hypocoagulant Effect of Fish Oil Intake in Humans: Modulation of Fibrinogen Level and Thrombin Generation." Arteriosclerosis, Thrombosis, and Vascular Biology. 2004;24:1734-1740. doi: 10.1161/01.ATV.0000137119.28893.0b

5.   https://www.nlm.nih.gov/medlineplus/druginfo/natural/807.html

6.   Cupp, M. J. "Herbal remedies: Adverse effects and drug interactions." *American Family Physician*. March 1, 1999;59(5):1239–1244. PMID 10088878.

7.   Elvin-Lewis, M. "Should we be concerned about herbal remedies." *Journal of Ethnopharmacology*. May 2001;75(2–3):141–164. doi: 10.1016/S0378-8741(00)00394-9. PMID 11297844.

8.   Saper, R. B. et al. "Lead, Mercury, and Arsenic in US- and Indian-Manufactured Ayurvedic Medicines Sold via the Internet." *JAMA*. 2008;300(8):915–923. doi: 10.1001/jama.300.8.915.

Chapter 9

1.   Grotenhermen, F. "The Therapeutic Potential of Cannabis and Cannabinoids." *Deutsches Arzteblatt International*. July 2012;109(29–30):495–501. doi: 10.3238/arztebl.2012.0495. PMC 3442177. PMID 23008748.

2. Ben Amar, M. "Cannabinoids in medicine: a review of their therapeutic potential." *Journal of Ethnopharmacology.* 2006;105(1–2):1–25. doi:10.1016/j.jep.2006.02.001. PMID 16540272.

3. Russo, E. B. et al. "Phytochemical and genetic analyses of ancient cannabis from Central Asia." *Journal of Experimental Botany.* 2008;59(15):4171–82. doi: 10.1093/jxb/ern260. PMC 2639026. PMID 19036842.

4. Abel, E. L. Chapter 1: "Cannabis in the Ancient World. India: The First Marijuana-Oriented Culture." *Marihuana – The First Twelve Thousand Years.* Berlin: Springer Nature; 2008.

5. Keel, R. "Drug Law Timeline, Significant Events in the History of our Drug Laws." Schaffer Library of Drug Policy. Accessed April 24, 2007.

6. McWilliams, John C. *The Protectors: Harry J. Anslinger and the Federal Bureau of Narcotics, 1930–1962.* Newark, DE: University of Delaware Press; 1990:183. ISBN 978-0-87413-352-3.

7. Marshall, D. "Notice of denial of petition to reschedule marijuana." *Federal Register.* Drug Enforcement Administration. March 20, 2001;66(75):20038–20076. Accessed June 13, 2013.

8. Thompson, G. R. et al. "Comparison of acute oral toxicity of cannabinoids in rats, dogs and monkeys." *Toxicology and Applied Pharmacology.* July 1973;25(3):363–372.

9. Silver, R. J. *Medical Marijuana and Your Pet: The Definitive Guide.* Morrisville, NC: Lulu Publishing Services; 2015:47.

10. Rosenberg, E. C. et al. "Cannabinoids and Epilepsy." *Neurotherapeutics.* October 2015;12(4):747–68. doi: 10.1007/s13311-015-0375-5.

11. Salim, K. et al. "Pain measurements and side effect profile of the novel cannabinoid ajulemic acid." *Neuropharmacology.* June 2005;48(8):1164–71.

12. Russo, E. B. "Clinical endocannabinoid deficiency (CECD): can this concept explain therapeutic benefits of cannabis in migraine, fibromyalgia, irritable bowel syndrome and other treatment-resistant conditions?" *Neuro Endocrinology Letters.* April 2008;29(2):192–200.

13. Aparisi Rey, A. et al. "Biphasic Effects of Cannabinoids in Anxiety Responses: CB1 and $GABA_B$ Receptors in the Balance of GABAergic and Glutamatergic Neurotransmission." *Neuropsychopharmacology.* November 2012;37(12): 2624–2634. doi. 10.1038/npp.2012.123. PMCID: PMC3473327.

14. Silver, R. J. *Medical Marijuana and Your Pet: The Definitive Guide.* Morrisville, NC: Lulu Publishing Services; 2015:52–53.

Chapter 10

1. Maffei, M. E. "Magnetic field effects on plant growth, development, and evolution." *Frontiers in Plant Science.* 2014;5:445. doi: 10.3389/fpls.2014.00445. PMCID: PMC4154392.

2. Sieroń-Stotny, K. et al. "The Influence of Electromagnetic Radiation Generated by a Mobile Phone on the Skeletal System of Rats." *Biomed Research International.* 2015;(2015): 896019. doi: 10.1155/2015/896019. PMCID: PMC4331479.

3. Ross, C. L. et al. "The effect of low-frequency electromagnetic field on human bone marrow stem/progenitor cell differentiation." *Stem Cell Research.* July 2015;15(1):96–108. doi: 10.1016/j.scr.2015.04.009. PMCID: PMC4516580. NIHMSID: NIHMS695721.

4. Pfeiffer, K., Dougados, M. and Doherty, M. "Pulsed electromagnetic field therapy in the management of knee OA." *Annals of the Rheumatic Diseases.* July 2001; 60(7):717. doi: 10.1136/ard.60.7.717. PMCID: PMC1753735.

5. Fioravanti, A. et al. "Biochemical and morphological study of human articular chondrocytes cultivated in the presence of pulsed signal therapy." *Annals of the Rheumatic Diseases.* November 2002;61(11):1032–1033. doi: 10.1136/ard.61.11.1032. PMCID: PMC1753927.

6. Fioravanti, A. et al. "Biochemical and morphological study of human articular chondrocytes cultivated in the presence of pulsed signal therapy." *Annals of the Rheumatic Diseases.* November 2002;61(11):1032–1033. doi: 10.1136/ard.61.11.1032. PMCID: PMC1753927.

7. Rohde, C. et al. 2015. "Pulsed Electromagnetic Fields Reduce Postoperative Interleukin-1β, Pain, and Inflammation: A Double-Blind, Placebo-Controlled Study in TRAM Flap Breast Reconstruction Patients." *Plastic and Reconstructive Surgery.* May 2015;135(5):808e-817e.

8. Strauch, B. et al. "Pulsed Electromagnetic Fields Increase Angiogenesis in a Rat Myocardial Ischemia Model." Bioelectromagnetic Society Meetings. June 2009; Davos, Switzerland.

9. Braswell, C. and Crowe, D. T. "Hyperbaric oxygen therapy." *Compendium:* Continuing Education of Veterinarians. March 2012;34(3):E1–5; quiz E6.

10. Kumar, M. A. et al. "Hyperbaric Oxygen Therapy—A Novel Treatment Modality in Oral Submucous Fibrosis: A Review." *Journal of Clinical & Diagnostic Research.* May 2015;9(5): ZE01–ZE04. doi: 10.7860/JCDR/2015/11500.5905. PMCID: PMC4484182.

11. http://www.livescience.com/53470-11-lab-grown-body-parts.html

12. http://discovermagazine.com/2014/jan-feb/05-stem-cell-future

13. Sánchez, M. et al. "Combination of Intra-Articular and Intraosseous Injections of Platelet-rich Plasma for Severe Knee Osteoarthritis: A Pilot Study." *BioMed Research International.* 2016;2016:4868613. doi: 10.1155/2016/4868613. Epub July 4, 2016.

14. Zanon, G. et al. "Platelet-rich plasma in the treatment of acute hamstring injuries in professional football players." *Joints.* June 13, 2016;4(1):17–23. doi: 10.11138/jts/2016.4.1.017.

15. Piras, L. A. et al. "Prolongation of survival of dogs with oral malignant melanoma treated by en bloc surgical resection and adjuvant CSPG4-antigen electrovaccination." *Veterinary and Comparative Oncology.* May 4, 2016. doi: 10.1111/vco.12239.

16. Bergman, P. J. "Canine oral melanoma." *Clinical Techniques in Small Animal Practice.* May 2007;22(2):55–60. 1.

17. Bergman, P. J. and Wolchok, J. K. "Of mice and men (and dogs): development of a xenogeneic DNA vaccine for canine oral malignant melanoma." *Cancer Therapy.* 2008;6:817–826.

18. Bergman, P. J. et al. "Development of a xenogeneic DNA vaccine program for canine malignant melanoma at the Animal Medical Center." *Vaccine.* May 22, 2006;24(21):4582–5. Epub Aug. 24, 2005.

19. Bergman, P. J. et al. "Long-term survival of dogs with advanced malignant melanoma after DNA vaccination with xenogeneic human tyrosinase: a phase I trial." *Clinical Cancer Research.* April 2003;9(4):1284–90.

Chapter 11

1. Hand, M. S. et al., eds. *Small Animal Clinical Nutrition*, 5th ed. Topeka, KS: Mark Morris Institute; 2002:609–635.

2. Vighi, G. et al. "Allergy and the Gastrointestinal System." *Clinical & Experimental Immunology.* September 2008;153(S1):3–6, doi: 10.1111/j.1365-2249.2008.03713.x

3. Quigley, E. M. "Leaky gut - concept or clinical entity?" *Current Opinion in Gastroenterology.* March 2016;32(2):74–9. doi: 10.1097/MOG.0000000000000243.

4. Fasano, A. "Leaky gut and autoimmune diseases." *Clinical Reviews in Allergy & Immunology.* February 2012;42(1):71–8. doi: 10.1007/s12016-011-8291-x.

5. Plumb, D. C. *Plumb's Veterinary Drug Handbook (Desk)*, 8th ed. Hoboken, NJ: John Wiley & Sons; 2015:200–202.

6. Plumb, D. C. *Plumb's Veterinary Drug Handbook (Desk)*, 8th ed. Hoboken, NJ: John Wiley & Sons; 2015:213–214.

7. Plumb, D. C. *Plumb's Veterinary Drug Handbook (Desk)*, 8th ed. Hoboken, NJ: John Wiley & Sons; 2015:342–343.

8. Plumb, D. C. *Plumb's Veterinary Drug Handbook (Desk)*, 8th ed. Hoboken, NJ: John Wiley & Sons; 2015:534–536.

9.   Tilford, G. L. and Wulff-Tilford, M. *Herbs for Pets: The Natural Way to Enhance Your Pet's Life*. Irvine, CA: BowTie Press; 2009:52–54.

10.   Tilford, G. L. and Wulff-Tilford, M. *Herbs for Pets: The Natural Way to Enhance Your Pet's Life*. Irvine, CA: BowTie Press; 2009:70–72.

11.   Tilford, G. L. and Wulff-Tilford, M. *Herbs for Pets: The Natural Way to Enhance Your Pet's Life*. Irvine, CA: BowTie Press; 2009:194–196.

12.   Tilford, G. L. and Wulff-Tilford, M. *Herbs for Pets: The Natural Way to Enhance Your Pet's Life*. Irvine, CA: BowTie Press; 2009:152–157.

13.   Tilford, G. L. and Wulff-Tilford, M. *Herbs for Pets: The Natural Way to Enhance Your Pet's Life*. Irvine, CA: BowTie Press; 2009:152–155.

14.   Tilford, G. L. and Wulff-Tilford, M. *Herbs for Pets: The Natural Way to Enhance Your Pet's Life*. Irvine, CA: BowTie Press; 2009:94–97.

15.   Tilford, G. L. and Wulff-Tilford, M. *Herbs for Pets: The Natural Way to Enhance Your Pet's Life*. Irvine, CA: BowTie Press; 2009: 52–54.

16.   Tilford, G. L. and Wulff-Tilford, M. *Herbs for Pets: The Natural Way to Enhance Your Pet's Life*. Irvine, CA: BowTie Press; 2009:196–198.

17.   Tilford, G. L. and Wulff-Tilford, M. *Herbs for Pets: The Natural Way to Enhance Your Pet's Life*. Irvine, CA: BowTie Press; 2009:142–145.

Chapter 12

1.   Plumb, D. C. *Plumb's Veterinary Drug Handbook (Desk)*, 8th ed. Hoboken, NJ: John Wiley & Sons; 2015:868–869.

2.   Slatter, D. *Textbook of Small Animal Surgery*, 2nd ed. Philadelphia: W.B. Saunders; 1993:1938–1976.

3.   Slatter, D. *Textbook of Small Animal Surgery*, 2nd ed. Philadelphia: W.B. Saunders; 1993:1921–1927.

4.   Welch Fossum, T. et al. *Small Animal Surgery*, 3rd ed. St. Louis: Mosby Elsevier; 2007:1143–1315.

5.   Plumb, D. C. *Plumb's Veterinary Drug Handbook (Desk)*, 8th ed. Hoboken, NJ: John Wiley & Sons; 2015:1052–1055.

6.   Plumb, D. C. *Plumb's Veterinary Drug Handbook (Desk)*, 8th ed. Hoboken, NJ: John Wiley & Sons; 2015:38–39.

7.   Plumb, D. C. *Plumb's Veterinary Drug Handbook (Desk)*, 8th ed. Hoboken, NJ: John Wiley & Sons; 2015:127–131.

8.   Plumb, D. C. *Plumb's Veterinary Drug Handbook (Desk)*, 8th ed. Hoboken, NJ: John Wiley & Sons; 2015:515–516.

9.   Roman-Blas, J. A. et al. "Chondroitin sulfate plus glucosamine sulfate shows no superiority over placebo in a randomized, double-blind, placebo-controlled clinical trial in patients with knee osteoarthritis." *Arthritis & Rheumatology*. Epub ahead of print: July 31, 2016. doi: 10.1002/art.39819.

10.   Kanzaki, N. et al. "Glucosamine-containing supplement improves locomotor functions in subjects with knee pain - a pilot study of gait analysis." *Clinical Interventions in Aging*. June 20, 2016;11:835–41. doi: 10.2147/CIA. S103943.

11.   Shaughnessy, A. F. "Chondroitin/Glucosamine Equal to Celecoxib for Knee Osteoarthritis." *American Family Physician*. June 15, 2016;93(12):1032.

12.   Plumb, D. C. *Plumb's Veterinary Drug Handbook (Desk)*, 8th ed. Hoboken, NJ: John Wiley & Sons; 2015:495–497.

13. Hassan, M. Q. et al. "The glutathione defense system in the pathogenesis of rheumatoid arthritis." *Journal of Applied Toxicology*. Jan-Feb 2001;21(1):69–73.

14. Abdollahzad, H. et al. "Effects of Coenzyme Q10 Supplementation on Inflammatory Cytokines (TNF-α, IL-6) and Oxidative Stress in Rheumatoid Arthritis Patients: A Randomized Controlled Trial." *Archives of Medical Research*. October 2015;46(7):527–33. Epub Sept. 3, 2015. doi: 10.1016/j.arcmed.2015.08.006.

15. Lee, E. Y. et al. "Alpha-lipoic acid suppresses the development of collagen-induced arthritis and protects against bone destruction in mice." *Rheumatology International*. January 2007;27(3):225–33. Epub Aug. 31, 2006.

16. Riveiro-Naveira, R.R. et al. "Resveratrol lowers synovial hyperplasia, inflammatory markers and oxidative damage in an acute antigen-induced arthritis model." *Rheumatology* (Oxford). Epub ahead of print: June 28, 2016. pii: kew255.

17. Zhang, Z. et al. "Curcumin slows osteoarthritis progression and relieves osteoarthritis-associated pain symptoms in a post-traumatic osteoarthritis mouse model." *Arthritis Research & Therapy*. June 3, 2016;18(1):128. doi: 10.1186/s13075-016-1025-y.

18. Siddiqui, M. Z. "Boswellia Serrata, A Potential Anti-inflammatory Agent: An Overview." *Indian Journal of Pharmaceutical Sciences*. May-June 2011;73(3):255–261.

19. Bartels, E. M. et al. "Efficacy and safety of ginger in osteoarthritis patients: a meta-analysis of randomized placebo-controlled trials." *Osteoarthritis and Cartilage*. 2015;23(1):13–21. doi: 10.1016/j.joca.2014.09.024. Epub Oct. 7, 2014

20. Conrozier, T. et al. "A complex of three natural anti-inflammatory agents provides relief of osteoarthritis pain." *Alternative Therapies in Health and Medicine*. Winter 2014;20(Suppl 1):32–7.

21. Tilford, G. L. and Wulff-Tilford, M. *Herbs for Pets: The Natural Way to Enhance Your Pet's Life*. Irvine, CA: BowTie Press; 2009:198–201.

Chapter 13

1. Markwell, P. J. and Buffington, C. A. T. "Feline Lower Urinary Tract Disease." Wills, J. M. *Waltham Book of Clinical Nutrition of the Dog and Cat*. Oxford: Pergamon Press; 1994:293–311.

2. Buffington, C. A. T. et al. "Clinical Evaluation of Cats with Nonobstructive Urinary Tract Diseases." *Journal of the American Veterinary Medical Association*. 1997;210(1):46–50.

3. Hoppe, A. E. "Canine Lower Urinary Tract Disease." Wills, J. M. *Waltham Book of Clinical Nutrition of the Dog and Cat*. Oxford: Pergamon Press; 1994:335–352.

4. Brooks, W. C. "Struvite Stones-Canine." The Pet Health Library. Feb. 21, 2002. http://www.veterinarypartner.com/Content.plx?P=A&S=0&C=0&A=460

5. Buffington, C. A. T. "Nutritional Aspects of Struvite Urolithiasis in Dogs and Cats." Nephrology and Urology: 16th Annual Waltham Symposium. Columbus, OH: Kal Kan Foods, Inc.; 1992:51–57.

6. Brooks, W. C. "Oxalate Bladder Stones (Canine)." The Pet Health Library. Jan. 1, 2001. http://www.veterinarypartner.com/Content.plx?P=A&S=0&C=0&A=662

7. Brooks, W. C. "Struvite Stones-Feline." The Pet Health Library. Oct. 27, 2011. http://www.veterinarypartner.com/Content.plx?P=A&S=0&C=0&A=3306

8. Brooks, W. C. "Oxalate Bladder Stones (Feline)." The Pet Health Library. Oct. 11, 2004. http://www.veterinarypartner.com/Content.plx?P=A&S=0&C=0&A=1741

9. Brooks, W. C. "Oxalate Bladder Stones (Canine)." The Pet Health Library. Jan. 1, 2001. http://www.veterinarypartner.com/Content.plx?P=A&S=0&C=0&A=662

10. Lulich, J. P. et al. "Calcium Oxalate Urolithiasis." Buffington, C. A. T. and Sokolowski, J. H. eds. Nephrology and Urology: 16th Annual Waltham Symposium. Columbus, OH: Kal Kan Foods, Inc.; 1992:69–74.

11. Kirk, C. A. et al. "Evaluation of Factors Associated with Development of Calcium Oxalate Urolithiasis in Cats." *Journal of the American Veterinary Medical Association*. December 1995;207(11):1429–1434.

12. Brooks, W. C. "Struvite Stones-Feline." The Pet Health Library. Oct. 27, 2011. http://www.veterinarypartner.com/Content.plx?P=A&S=0&C=0&A=3306

13. Brooks, W. C. "Oxalate Bladder Stones (Feline)." The Pet Health Library. Oct. 11, 2004. http://www.veterinarypartner.com/Content.plx?P=A&S=0&C=0&A=1741

14. Brooks, W. C. "Oxalate Bladder Stones (Canine)." The Pet Health Library. Jan. 1, 2001. http://www.veterinarypartner.com/Content.plx?P=A&S=0&C=0&A=662

15. Lulich, J. P. et al. "Calcium Oxalate Urolithiasis." Buffington, C. A. T. and Sokolowski, J. H. eds. Nephrology and Urology: 16th Annual Waltham Symposium. Columbus, OH: Kal Kan Foods, Inc.; 1992:69–74.

16. Kirk, C. A. et al. "Evaluation of Factors Associated with Development of Calcium Oxalate Urolithiasis in Cats." *Journal of the American Veterinary Medical Association.* December 1995;207(11):1429–1434.

17. Tilford, G. L. and Wulff-Tilford, M. *Herbs for Pets: The Natural Way to Enhance Your Pet's Life.* Irvine, CA: BowTie Press; 2009:188–190.

18. Tilford, G. L. and Wulff-Tilford, M. *Herbs for Pets: The Natural Way to Enhance Your Pet's Life.* Irvine, CA: BowTie Press; 2009:145–148.

19. Tilford, G. L. and Wulff-Tilford, M. *Herbs for Pets: The Natural Way to Enhance Your Pet's Life.* Irvine, CA: BowTie Press; 2009:194–196.

20. Tilford, G. L. and Wulff-Tilford, M. *Herbs for Pets: The Natural Way to Enhance Your Pet's Life.* Irvine, CA: BowTie Press; 2009:164–166.

21. Tilford, G. L. and Wulff-Tilford, M. *Herbs for Pets: The Natural Way to Enhance Your Pet's Life.* Irvine, CA: BowTie Press; 2009:184–186.

22. Tilford, G. L. and Wulff-Tilford, M. *Herbs for Pets: The Natural Way to Enhance Your Pet's Life.* Irvine, CA: BowTie Press; 2009:91–94.

23. Tilford, G. L. and Wulff-Tilford, M. *Herbs for Pets: The Natural Way to Enhance Your Pet's Life.* Irvine, CA: BowTie Press; 2009:99–104.

24. Tilford, G. L. and Wulff-Tilford, M. *Herbs for Pets: The Natural Way to Enhance Your Pet's Life.* Irvine, CA: BowTie Press; 2009:157–160.

25. Wojnicz, D. et al. "Study of the impact of cranberry extract on the virulence factors and biofilm formation by Enterococcus faecalis strains isolated from urinary tract infections." *International Journal of Food Sciences and Nutrition.* Epub ahead of print: July 26, 2016:1–12.

26. Singh, I., Gautam, L. K., and Kaur, I. R. "Effect of oral cranberry extract (standardized proanthocyanidin-A) in patients with recurrent UTI by pathogenic E. coli: a randomized placebo-controlled clinical research study." *International Urology and Nephrology.* September 2016;48(9):1379–86. doi: 10.1007/s11255-016-1342-8. Epub June 17, 2016.

27. Tilford, G. L. and Wulff-Tilford, M. *Herbs for Pets: The Natural Way to Enhance Your Pet's Life.* Irvine, CA: BowTie Press; 2009:182–184.

28. Tilford, G. L. and Wulff-Tilford, M. *Herbs for Pets: The Natural Way to Enhance Your Pet's Life.* Irvine, CA: BowTie Press; 2009:190–192.

29. Jawna-Zboińska, K. et al. "Passiflora incarnata L. Improves Spatial Memory, Reduces Stress, and Affects Neurotransmission in Rats." *Phytotherapy Research.* May 2016;30(5):781–9. doi: 10.1002/ptr.5578. Epub Jan. 27, 2016

Chapter 14

1. Vighi, G. et al. "Allergy and the Gastrointestinal System." *Clinical & Experimental Immunology.* September 2008;153(S1):3–6, doi: 10.1111/j.1365-2249.2008.03713.x

2. Guarner, F. and Malagelada, J. "Gut flora in health and disease." *The Lancet.* Feb. 8, 2003; 361(9356):512–519. doi: 10.1016/S0140-6736(03)12489-0.

3. Nelson, R. W. and Couto, C. G. *Essentials of Small Animal Internal Medicine.*
    St. Louis: Mosby-Year Book; 1992:255–366.

4. Quigley, E. M. "Leaky gut - concept or clinical entity?" *Current Opinion in Gastroenterology.* March
    2016;32(2):74–9. doi: 10.1097/MOG.0000000000000243.

5. Fasano, A. "Leaky gut and autoimmune diseases." *Clinical Reviews in Allergy & Immunology.* February
    2012;42(1):71–8. doi: 10.1007/s12016-011-8291-x.

6. Hand, M. S. et al., eds. *Small Animal Clinical Nutrition,* 5th ed. Topeka, KS:
    Mark Morris Institute; 2002:619–625.

7. Hand, M. S. et al., eds. *Small Animal Clinical Nutrition,* 5th ed. Topeka, KS:
    Mark Morris Institute; 2002:619–621.

8. Plumb, D. C. *Plumb's Veterinary Drug Handbook (Desk),* 8th ed. Hoboken, NJ:
    John Wiley & Sons; 2015:715–718.

9. Menchetti, L. et al. "Potential benefits of colostrum in gastrointestinal diseases." *Frontiers in Bioscience* (Schol
    edition). June 1, 2016;8:331–51.

10. Kanwar, J. R. et al. "Comparative activities of milk components in reversing chronic colitis." *Journal of Dairy
    Science.* April 2016;99(4):2488–501. doi: 10.3168/jds.2015-10122. Epub Jan. 21, 2016.

11. Playford, R. et al. "Bovine colostrum is a health food supplement which prevents NSAID induced gut damage."
    Gut. May 1999;44(5):653–658. PMCID: PMC1727496

12. Williams, L. B., Haydel, S. E., and Ferrell, R. E. "Bentonite, Bandaids, and Borborygmi." *Elements-
    GeoScienceWorld.* April 2009;5(2)99–104. doi: 10.2113/gselements.5.2.99

13. Williams, L. B. and Haydel, S. E. "Evaluation of the medicinal use of clay minerals as antibacterial agents."
    International Geology Review. July 2010;52(7/8):745–770. doi: 10.1080/00206811003679737.

14. Otto, C. C. and Haydel, S. E. "Exchangeable Ions Are Responsible for the *In Vitro* Antibacterial Properties of
    Natural Clay Mixtures." *PLoS One.* May 17, 2013. doi: 10.1371/journal.pone.0064068.

15. Tilford, G. L. and Wulff-Tilford, M. *Herbs for Pets: The Natural Way to Enhance Your Pet's Life.* Irvine, CA:
    BowTie Press; 2009:52–54.

16. Valussi, M. "Functional foods with digestion-enhancing properties." International Journal of Food Sciences and
    Nutrition. March 2012;63(Suppl 1):82–9. doi: 10.3109/09637486.2011.627841. Epub Oct. 19, 2011.

17. Langner, E., Greifenberg, S., and Gruenwald, J. "Ginger: history and use." Advances in Therapy. Jan.-Feb.
    1998;15(1):25–44.

18. Fujita, T. and Sakurai, K. "Efficacy of glutamine-enriched enteral nutrition in an experimental model of mucosal
    ulcerative colitis." *British Journal of Surgery.* June 1995;82(6):749–51.

19. Tilford, G. L. and Wulff-Tilford, M. *Herbs for Pets: The Natural Way to Enhance Your Pet's Life.* Irvine, CA:
    BowTie Press; 2009:142–145.

20. Tilford, G. L. and Wulff-Tilford, M. *Herbs for Pets: The Natural Way to Enhance Your Pet's Life.* Irvine, CA:
    BowTie Press; 2009:145–148.

21. Zhu, A. Z. X. et al. "N-Acetylglucosamine for Treatment of Inflammatory Bowel Disease: A real-world pragmatic
    clinical trial." *Natural Medicine Journal.* April 2015;7(4).

22. Tilford, G. L. and Wulff-Tilford, M. *Herbs for Pets: The Natural Way to Enhance Your Pet's Life.* Irvine, CA:
    BowTie Press; 2009:157–160.

23. Tilford, G. L. and Wulff-Tilford, M. *Herbs for Pets: The Natural Way to Enhance Your Pet's Life.* Irvine, CA:
    BowTie Press; 2009:164–166.

24. Tilford, G. L. and Wulff-Tilford, M. *Herbs for Pets: The Natural Way to Enhance Your Pet's Life.* Irvine, CA:
    BowTie Press; 2009:184–186.

25. Rubin, D. T. "Fecal Microbiota Transplantation for the Treatment of Inflammatory Bowel Disease."
    Gastroenterology & Hepatology. September 2015;11(9):618–620. PMCID: PMC4965622.

Chapter 15

1. Hand, M. S. et al., eds. *Small Animal Clinical Nutrition,* 5th ed. Topeka, KS: Mark Morris Institute; 2002:1135–1154.

2. Ettinger, S. E. and Feldman, E. C. *Textbook of Veterinary Internal Medicine,* 6th ed. St. Louis: Elsevier Saunders; 2005:1482–1497.

3. Nelson, R. W. and Couto, C. G. *Essentials of Small Animal Internal Medicine.* St. Louis: Mosby-Year Book; 1992:432–445.

4. Hand, M. S. et al., eds. *Small Animal Clinical Nutrition,* 5th ed. Topeka, KS: Mark Morris Institute; 2002:1135–1154.

5. Ettinger, S. E. and Feldman, E. C. *Textbook of Veterinary Internal Medicine,* 6th ed. St. Louis: Elsevier Saunders; 2005:1482–1497.

6. Nelson, R. W. and Couto, C. G. *Essentials of Small Animal Internal Medicine.* St. Louis: Mosby-Year Book; 1992:432–445.

7. Nelson, R. W. and Couto, C. G. *Essentials of Small Animal Internal Medicine.* St. Louis: Mosby-Year Book; 1992:432–445.

8. Ettinger, S. E. and Feldman, E. C. *Textbook of Veterinary Internal Medicine,* 6th ed. St. Louis: Elsevier Saunders; 2005:1482–1497.

9. Hand, M. S. et al., eds. *Small Animal Clinical Nutrition,* 5th ed. Topeka, KS: Mark Morris Institute; 2002:1135–1154.

10. Braswell, C. and Crowe, D. T. "Hyperbaric oxygen therapy." *Compendium:* Continuing Education of Veterinarians. March 2012;34(3):E1–5; quiz E6.

11. Williams, L. B., Haydel, S. E., and Ferrell, R. E. "Bentonite, Bandaids, and Borborygmi." *Elements-GeoScienceWorld.* April 2009;5(2)99–104. doi: 10.2113/gselements.5.2.99

12. Williams, L. B. and Haydel, S. E. "Evaluation of the medicinal use of clay minerals as antibacterial agents." *International Geology Review.* July 2010;52(7/8):745–770. doi: 10.1080/00206811003679737.

13. Otto, C. C. and Haydel, S. E. "Exchangeable Ions Are Responsible for the *In Vitro* Antibacterial Properties of Natural Clay Mixtures." *PLoS One.* May 17, 2013. doi: 10.1371/journal.pone.0064068.

14. Menchetti, L. et al. "Potential benefits of colostrum in gastrointestinal diseases." *Frontiers in Bioscience* (Schol edition). June 1, 2016;8:331–51.

15. Kanwar, J. R. et al. "Comparative activities of milk components in reversing chronic colitis." *Journal of Dairy Science.* April 2016;99(4):2488–501. doi: 10.3168/jds.2015-10122. Epub Jan. 21, 2016.

16. Playford, R. et al. "Bovine colostrum is a health food supplement which prevents NSAID induced gut damage." *Gut.* May 1999;44(5):653–658. PMCID: PMC1727496

Chapter 16

1. Ettinger, S. E. and Feldman, E. C. *Textbook of Veterinary Internal Medicine,* 6th ed. St. Louis: Elsevier Saunders; 2005:1482–1497.

2. Nelson, R. W. and Couto, C. G. *Essentials of Small Animal Internal Medicine.* St. Louis: Mosby-Year Book; 1992:432–445.

3. Hand, M. S. et al., eds. *Small Animal Clinical Nutrition,* 5th ed. Topeka, KS: Mark Morris Institute; 2002:1135–1154.

4. Kahn, S. E., Hull, R. L., and Utzschneider, K. M. "Mechanisms linking obesity to insulin resistance and type 2 diabetes." *Nature.* Dec. 14, 2006:840–846.

5. Ettinger, S. E. and Feldman, E. C. *Textbook of Veterinary Internal Medicine,* 6th ed. St. Louis: Elsevier Saunders; 2005:1563–1591.

6. Nelson, R. W. and Couto, C. G. *Essentials of Small Animal Internal Medicine.* St. Louis: Mosby-Year Book; 1992:561–586.

7. Plumb, D. C. *Plumb's Veterinary Drug Handbook (Desk),* 8th ed. Hoboken, NJ: John Wiley & Sons; 2015:552–558.

8. Plumb, D. C. *Plumb's Veterinary Drug Handbook (Desk),* 8th ed. Hoboken, NJ: John Wiley & Sons; 2015:552–558.

9. Plumb, D. C. *Plumb's Veterinary Drug Handbook (Desk),* 8th ed. Hoboken, NJ: John Wiley & Sons; 2015:490–491.

10. Hand, M. S. et al., eds. *Small Animal Clinical Nutrition,* 5th ed. Topeka, KS: Mark Morris Institute; 2002:559–586.

11. Hand, M. S. et al., eds. *Small Animal Clinical Nutrition,* 5th ed. Topeka, KS: Mark Morris Institute; 2002:559–586.

Chapter 17

1. "Target Heart Rates – AHA." American Heart Association. April 4, 2014. Accessed May 21, 2014. http://www.heart.org/HEARTORG/HealthyLiving/PhysicalActivity/Target-Heart-Rates_UCM_434341_Article.jsp#.WKQUITsrJPY

2. Ettinger, S. E. and Feldman, E. C. *Textbook of Veterinary Internal Medicine,* 6th ed. St. Louis: Elsevier Saunders; 2005:914–1167.

3. Nelson, R. W. and Couto, C. G. *Essentials of Small Animal Internal Medicine.* St. Louis: Mosby-Year Book; 1992:3–152.

4. Nelson, R. W. and Couto, C. G. *Essentials of Small Animal Internal Medicine.* St. Louis: Mosby-Year Book; 1992:3–152.

5. Ettinger, S. E. and Feldman, E. C. *Textbook of Veterinary Internal Medicine,* 6th ed. St. Louis: Elsevier Saunders; 2005:914–1167.

6. MacDonald, K. A. et al. "The effect of ramipril on left ventricular mass, myocardial fibrosis, diastolic function, and plasma neurohormones in Maine Coon cats with familial hypertrophic cardiomyopathy without heart failure." *Journal of Veterinary Internal Medicine.* 2006;20(5):1093–1105.

7. MacDonald, K. A. et al. "Effect of spironolactone on diastolic function and left ventricular mass in Maine Coon cats with familial hypertrophic cardiomyopathy." *Journal of Veterinary Internal Medicine.* 2008;22(2):335–41.

8. Plumb, D. C. *Plumb's Veterinary Drug Handbook (Desk),* 8th ed. Hoboken, NJ: John Wiley & Sons; 2015:86–88.

9. Killingsworth, C. R. et al. "Streptokinase treatment of cats with experimentally induced aortic thrombosis." *American Journal of Veterinary Research.* 1986;47(6):1351–59.

10. Hogan, D. F. et al. "Secondary prevention of cardiogenic arterial thromboembolism in the cat: The double-blind, randomized, positive-controlled feline arterial thromboembolism; clopidogrel vs. aspirin trial (FAT CAT)." *Journal of Veterinary Cardiology.* December 2015;17(Suppl 1):S306–17. doi: 10.1016/j.jvc.2015.10.004.

11. Plumb, D. C. *Plumb's Veterinary Drug Handbook (Desk),* 8th ed. Hoboken, NJ: John Wiley & Sons; 2015:249–251.

12. O'Grady, M. R. et al. "Efficacy of benazepril hydrochloride to delay the progression of occult dilated cardiomyopathy in Doberman Pinschers." *Journal of Veterinary Internal Medicine.* Sept.-Oct. 2009;23(5):977–83. doi: 10.1111/j.1939-1676.2009.0346.x. Epub July 1, 2009.

13. Plumb, D. C. *Plumb's Veterinary Drug Handbook (Desk),* 8th ed. Hoboken, NJ: John Wiley & Sons; 2015:374–377.

14. Plumb, D. C. *Plumb's Veterinary Drug Handbook (Desk),* 8th ed. Hoboken, NJ: John Wiley & Sons; 2015:107–109.

15. O'Sullivan, M. L. and O'Grady, M. R. "Treatment of Dilated Cardiomyopathy." ACVIM Forum 2012. University of Guelph. Ontario, Canada.

16. Plumb, D. C. *Plumb's Veterinary Drug Handbook (Desk)*, 8th ed. Hoboken, NJ: John Wiley & Sons; 2015:969–970.

17. Summerfield, N. J. et al. "Efficacy of pimobendan in the prevention of congestive heart failure or sudden death in Doberman Pinschers with preclinical dilated cardiomyopathy (The PROTECT Study)." *Journal of Veterinary Internal Medicine*. Nov.-Dec. 2012;26(6):1337–49. doi: 10.1111/j.1939-1676.2012.01026.x. Epub Oct. 18, 2012.

18. Plumb, D. C. *Plumb's Veterinary Drug Handbook (Desk)*, 8th ed. Hoboken, NJ: John Wiley & Sons; 2015:858–861.

19. Plumb, D. C. *Plumb's Veterinary Drug Handbook (Desk)*, 8th ed. Hoboken, NJ: John Wiley & Sons; 2015:475–478.

20. Plumb, D. C. *Plumb's Veterinary Drug Handbook (Desk)*, 8th ed. Hoboken, NJ: John Wiley & Sons; 2015:974–976.

21. Plumb, D. C. *Plumb's Veterinary Drug Handbook (Desk)*, 8th ed. Hoboken, NJ: John Wiley & Sons; 2015:374–377.

22. Plumb, D. C. *Plumb's Veterinary Drug Handbook (Desk)*, 8th ed. Hoboken, NJ: John Wiley & Sons; 2015:325–328.

23. Plumb, D. C. *Plumb's Veterinary Drug Handbook (Desk)*, 8th ed. Hoboken, NJ: John Wiley & Sons; 2015:858–861.

24. Plumb, D. C. *Plumb's Veterinary Drug Handbook (Desk)*, 8th ed. Hoboken, NJ: John Wiley & Sons; 2015:52–52.

25. Hand, M. S. et al., eds. *Small Animal Clinical Nutrition*, 5th ed. Topeka, KS: Mark Morris Institute; 2002:733–764.

26. Kittelson, M. D. et al. "Results of the multicenter spaniel trial (MUST): taurine- and carnitine-responsive dilated cardiomyopathy in American cocker spaniels with decreased plasma taurine concentration." *Journal of Veterinary Internal Medicine*. July-Aug. 1997;11(4):204–211.

27. Pion, P. D., Sanderson, S. L., and Kittelson, M. D. "The effectiveness of taurine and levocarnitine in dogs with heart disease." *Veterinary Clinics of North America. Small Animal Practice*. November 1998;28(6):1495–1514.

28. Kris-Etherton, P. M., Harris, W. S., and Appel, L. J., American Heart Association Nutrition Committee. "Fish consumption, fish oil, omega-3 fatty acids, and cardiovascular disease." *Arteriosclerosis, Thrombosis, and Vascular Biology*. 2003;23(2):e20–30.

29. Mayor, S. "Fish oil omega 3 fatty acids improve heart muscle recovery after MI, trial shows." *BMJ*. Aug. 1, 2016;354:i4240. doi: 10.1136/bmj.i4240.

30. Firuzi, O. et al. "Effects of omega-3 polyunsaturated Fatty acids on heart function and oxidative stress biomarkers in pediatric patients with dilated cardiomyopathy." *International Cardiovascular Research Journal*. March 2013;7(1):8–14. Epub March 15, 2013.

31. Zhukovska, A. et al. "Heart-protective effect of n-3 PUFA demonstrated in a rat model of diabetic cardiomyopathy." *Molecular and Cellular Biochemistry*. April 2014;389(1-2):219–27. doi: 10.1007/s11010-013-1943-9. Epub Dec. 31, 2013.

32. Gompf, R. E. "Nutritional and herbal therapies in the treatment of heart disease in cats and dogs." *Journal of the American Animal Hospital Association*. Nov.-Dec., 2005;41(6):355–67.

33. Dove, R. S. "Nutritional therapy in the treatment of heart disease in dogs." *Alternative Medicine Review*. September 2001;6(Suppl):S38–45.

34. Dove, R. S. "Nutritional therapy in the treatment of heart disease in dogs." *Alternative Medicine Review*. September 2001;6(Suppl):S38–45.

35. Tilford, G. L. and Wulff-Tilford, M. *Herbs for Pets: The Natural Way to Enhance Your Pet's Life*. Irvine, CA: BowTie Press; 2009:94–97.

36. Tilford, G. L. and Wulff-Tilford, M. *Herbs for Pets: The Natural Way to Enhance Your Pet's Life.* Irvine, CA: BowTie Press; 2009:118–120.

37. Tilford, G. L. and Wulff-Tilford, M. *Herbs for Pets: The Natural Way to Enhance Your Pet's Life.* Irvine, CA: BowTie Press; 2009:194–196.

Chapter 18

1. "Anatomy and Physiology of the Liver." Canadian Cancer Society. http://www.cancer.ca/en/cancer-information/cancer-type/liver/anatomy-and-physiology/?region=on

2. Gow, A. G. "Pathophysiology of Hepatic Encephalopathy in Companion Animals: New Information." ACVIM Forum 2012.

3. Berent, A. C. and Weisse, C. "Hepatic Vascular Anomalies." Ettinger, S. E. and Feldman, E. C. *Textbook of Veterinary Internal Medicine,* 7th ed. St. Louis: Elsevier Saunders; 2010:1649–1672.

4. Plumb, D. C. *Plumb's Veterinary Drug Handbook (Desk),* 8th ed. Hoboken, NJ: John Wiley & Sons; 2015:883–886.

5. Plumb, D. C. *Plumb's Veterinary Drug Handbook (Desk),* 8th ed. Hoboken, NJ: John Wiley & Sons; 2015:99–101.

6. Plumb, D. C. *Plumb's Veterinary Drug Handbook (Desk),* 8th ed. Hoboken, NJ: John Wiley & Sons; 2015:269–273.

7. Plumb, D. C. *Plumb's Veterinary Drug Handbook (Desk),* 8th ed. Hoboken, NJ: John Wiley & Sons; 2015:258–259.

8. Plumb, D. C. *Plumb's Veterinary Drug Handbook (Desk),* 8th ed. Hoboken, NJ: John Wiley & Sons; 2015:1073–1074.

9. Plumb, D. C. *Plumb's Veterinary Drug Handbook (Desk),* 8th ed. Hoboken, NJ: John Wiley & Sons; 2015:822–823.

10. Plumb, D. C. *Plumb's Veterinary Drug Handbook (Desk),* 8th ed. Hoboken, NJ: John Wiley & Sons; 2015:715–718.

11. Plumb, D. C. *Plumb's Veterinary Drug Handbook (Desk),* 8th ed. Hoboken, NJ: John Wiley & Sons; 2015:608–609.

12. Plumb, D. C. *Plumb's Veterinary Drug Handbook (Desk),* 8th ed. Hoboken, NJ: John Wiley & Sons; 2015:1073–1074.

13. Rutgers, H., Carolien, C., and Harte, J. G. "Hepatic Disease." Wills, J. M. *Waltham Book of Clinical Nutrition of the Dog and Cat.* Oxford: Pergamon Press; 1994:239–276.

14. Price, W. D., Lovell, R. A., and McChesney, D. G. "Naturally occurring toxins in feedstuffs: Center for Veterinary Medicine Perspective." *Journal of Animal Science.* September 1993:2556–2562.

15. Scudamore, K. A. et al. "Determination of mycotoxins in pet foods sold for domestic pets and wild birds using linked-column immunoassay clean-up and HPLC." *Food Additives and Contaminants.* 1997:175–86.

16. Leung, M. C., Díaz-Llano, G., and Smith, T. K. "Mycotoxins in pet food: a review on worldwide prevalence and preventive strategies." *Journal of Agricultural and Food Chemistry.* December 2006;54(26):9623–35. doi: 10.1021/jf062363+

17. Boermans, H. J. and Leung, M. C. "Mycotoxins and the pet food industry: toxicological evidence and risk assessment." *International Journal of Food Microbiology.* October 2007;119(1-2):95–102, doi: 10.1016/j.ijfoodmicro.2007.07.063

18. Böhm, J. et al. "Survey and risk assessment of the mycotoxins deoxynivalenol, zearalenone, fumonisins, ochratoxin A, and aflatoxins in commercial dry dog food." *Mycotoxin Research.* August 2010;26(3):147–153. doi: 10.1007/s12550-010-0049-4

19. Marks, S. L., Rogers, Q. R., and Strombeck, D. R. "Nutritional Support in Hepatic Disease. Part I. Metabolic Alterations and Nutritional Considerations in Dogs and Cats." *Compendium: Continuing Education Practicing Veterinarians*. 1994:971–979.

20. Marks, S. L., Rogers, Q. R., and Strombeck, D. R. "Nutritional Support in Hepatic Disease. Part II. Dietary Management of Common Liver Disorders in Dogs and Cats." *Compendium: Continuing Education Practicing Veterinarians*. 1994:1287–1296.

21. Tilford, G. L. and Wulff-Tilford, M. *Herbs for Pets: The Natural Way to Enhance Your Pet's Life*. Irvine, CA: BowTie Press; 2009:148–150.

22. Bosisio, E., Benelli, C., and Pirola, O. "Effect of the flavanolignans of Silybum marianum L. on lipid peroxidation in rat liver microsomes and freshly isolated hepatocytes." *Pharmacological Research*. Feb-Mar 1992;25(2):147–54.

23. Deulofeu, R. et al. "S-adenosylmethionine prevents hepatic tocopherol depletion in carbon tetrachloride-injured rats." *Clinical Science* (London). October 2000;99(4):315–20.

24. Garg, M. C. and Bansal, D. D. "Protective antioxidant effect of vitamins C and E in streptozotocin induced diabetic rats." *Indian Journal of Experimental Biology*. February 2000;38(2):101–4.

25. Genova, M. L. et al. "Protective effect of exogenous coenzyme Q in rats subjected to partial hepatic ischemia and reperfusion." *Biofactors*. 1999;9(2-4):345–9.

26. Biewenga, G. P., Haenen, G. R., and Bast, A. "The pharmacology of the antioxidant lipoic acid." *General Pharmacology*. September 1997;29(3):315–31.

27. Rivera-Espinoza, Y. and Muriel, P. "Pharmacological actions of curcumin in liver diseases or damage." *Liver International*. November 2009;29(10):1457-66. doi: 10.1111/j.1478-3231.2009.02086.x.

28. Silveira, M. R. et al. "Effects of hyperbaric oxygen therapy on the liver after injury caused by the hepatic ischemia-reperfusion process." Acta Cirurgica Brasileira. 2014;29(Suppl 1):29–33.

29. Taslipinar, M. Y. et al. "Hyperbaric oxygen treatment and N-acetylcysteine ameliorate acetaminophen-induced liver injury in a rat model." *Human & Experimental Toxicology*. October 2013;32(10):1107–16. doi: 10.1177/0960327113499167. Epub Aug. 7, 2013.

Chapter 19

1. Nelson, R. W. and Couto, C. G. *Essentials of Small Animal Internal Medicine*. St. Louis: Mosby-Year Book; 1992:481–494.

2. Hand, M. S. et al., eds. *Small Animal Clinical Nutrition*, 5th ed. Topeka, KS: Mark Morris Institute; 2002:765–812.

3. Grauer, G. F. and Lane, I. F. "Acute Renal Failure: Strategies for its Prevention." *Nephrology and Urology*. 1994.

4. Plumb, D. C. *Plumb's Veterinary Drug Handbook (Desk)*, 8th ed. Hoboken, NJ: John Wiley & Sons; 2015:374–377.

5. Plumb, D. C. *Plumb's Veterinary Drug Handbook (Desk)*, 8th ed. Hoboken, NJ: John Wiley & Sons; 2015:107–109.

6. Plumb, D. C. *Plumb's Veterinary Drug Handbook (Desk)*, 8th ed. Hoboken, NJ: John Wiley & Sons; 2015:52–52.

7. Plumb, D. C. *Plumb's Veterinary Drug Handbook (Desk)*, 8th ed. Hoboken, NJ: John Wiley & Sons; 2015:374–377.

8. Plumb, D. C. *Plumb's Veterinary Drug Handbook (Desk)*, 8th ed. Hoboken, NJ: John Wiley & Sons; 2015:107–109.

9. Plumb, D. C. *Plumb's Veterinary Drug Handbook (Desk)*, 8th ed. Hoboken, NJ: John Wiley & Sons; 2015:37–38.

10. Plumb, D. C. *Plumb's Veterinary Drug Handbook (Desk)*, 8th ed. Hoboken, NJ: John Wiley & Sons; 2015:146–147.

11. Nelson, R. W. and Couto, C. G. *Essentials of Small Animal Internal Medicine.* St. Louis: Mosby-Year Book; 1992:487–493.

12. Plumb, D. C. *Plumb's Veterinary Drug Handbook (Desk),* 8th ed. Hoboken, NJ: John Wiley & Sons; 2015:390–392.

13. Polzin, D. J., Osborne, C. A., and Adams, L. G. "Effect of Modified Protein Diets in Dogs and Cats with Chronic Renal Failure: Current Status." *Journal of Nutrition* 1991:S140–S144.

14. Plantinga, E. A. et al. "Retrospective study of the survival of cats with acquired chronic renal insufficiency offered different commercial diets." *Veterinary Record.* Aug. 13, 2005;157(7):185–7.

15. Lauretani, F. et al. "Omega-3 and Renal Function in Older Adults." *Current Pharmaceutical Design.* 2009; 15(36): 4149–4156. PMCID: PMC2863302. NIHMSID: NIHMS196923.

16. Zhang, H. W. et al. "Astragalus (a traditional Chinese medicine) for treating chronic kidney disease." Cochrane Database of Systematic Reviews. Oct 22, 2014;(10):CD008369. doi: 10.1002/14651858.CD008369.pub2.

17. Yonghong, L. et al. "Effects of an astragalus polysaccharide and rhein combination on apoptosis in rats with chronic renal failure." *Evidence-Based Complementary and Alternative Medicine.* January 2014;2014(0):271862.

18. Klahr, S. and Morrissey, J. "L-arginine as a therapeutic tool in kidney disease." *Seminars in Nephrology.* July 2004;24(4):389-94. 1,

19. Du, F. et al. "Cordyceps sinensis attenuates renal fibrosis and suppresses BAG3 induction in obstructed rat kidney." *American Journal of Translational Research.* May 15, 2005;7(5):932–40. eCollection 2015.

20. Zhang, Z. "Effect of Cordyceps sinensis on renal function of patients with chronic allograft nephropathy." Urologie Internationalis. 2011;86(3):298–301. doi: 10.1159/000323655. Epub Feb. 19, 2011.

21. Zhong, Y. et al. "Therapeutic use of traditional Chinese herbal medications for chronic kidney diseases." *Kidney International.* December 2013;84(6):1108–1118. Published online July 17, 2013. doi: 10.1038/ki.2013.276. PMCID: PMC3812398. NIHMSID: NIHMS496924.

22. Lu, Q. et al. "Ethanolic Ginkgo biloba leaf extract prevents renal fibrosis through Akt/mTOR signaling in diabetic nephropathy." *Phytomedicine.* Nov. 15, 2015;22(12):1071–8. doi: 10.1016/j.phymed.2015.08.010. Epub Sept. 6, 2015. Lu Q1, Zuo WZ1, Ji XJ1, Zhou YX1, Liu YQ1, Yao XQ1, Zhou XY1, Liu YW1, Zhang F1, Yin XX2.

23. Sener, G. "Ginkgo biloba extract ameliorates ischemia reperfusion-induced renal injury in rats." *Pharmacological Research.* September 2005;52(3):216–22.

24. Buijs, N. et al. "Intravenous glutamine supplementation enhances renal de novo arginine synthesis in humans: a stable isotope study." *American Journal of Clinical Nutrition.* November 2014;100(5):1385–91. doi: 10.3945/ajcn.113.081547. Epub Oct. 1, 2014.

25. Wang, H. et al. "Protective Effects of Green Tea Polyphenol Against Renal Injury Through ROS-Mediated JNK-MAPK Pathway in Lead Exposed Rats." *Molecules and Cells.* Jun 30, 2016;39(6):508–13. doi: 10.14348/molcells.2016.2170. Epub May 26, 2016.

26. Yokozawa, T., Noh, J. S., and Park, C. H. "Green Tea Polyphenols for the Protection against Renal Damage Caused by Oxidative Stress." *Evidence-Based Complementary and Alternative Medicine.* 2012;(2012):845917. doi: 10.1155/2012/845917. Epub July 10, 2012.

27. Parlakpinar, H. et al. "Protective effects of melatonin on renal failure in pinealectomized rats." *International Journal of Urology.* August 2007;14(8):743–8.

28. Post-White, J., Ladas, E. J., and Kelly, K. M. "Advances in the use of milk thistle (Silybum marianum)." *Integrative Cancer Therapies.* June 2007;6(2):104–9.

29. Shimizu, M. H. et al. "N-acetylcysteine attenuates the progression of chronic renal failure." *Kidney International.* November 2005;68(5):2208–17.

30. Kang, D. G. et al. "Rehmannia glutinose ameliorates renal function in the ischemia/reperfusion-induced acute renal failure rats." *Biological & Pharmaceutical Bulletin.* September 2005;28(9):1662–7.

31. Lee, B. C. et al. "Rehmannia glutinosa ameliorates the progressive renal failure induced by 5/6 nephrectomy." *Journal of Ethnopharmacology.* Feb. 25, 2009;122(1):131–5. doi: 10.1016/j.jep.2008.12.015. Epub Dec. 25, 2008.

32. Khan, I. A. et al. "Evaluation of Rhubarb Supplementation in Stages 3 and 4 of Chronic Kidney Disease: A Randomized Clinical Trial." *International Journal of Chronic Diseases*. 2014;2014:789340. Published online Sept. 11, 2014. doi: 10.1155/2014/789340. PMCID: PMC4590915.

33. An, P. et al. "Effect of acupuncture on renal function and pathologic changes of kidney in rabbits with nephritis." [Article in Chinese] *Zhongguo Zhen Jiu*. September 2012;32(9):819–23.

34. Garcia, G. E., Ma, S. X., and Feng, L. "Acupuncture and kidney disease." *Advances in Chronic Kidney Disease*. July 2005;12(3):282–91.

Chapter 20

1. Visvader, J. E. "Cells of origin in cancer." *Nature*. Jan. 20, 2011:314–322. doi: 10.1038/nature09781

2. Burstein, H. J. and Schwartz, R. S. "Molecular Origins of Cancer." *New England Journal of Medicine*. Jan. 31, 2008:527. doi: 10.1056/NEJMe0800065

3. Seyfried, T. N. et al. "Cancer as a metabolic disease: implications for novel therapeutics." *Carcinogenesis*. March 2014:515–27. doi: 10.1093/carcin/bgt480.

4. Swann, J. B. and Smyth, M. J. "Immune surveillance of tumors." *Journal of Clinical Investigation*. May 1, 2007;117(5):1137–1146. Published online May 1, 2007. doi: 10.1172/JCI31405. PMCID: PMC1857231.

5. Ryungsa, K., Manabu, E., and Kazuaki, T. "Cancer immunoediting from immune surveillance to immune escape." *Immunology*. May 2007;121(1): 1–14. doi: 10.1111/j.1365-2567.2007.02587.x. PMCID: PMC2265921. 2

6. Sersa, G., Cemazar, M., and Snoj, M. "Electrochemotherapy of tumours." *Current Oncology*. March 2009;16(2):34–35. PMCID: PMC2669236.

7. Bergman, P. J. et al. "Development of a xenogeneic DNA vaccine program for canine malignant melanoma at the Animal Medical Center." *Vaccine*. May 22, 2006;24(21):4582–5. Epub Aug. 24, 2005.

8. Bergman, P. J. et al. "Long-term survival of dogs with advanced malignant melanoma after DNA vaccination with xenogeneic human tyrosinase: a phase I trial." *Clinical Cancer Research*. April 2003;9(4):1284–90.

9. Vander Heiden, M. G., Cantley, L. C., and Thompson, C. B. "Understanding the Warburg Effect: The Metabolic Requirements of Cell Proliferation." *Science*. May 22, 2009;324(5930):1029–1033. doi: 10.1126/science.1160809. PMCID: PMC2849637. NIHMSID: NIHMS165713.

10. Ogilvie, G. K. "Nutrition and Cancer—Are Eicosanoids the Answer?" *Veterinary Clinical Nutrition*. 1996:78–82.

11. Bauer, J. E. "Therapeutic use of fish oils in companion animals." *Journal of the American Veterinary Medical Association*. Dec. 1, 2011:1441–1451.

12. Rakoff-Nahoum, S. "Why Cancer and Inflammation?" *Yale Journal of Biology and Medicine*. December 2006;79(3-4):123–130.

13. *Food, Nutrition, Physical Activity, and the Prevention of Cancer: a Global Perspective*. World Cancer Research Fund. American Institute for Cancer Research. 2007:30–62.

14. "Nutrition and Cancer." Pet Cancer Center. http://www.petcancercenter.org/files/Nutrition_and_cancer_by_Dr_Ogilvie.pdf

15. Narayanan, Amoolya, et al. "Anticarcinogenic Properties of Medium Chain Fatty Acids on Human Colorectal, Skin and Breast Cancer Cells *in Vitro*." *International Journal of Molecular Sciences*. Mar. 2015; 16(3): 5014–5027. doi: 10.3390/ijms16035014 PMCID: PMC4394462

16. Ogilvie, G. K. "Nutrition and Cancer—Are Eicosanoids the Answer?" *Veterinary Clinical Nutrition*. 1996:78–82.

17. Bauer, J. E. "Therapeutic use of fish oils in companion animals." *Journal of the American Veterinary Medical Association*. Dec. 1, 2011:1441–1451.

18. Roudebush, P., Davenport, D. J., and Novotny, B. J. "The use of nutraceuticals in cancer therapy." *Veterinary Clinics of North America: Small Animal Practice*. January 2004;34(1):249–69, viii.

19. Ogilvie, G. K. et a. "Effect of fish oil, arginine, and doxorubicin chemotherapy on remission and survival time for dogs with lymphoma: a double-blind, randomized placebo-controlled study." *Cancer.* April 15, 2000;88(8):1916–28.

20. Yoon, T. J., Koppula, S., and Lee, K. H. "The effects of β-glucans on cancer metastasis." *Anticancer Agents in Medicinal Chemistry.* June 2013;13(5):699–708.

21. Chan, G. C. H., Chan, W. K., and Sze, D. M. Y. "The effects of β-glucan on human immune and cancer cells." *Journal of Hematology & Oncology.* 2009;2:25. Published online June 10, 2009. doi: 10.1186/1756-8722-2-25 PMCID: PMC2704234.

22. Brown, D. C. and Reetz, J. "Single Agent Polysaccharopeptide Delays Metastases and Improves Survival in Naturally Occurring Hemangiosarcoma." *Evidence-Based Complementary and Alternative Medicine.* 2012; (2012):384301. Published online 2012 Sep 5. doi: 10.1155/2012/384301. PMCID: PMC3440946.

23. Marsden, S. *Dr. Steve Marsden's Essential Guide to Chinese Herbal Formulas: Bridging Science and Tradition in Integrative Veterinary Medicine.* 2014:201.

24. Grant, W. B. "A critical review of *Vitamin D and Cancer.* A report of the IARC Working Group." *Dermato-Endocrinology.* Jan-Feb 2009;1(1):25–33. PMCID: PMC2715207.

25. Zhang, X. K. "Vitamin A and apoptosis in prostate cancer." *Endocrine-Related Cancer.* June 2002;9(2):87–102.

26. Yan, B. et al. "Mitochondrially targeted vitamin E succinate efficiently kills breast tumour-initiating cells in a complex II-dependent manner." *BMC Cancer.* May 13, 2015;15:401. doi: 10.1186/s12885-015-1394-7.

27. Padayatty, S. J. et a. "Intravenously administered vitamin C as cancer therapy: three cases." *CMAJ.* Mar 28, 2006;174(7):937–942. doi: 10.1503/cmaj.050346. PMCID: PMC1405876. ,

28. Chen, Y. C., Prabhu, K. S., and Mastro, A. M. "Is Selenium a Potential Treatment for Cancer Metastasis?" *Nutrients.* April 2013;5(4):1149–1168. Published online April 8, 2013. doi: 10.3390/nu5041149. PMCID: PMC3705340.

29. Costello, L. C. and Franklin, R. B. "Cytotoxic/tumor suppressor role of zinc for the treatment of cancer: an enigma and an opportunity." *Expert Review of Anticancer Therapy.* January 2012;12(1):121–128.. doi: 10.1586/era.11.190. PMCID: PMC3291177. NIHMSID: NIHMS356002.

30. Roudebush, P., Davenport, D. J., and Novotny, B. J. "The use of nutraceuticals in cancer therapy." *Veterinary Clinics of North America: Small Animal Practice.* January 2004;34(1):249–69, viii.

31. Kuhn, K. S. et al. "Glutamine as indispensable nutrient in oncology: experimental and clinical evidence." *European Journal of Nutrition.* June 2010;49(4):197–210. doi: 10.1007/s00394-009-0082-2. Epub Nov. 21, 2009.

32. Lee, H. E. et al. "Anticancer activity of Ashwagandha against human head and neck cancer cell lines." *Journal of Oral Pathology & Medicine.* March 2016;45(3):193–201. doi: 10.1111/jop.12353. Epub Aug. 31, 2015.

33. Wang, T. et al. "Astragalus saponins affect proliferation, invasion and apoptosis of gastric cancer BGC-823 cells." *Diagnostic Pathology.* 2013;8:179. Published online Oct. 24, 2013. doi: 10.1186/1746-1596-8-179. PMCID: PMC3818446.

34. Frank, M. B. et al. "Frankincense oil derived from Boswellia carteri induces tumor cell specific cytotoxicity." *BMC Complementary and Alternative Medicine.* March 18, 2009;9:6. doi: 10.1186/1472-6882-9-6.

35. Ravindran, J. et al. "Curcumin and Cancer Cells: How Many Ways Can Curry Kill Tumor Cells Selectively?" *AAPS Journal.* September 2009;11(3):495–510. Published online Jul 10, 2009. doi: 10.1208/s12248-009-9128-x. PMCID: PMC2758121.

36. Kahn, N. and Mukhtar, H. "Cancer and metastasis: prevention and treatment by green tea." *Cancer Metastasis Reviews.* September 2010;29(3):435–445. doi: 10.1007/s10555-010-9236-1. PMCID: PMC3142888. NIHMSID: NIHMS311687.

37. Vucenik, I. and Shamsuddin, A.M. "Cancer inhibition by inositol hexaphosphate (IP6) and inositol: from laboratory to clinic." *Journal of Nutrition.* November 2003;133(11 Suppl 1):3778S–3784S.

38. Angst, E. et al. "The flavonoid quercetin inhibits pancreatic cancer growth in vitro and in vivo." *Pancreas.* March 2013;42(2):223–9. doi: 10.1097/MPA.0b013e318264ccae.

39. Aluyen, J. K. et al. "Resveratrol: potential as anticancer agent." *Journal of Dietary Supplements*. March 2012;9(1):45–56. doi: 10.3109/19390211.2011.650842.

40. Hileman, E. A., Achanta, G., and Huang, P. "Superoxide dismutase: an emerging target for cancer therapeutics." *Expert Opinion on Therapeutic Targets*. December 2001;5(6):697–710.

41. Cannabis and Cannabinoids (PDQ®)-Health Professional Version. PDQ Integrative, Alternative, and Complementary Therapies Editorial Board. Published online May 27, 2016. Created March 16, 2011.

42. Lu, W. and Rosenthal, D. S. "Acupuncture for Cancer Pain and Related Symptoms." *Current Pain and Headache Reports*. March 2013;17(3):321. doi: 10.1007/s11916-013-0321-3. PMCID: PMC4008096. NIHMSID: NIHMS438040.

43. Lu, W. et al. "The Value of Acupuncture in Cancer Care." *Hematology/Oncology Clinics of North America*. August 2008;22(4):631–viii. doi: 10.1016/j.hoc.2008.04.005. PMCID: PMC2642987. NIHMSID: NIHMS65572.

44. Safarzadeh, E. et al. "Herbal Medicine as Inducers of Apoptosis in Cancer Treatment." *Advanced Pharmaceutical Bulletin*. October 2014;4(Suppl 1):421–427. Published online Aug. 25, 2014. doi: 10.5681/apb.2014.062. PMCID: PMC4213780.

45. Yin, S. Y. et al. "Therapeutic Applications of Herbal Medicines for Cancer Patients." *Evidence-Based Complementary and Alternative Medicine*. 2013;(2013):302426. Published online July 11, 2013. doi: 10.1155/2013/302426. PMCID: PMC3727181.

46. Bhutani, S. and Vishwanath, G. "Hyperbaric oxygen and wound healing." *Indian Journal of Plastic Surgery*. May-Aug 2012;45(2):316–324. doi: 10.4103/0970-0358.101309. PMCID: PMC3495382.

Chapter 21

1. Dodds, W. J. and Laverdure, D. R. (2011). *The Canine Thyroid Epidemic: Answers You Need for Your Dog*. Wenatchee, WA: Dogwise Publishing; 2011:7.

2. Dodds, W. J. and Laverdure, D. R. (2011). *The Canine Thyroid Epidemic: Answers You Need for Your Dog*. Wenatchee, WA: Dogwise Publishing; 2011:12–14.

3. Dodds, W. J. and Laverdure, D. R. (2011). *The Canine Thyroid Epidemic: Answers You Need for Your Dog*. Wenatchee, WA: Dogwise Publishing; 2011:10.

4. Peterson, M. "Hyperthyroidism in cats: what's causing this epidemic of thyroid disease and can we prevent it?" *Journal of Feline Medicine and Surgery*. November 2012;14(11):804–18. doi: 10.1177/1098612X12464462.

5. Kass, P. H. et al. "Evaluation of environmental, nutritional, and host factors in cats with hyperthyroidism." *Journal of Veterinary Internal Medicine*. Jul-Aug 1999;13(4):323–9.

6. Potera, C. "Chemical Exposures: Cats as Sentinel Species." *Environmental Health Perspectives*. December 2007;115(12):A580. PMCID: PMC2137107.

7. Plumb, D. C. *Plumb's Veterinary Drug Handbook (Desk)*, 8th ed. Hoboken, NJ. John Wiley & Sons; 2015:619–622.

8. Dodds, W. J. and Laverdure, D. R. (2011). *The Canine Thyroid Epidemic: Answers You Need for Your Dog*. Wenatchee, WA: Dogwise Publishing; 2011:109–110.

9. Dodds, W. J. and Laverdure, D. R. (2011). *The Canine Thyroid Epidemic: Answers You Need for Your Dog*. Wenatchee, WA: Dogwise Publishing; 2011:84–110.

10. Dodds, W. J. and Laverdure, D. R. (2011). *The Canine Thyroid Epidemic: Answers You Need for Your Dog*. Wenatchee, WA: Dogwise Publishing; 2011:84–110.

11. Plumb, D. C. *Plumb's Veterinary Drug Handbook (Desk)*, 8th ed. Hoboken, NJ: John Wiley & Sons; 2015:693–695.

12. Peterson, M. E. and Becker, D. V. "Radioiodine treatment of 524 cats with hyperthyroidism." *Journal of the American Veterinary Medical Association*. Dec 1, 1995;207(11):1422–8.

13. Plumb, D. C. *Plumb's Veterinary Drug Handbook (Desk)*, 8th ed. Hoboken, NJ: John Wiley & Sons; 2015:52–53.

14. Wynn, S. G. and Marsden, S. *Manual of Natural Veterinary Medicine: Science and Tradition*. St. Louis: Mosby; 2003:255–258.

15. Wynn, S. G. and Marsden, S. *Manual of Natural Veterinary Medicine: Science and Tradition*. St. Louis: Mosby; 2003:249–255.

Chapter 22

1. Côté, E. *Clinical Veterinary Advisor: Dogs and Cats*. St. Louis: Elsevier Mosby; 2011:573–575.

2. Côté, E. *Clinical Veterinary Advisor: Dogs and Cats*. St. Louis: Elsevier Mosby; 2011:548–551.

3. Plumb, D. C. *Plumb's Veterinary Drug Handbook (Desk)*, 8th ed. Hoboken, NJ: John Wiley & Sons; 2015:297–299.

4. Plumb, D. C. *Plumb's Veterinary Drug Handbook (Desk)*, 8th ed. Hoboken, NJ: John Wiley & Sons; 2015:737–739.

5. Plumb, D. C. *Plumb's Veterinary Drug Handbook (Desk)*, 8th ed. Hoboken, NJ: John Wiley & Sons; 2015:1063–1065.

6. Wynn, S. G. and Marsden, S. *Manual of Natural Veterinary Medicine: Science and Tradition*. St. Louis: Mosby; 2003:247.

7. Wynn, S. G. and Marsden, S. *Manual of Natural Veterinary Medicine: Science and Tradition*. St. Louis: Mosby; 2003:245.

Chapter 23

1. Gershwin, L. J. "Veterinary autoimmunity: autoimmune diseases in domestic animals." *Annals of the New York Academy of Sciences*. August 2007;1109:109–16.

2. Hess, E. V. "Environmental chemicals and autoimmune disease: cause and effect." *Toxicology*. Dec 27, 2002;181-182:65–70.

3. Fujinami, R. S. et al. "Molecular Mimicry, Bystander Activation, or Viral Persistence: Infections and Autoimmune Disease." *Clinical & Experimental Immunology*. 1991 Nov; 86(2):322–327.

4. Shoenfeld, Y. and Aron-Maor, A. "Vaccination and autoimmunity-'vaccinosis': a dangerous liaison?" *Journal of Autoimmunity*. February 2000;14(1):1–10.

5. Duval, D. and Giger, U. "Vaccine-associated immune-mediated hemolytic anemia in the dog." *Journal of Veterinary Internal Medicine*. Sep-Oct 1996;10(5):290–5.

6. Fasano, A. "Leaky gut and autoimmune diseases." *Clinical Reviews in Allergy & Immunology*. February 2012;42(1):71–8. doi: 10.1007/s12016-011-8291-x.

7. Côté, E. *Clinical Veterinary Advisor: Dogs and Cats*. St. Louis: Elsevier Mosby; 2011:71–75.

8. Côté, E. *Clinical Veterinary Advisor: Dogs and Cats*. St. Louis: Elsevier Mosby; 2011:1091–1093.

9. Scott, D. W. et al. *Muller & Kirk's Small Animal Dermatology*. Philadelphia: W.B. Saunders; 2001:678–680.

10. Scott, D. W. et al. *Muller & Kirk's Small Animal Dermatology*. Philadelphia: W.B. Saunders; 2001:704–705.

11. Plumb, D. C. *Plumb's Veterinary Drug Handbook (Desk)*, 8th ed. Hoboken, NJ: John Wiley & Sons; 2015:883–887.

12. Plumb, D. C. *Plumb's Veterinary Drug Handbook (Desk)*, 8th ed. Hoboken, NJ: John Wiley & Sons; 2015:102–104.

13. Plumb, D. C. *Plumb's Veterinary Drug Handbook (Desk)*, 8th ed. Hoboken, NJ: John Wiley & Sons; 2015:365–369.

14. Plumb, D. C. *Plumb's Veterinary Drug Handbook (Desk)*, 8th ed. Hoboken, NJ:]John Wiley & Sons; 2015:768–769.

15. Plumb, D. C. *Plumb's Veterinary Drug Handbook (Desk)*, 8th ed. Hoboken, NJ:]John Wiley & Sons; 2015:836–838.

16. Maggs, D. and Miller, P. *Slatter's Fundamentals of Veterinary Ophthalmology*, 4th ed. St. Louis: Elsevier Saunders; 2008:194–195.

17. Plumb, D. C. *Plumb's Veterinary Drug Handbook (Desk)*, 8th ed. Hoboken, NJ:]John Wiley & Sons; 2015:1133–1134.

18. Plumb, D. C. *Plumb's Veterinary Drug Handbook (Desk)*, 8th ed. Hoboken, NJ:]John Wiley & Sons; 2015:1172–1173.

19. Wynn, S. G. and Marsden, S. *Manual of Natural Veterinary Medicine: Science and Tradition*. St. Louis: Mosby; 2003:271.

20. Wynn, S. G. and Marsden, S. *Manual of Natural Veterinary Medicine: Science and Tradition*. St. Louis: Mosby; 2003:271.

21. Harbige, L. S. "Dietary n-6 and n-3 fatty acids in immunity and autoimmune disease." *Proceedings of the Nutrition Society.* November 1998;57(4):555–62.

22. Swails, W. S. et al. "Fish-oil-containing diet and platelet aggregation." *Nutrition.* May-June 1993;9(3):211–7.

23. Wynn, S. G. and Marsden, S. *Manual of Natural Veterinary Medicine: Science and Tradition*. St. Louis: Mosby; 2003:285–286.

24. Saito, K. et al. "Suppressive effect of hyperbaric oxygenation on immune responses of normal and autoimmune mice." *Clinical & Experimental Immunology.* November 1991;86(2):322–7.

25. Chen, S. Y. et al. "Early hyperbaric oxygen therapy attenuates disease severity in lupus-prone autoimmune (NZB x NZW) F1 mice." *Clinical Immunology.* August 2003;108(2):103–10.

26. Kaplan, B. L., Springs, A. E., and Kaminski, N. E. "The Profile of Immune Modulation by Cannabidiol (CBD) Involves Deregulation of Nuclear Factor of Activated T Cells (NFAT)." *Biochemical Pharmacology.* Sept. 15, 2008;76(6): 726–737. Published online July 8, 2008. doi: 10.1016/j.bcp.2008.06.022. PMCID: PMC2748879. NIHMSID: NIHMS131165.

27. Pandey, R. et al. "Use of Cannabinoids as a Novel Therapeutic Modality Against Autoimmune Hepatitis." *Vitamins and Hormones.* 2009;81:487–504. doi: 10.1016/S0083-6729(09)81019-4. PMCID: PMC4139007. NIHMSID: NIHMS617536.

Appendix C

1. R. C. Nap, H.A. Hazewinkel, G. Voorhout, et al, "Growth and skeletal development in Great Dane pups fed different levels of protein intake," Journal Nutrition, Nov. 1991, S107-13.

2. J. Grondalen, A. Hedhammar, "Nutrition of the rapidly growing dog with special reference to skeletal disease," in *Nutrition and Behaviour in dogs and cats* by R.S. Anderson ed., (Oxford: Pergamon Press,1982), 81-88.

3. R.D. Kealy, D.F. Lawler DF, J.M. Ballam, et al., "Effects of diet restriction on life span and age-related changes in dogs," *Journal of American Vet Med Assoc*, May 1, 2002, 1315-20.

4. A. Hedhammar, L. Krook, B.E. Sheffy, et al., "Overnutrition and skeletal disease. An experimental study in growing Great Dane dogs. I-IX. Design of experiment," *Cornell Vet.* April 1974, 11-22.

Further Works Consulted

Arlian, L. G. et al. "Serum immunoglobulin E against storage mites in dogs with atopic dermatitis." *American Journal of Veterinary Research*. 2003;64(1):32–36.

Bauer, J. E. "Fatty acid metabolism in domestic cats (*Felis catus*) and cheetahs (*Acinoyx jubatas*)." *Proceedings of the Nutrition Society*. December 1997;56(3):1013–1024.

Butterwick, R. F. et al. "Challenges in Developing Nutrient Guidelines for Companion Animals." *British Journal of Nutrition*. Oct. 12, 2011;106:S24–S31.

Dunbar, B. L. and Bauer, J. E. "Conversion of essential fatty acids by delta 6-desaturase in dog liver microsomes." *Journal of Nutrition*. 2002;132(6):1701S–1703S.

Favrot, C. et al. "A prospective study on the clinical features of chronic atopic dermatitis and its diagnosis." *Veterinary Dermatology*. 2010;21(1):23–31. doi: 10.1111/j.1365-3164.2009.00758.x

Finke, M. D. "Evaluation of the Energy Requirements of Adult Kennel Dogs." *Journal of Nutrition*. November 1991:S22–S28.

Forrester, S. D. and Kirk, C. A. "Cats and Carbohydrates—What Are the Concerns?" Hills Pet Nutrition. 2009. http://www.hillsvet.com/conference-documents/Proceedings/Myth_Symposium/1_Cats_and_Carbs.pdf

Jackson, H. A. "Dermatologic manifestations and nutritional management of adverse food reactions." *Veterinary Medicine*. 2007;102(1):51–64.

Kennis, R. A. "Food allergies: Update of pathogenesis, diagnosis, and management." *Veterinary Clinics of North America, Small Animal Practice*. 2006;36(1):175–184.

Kienzle, E. and Rainbird, A. "Maintenance Energy Requirement of Dogs: What is the Correct Value for the Calculation of Metabolic Body Weight in Dogs?" *Journal of Nutrition*. November 1991:S39–S40. http://www.ncbi.nlm.nih.gov/pubmed/1941233

Laflamme, D. P. "Focus on Nutrition: Cats and Carbohydrates: Implications for Health and Disease." *Compendium*. January 2010;32(1).

Landry, S. M. "Food Habits of Feral Carnivores: A Review of Stomach Content Analysis." *Journal of the American Animal Hospital Association*. 1979;15:775–782.

Lewis, L. D. *Small Animal Clinical Nutrition*, 3rd ed. Topeka, KS: Mark Morris Associates; 1987.

Morris, J. G. and Rogers, Q. R. "Assessment of the Nutritional Adequacy of Pet Foods Through the Life Cycle." *Journal of Nutrition*. 1994;124(12):2520S–2534S.

Picco, F. et al. "A prospective study on canine atopic dermatitis and food-induced allergic dermatitis in Switzerland." *Veterinary Dermatology*. 2008;19(3):150–155.

Pierson, L. "Transitioning Feline Dry Food Addicts to Canned Food." Veterinary Information Network. Jan. 14, 2010. http://www.veterinarypartner.com/Content.plx?A=3041

Smith, C. A. "Changes and Challenges in Feline Nutrition," *Journal of the American Veterinary Medical Association*. Nov. 15, 1993;203(10):1395–1400.

Thalmann, O. et al. "Complete Mitochondrial Genomes of Ancient Canids Suggest a European Origin of Domestic Dogs." *Science*. 2013;342(6160):871–874. doi: 10.1126/science.1243650. Refer to supplementary material: page 27, Table S1.

Wayne, R. K. "Molecular Evolution of the Dog Family." *Trends in Genetics*. 1993;9(6):218–224. doi: 10.1016/0168-9525(93)90122-X.

Wolpert, S. "Dogs likely originated in Europe more than 18,000 years ago, UCLA biologists report." UCLA Newsroom. Nov. 14, 2013. http://newsroom.ucla.edu/releases/dogs-likely-originated-in-europe-249325

INDEX

Note: Page references in *italics indicate recipes.*

ACKNOWLEDGMENTS

A former employer once told me that his philosophy was to surround himself with people smarter than him. I took the axiom to heart, and it is no accident that I find myself in the company of outstanding people who are both teachers and partners in patient care. I have the great fortune to work with brilliant medical minds like Jean Dodds, D.V.M.; Lisa Koenig, D.C.; and Kaylah Sterling, L.Ac. Special thanks go to Susan Lauten, Ph.D., who spent tireless hours formulating and perfecting recipes for this book. Equally invaluable is the support from the veterinary technicians, receptionists, and managers who allow me to focus on medical care. Without people like Kristie Austin, R.V.T.; Ashley Crnkovich; and, of course, my wife, Lee, there would be no veterinary practice to work from.

As with any scientific discipline, modern medicine is built upon the successes and failures of those who came before us. The inherited knowledge from great minds dating back thousands of years combined with modern discoveries allow today's healers to help patients in ways that could only have been dreamed of in the past. All medical practitioners owe a great debt of gratitude to our predecessors. We are standing on the shoulders of giants.

At the end of the day, it is the human–animal bond that binds us. The age-old connection is stronger than most people realize, and we humans are better for it. And so, to every human who has ever extended, begged, borrowed, or stolen to care for an animal, I thank you. What we get is always more than what we give.

ABOUT THE AUTHOR

Dr. Gary Richter is a graduate of the University of Florida with a B.S. in animal science, an M.S. in veterinary medical science, and a doctorate of veterinary medicine with honors. Since 2002, he has been the owner and medical director of Montclair Veterinary Hospital in Oakland, California, and he launched Holistic Veterinary Care in 2009.

Dr. Richter is certified in veterinary acupuncture as well as veterinary chiropractic and uses these therapies along with his veterinary medical education to achieve better outcomes for his patients. His primary focus is promoting health and treating disease through integration of Western and complementary therapies. The use of appropriate fresh, whole food diets is a cornerstone of treatment in many of these patients.

Dr. Richter has published numerous articles educating pet owners on the benefits of complementary and integrative healthcare options for their pets. Dr. Richter and his two animal hospitals have received more than 30 local and national awards, including Best Veterinary Hospital, Best Veterinarian, Best Canine Therapy Facility and Best Alternative Medicine Provider. Montclair Veterinary Hospital was named one of the top ten veterinary hospitals in 2013 while Dr. Richter was named one of the top ten veterinarians in the United States for 2012, and America's Favorite Veterinarian in 2015.

For more information on Gary's work, as well as pet health resources to complement the book, please visit: PetVetExpert.com.

Hay House Titles of Related Interest

YOU CAN HEAL YOUR LIFE, *the movie,* starring Louise Hay & Friends
(available as a 1-DVD program, an expanded
2-DVD set, and an online streaming video)
Learn more at www.hayhouse.com/louise-movie

THE SHIFT, *the movie,*
starring Dr. Wayne W. Dyer
(available as a 1-DVD program, an expanded
2-DVD set, and an online streaming video)
Learn more at www.hayhouse.com/the-shift-movie

THE ANIMAL COMMUNICATOR'S GUIDE THROUGH
LIFE, LOSS AND LOVE, by Pea Horsley

THE ANIMAL HEALER: *A Unique Insight into the Healing,
Care and Wellbeing of Animals,* by Elizabeth Whiter

NATURAL NUTRITION FOR DOGS AND CATS: *The Ultimate Diet,*
by Kymythy Schultze, C.C.N., A.H.I.

WHOLE-PET HEALING: *A Head-to-Tail Guide to Caring for and
Connecting with Your Animal Companion,* by Dennis W. Thomas, D.V.M.

YOU CAN HEAL YOUR PET: *The Practical Guide to Holistic Health
and Veterinary Care,* by Elizabeth Whiter and Dr. Rohini Sathish, M.R.C.V.S.

Please visit:

Gary's website: www.PetVetExpert.com
Hay House USA: www.hayhouse.com®
Hay House Australia: www.hayhouse.com.au
Hay House UK: www.hayhouse.co.uk
Hay House South Africa: www.hayhouse.co.za
Hay House India: www.hayhouse.co.in

We hope you enjoyed this Hay House book.
If you'd like to receive our online catalog featuring additional information
on Hay House books and products, or if you'd like to find out more
about the Hay Foundation, please contact:

Hay House, Inc., P.O. Box 5100, Carlsbad, CA 92018-5100
(760) 431-7695 or (800) 654-5126
(760) 431-6948 (fax) or (800) 650-5115 (fax)
www.hayhouse.com® • www.hayfoundation.org

Published and distributed in Australia by: Hay House Australia Pty. Ltd.,
18/36 Ralph St., Alexandria NSW 2015 • *Phone:* 612-9669-4299 • *Fax:* 612-9669-4144
www.hayhouse.com.au

Published and distributed in the United Kingdom by: Hay House UK, Ltd.,
Astley House, 33 Notting Hill Gate, London W11 3JQ • *Phone:* 44-20-3675-2450
Fax: 44-20-3675-2451 • www.hayhouse.co.uk

Published and distributed in the Republic of South Africa by: Hay House SA
(Pty), Ltd., P.O. Box 990, Witkoppen 2068 • info@hayhouse.co.za • www.hayhouse.co.za

Published in India by: Hay House Publishers India, Muskaan Complex, Plot No. 3,
B-2, Vasant Kunj, New Delhi 110 070 • *Phone:* 91-11-4176-1620 • *Fax:* 91-11-4176-1630
www.hayhouse.co.in

Distributed in Canada by: Raincoast Books, 2440 Viking Way, Richmond,
B.C. V6V 1N2 • *Phone:* 1-800-663-5714 • *Fax:* 1-800-565-3770 • www.raincoast.com

<u>Access New Knowledge.</u>
<u>Anytime. Anywhere.</u>

Learn and evolve at your own pace with the world's leading experts.

www.hayhouseU.com

HEAL YOUR LIFE

you can

make your soul smile

Visit HealYourLife.com daily and meet the world's best-selling Hay House authors; leading intuitive, health, and success experts; inspirational writers; and like-minded friends who will share their insights, experiences, personal stories, and wisdom.

- ♥ DAILY AFFIRMATIONS
- ♥ UPLIFTING ARTICLES
- ♥ VIDEO AND AUDIO LESSONS
- ♥ GUIDED MEDITATIONS
- ♥ FREE ORACLE CARD READINGS

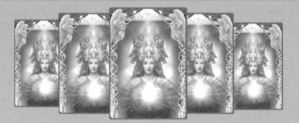

FEEL THE LOVE...

Join our community on Facebook.com/HealYourLife

www.HealYourLife.com®

Free e-newsletters from Hay House, the Ultimate Resource for Inspiration

Be the first to know about Hay House's dollar deals, free downloads, special offers, affirmation cards, giveaways, contests, and more!

 Get exclusive excerpts from our latest releases and videos from **Hay House Present Moments**.

 Enjoy uplifting personal stories, how-to articles, and healing advice, along with videos and empowering quotes, within **Heal Your Life**.

 Have an inspirational story to tell and a passion for writing? Sharpen your writing skills with insider tips from **Your Writing Life**.

Sign Up Now!

Get inspired, educate yourself, get a complimentary gift, and share the wisdom!

http://www.hayhouse.com/newsletters.php

Visit www.hayhouse.com to sign up today!

 HAY HOUSE

HealYourLife.com ♥